A Y U R V E D A

Secrets
of
Healing

Critical Reviews of Ayurveda: Secrets of Healing
Bri. Maya Tiwari

To have this book in your hands is to have the oceanic presence of Bri. Maya Tiwari in your home, is to have the cosmos in your soul...remembered. Read it at your own risk, for you may lose your false self in the process, and find true health and happiness.

DIRK BENEDICT
ACTOR AND AUTHOR, *Kamakazi Cowboy*

Ayurveda: Secrets of Healing is an excellent book for the serious practitioner and layperson who wish to learn the Ayurvedic healing practices. Maya Tiwari has clearly and beautifully written an in-depth, detailed manual on this timeless, ancient form of healing.

MARGARET PAUL, PH.D.
AUTHOR, *Healing Your Aloneness*

Maya Tiwari brought together ancient concepts of Ayurveda in such a way that they are comprehensible and useable in our modern western culture. This book is valuable in its overall discussion of philosophy and then in its ability to adapt the philosophy to practical day by day activities which can be used by people in their own home and also by health care practitioners. The way we as humans relate to the world around us including the seasons of the year and the phases of the sun and moon is presented in interesting ways. I recommend this book not for casual reading but for in-depth study.

GLADYS TAYLOR MCGAREY, M.D., M.D.(H)
Scottsdale Holistic Medical Group, P.A.

Since the beginning of time, some of us search for growth—personal and humanitary development. On that path, we need tools and guidance to mirror back to us our progress or our obstacles. This book is one of those precious tools that one will keep, refer to, return to, to continuously find in it that important vibration emanating from someone in mastery and willing to share it with us. This is a rich manual to empower all aspects of our being: mental, physical and spiritual.

NIRO MARKOFF ASISTENT
AUTHOR, *Why I Survived Aids*

Bri. Maya Tiwari is one of the most beloved and inspiring teachers of Ayurveda in the country today.

New York Open Center

NOTE ON THE COVER

The Vedic lore is rich with stories of beings from the celestial plane and their gifts to Earth. It is said in the Vedas that all life emanated from the lotus flower which sprang from the navel of Lord Vishnu as He reclined on the primeval water of the causal plane. The lotus plant is considered the cradle of the universe, unfolding from formlessness into resplendent life. The seeds of all plants are believed to have been brought to Earth by the celestials. The sesame plant is said to have grown when a drop of sweat from Lord Vishnu's body fell to Earth and seeded itself.

In a recent re-visiting of the psychic plane through a dream, I came upon a celestial child whose transport was the trunk of a tree. I awakened with a vision which became the cover art, entitled *Celestial Grace*. In keeping with the vast and stupendous symbology of Vedic literature, the cover art depicts the ceaseless psychic communion among the three planes of existence: causal, psychic and physical. The entire universe is formed from the relationship between the divine forces of *Shiva*, solar memory, and *Shakti*, lunar memory. In *Celestial Grace*, a cosmic chariot glides through boundless space, illuminated by the waxing moon, luminous stars and the rainbow.

The chariot is empowered by Shiva, who embodies masculinity and strength, symbolized by the two young, tusked rainbow elephants propelling forward the chakras, or wheels, of the chariot. The chakras propagate the cosmic energy of space, represented by the sixteen spokes of each wheel. The energy of space is born of the cosmic sound, *Om*. Carrying the cosmic memory of plants on Earth, the elephants progress the chakras through the celestial river of boundless life, effortlessly transporting the force of Shakti to Earth in the form of four numinous, celestial beings, *Artha, Kama, Dharma* and *Moksha*. They bring to Earth reminders of the four gifts of life: Artha being wealth and wellness, symbolized by the plant; Kama being desires and happiness, symbolized by the seed; Dharma being devotion to the divine, symbolized by the fruit; and Moksha being wisdom of our boundless nature, symbolized by the prayer.

May the rainbow elephants and the celestials bless us with the wisdom to render self-healing through the harmonious use of the healing herbs, grains and seeds, and may our spirit turn towards the Divine Love.

ABOUT THE AUTHOR

*O*ver twenty years ago, Maya Tiwari healed herself of cancer through her fortitude and spiritual strength. As a result, she re-directed her life, beginning her holistic studies in Oriental medicine. She later returned to her roots in the Vedas and was carefully tutored by Swami Dayananda, one of India's few living masters of the traditional teaching of Vedanta and Sanskrit. She has been trained to preserve the precious oral teachings of the most ancient spiritual heritage, the Vedas—and has since devoted her life to the study and teaching of Ayurveda and Vedanta.

In 1992, Maya Tiwari was initiated by her teacher as a *brahmacarini*, one whose life is committed to the study of the Vedas. Being a traditional Vedic monk, Bri. Maya lives a simple life in Asheville, North Carolina, and teaches with love and selflessness the ancient wisdom of *sadhanas*, the art of consciously participating in the wholesome activities of nature. Over the years she has assisted hundreds of cancer patients, and more recently AIDS patients, through their "dark night of the soul" into good health.

Bri. Maya co-authored *Diet for Natural Beauty* with Aveline Kushi and has written the current best-selling *Ayurveda: A Life of Balance*, the definitive work on Ayurvedic nutrition.

A Y U R V E D A

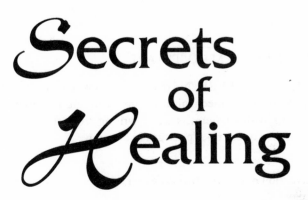

Secrets
of
Healing

The complete Ayurvedic guide to healing
through Pancha Karma seasonal therapies,
diet, herbal remedies and memory.

Maya Tiwari

LOTUS PRESS
Twin Lakes, Wisconsin

Cover illustration of *Celestial Grace*, design by Maya Tiwari and illustrated by Franzi Talley

Line drawings design by Maya Tiwari and illustrated by Marnie Mikell

Photograph of Maya Tiwari by Ron Reuhl

Jacket and book design by Jancis Salerno

Page composition by Susan Tinkle

Art and editorial directions by Maya Tiwari

First printing 1995

Printed in the United States of America

Library of Congress Cataloging-in-Publication Data
Tiwari, Maya,
    Ayurveda: Secrets of Healing / by Maya Tiwari
    includes bibliographical references.
    ISBN 0-914955-15-2   95-75338
                                                                 CIP

Published in 1995 by
Lotus Press, P.O. Box 325, Twin Lakes, Wisconsin 53181

To my beloved teacher, Swami Dayananda Saraswati

The One who gives happiness and knowledge
And is beyond duality and extremes,
boundless like space, He is without a second
Pure and timeless, He is beyond samsara,
free from the bondage of maya
I salute my teacher who is Truth.

To the Goddess forces of my life

Stella Adler and Helena Monbo,
two powerful teachers of my early life...
Kalayi and Jeerah, my two beautiful mothers...

Thank thee for thy nurturing wisdom
and eternal love.

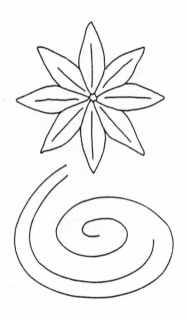

CONTENTS

FOREWORD

*O*n the surface, the author of this book, a descendant of Indian Hindus transplanted to British Guiana (now Guyana), and the writer of this foreword, born of Swiss/German parents in Helena, Montana, would seem to have little, if anything, in common. One from the fertile rice fields and redwood forests on the salty shores of South America; the other from the mountainous ranch country on the eastern slope of the Rocky Mountains of North America. One a *Brahmacarini* who has stood in the cool waters of the Ganges, walked the Himalayas and lives her life in Shiva according to the knowledge of the Vedas; the other an actor/writer who has fished the Missouri, climbed the Crazy Mountains and floundered through his life, both public and private, with only a curious soul and boundless hunger for Truth to guide him. But beneath the surface of all this biographical detail, all these "differences" (by which we are all taught to revel in our uniqueness and jump to the conclusions that make us unhappy, disenchanted and divided), beneath and beyond all this lies the "real nature" that is the cosmic Truth of Maya Tiwari and Dirk Benedict—and indeed, of all of us. For no matter how unique, how different, our life experiences, we are all brothers and sisters, born of the same universe and sharing the same cosmic dream.

I know this is true because a little thing called cancer told me so; and it is there, in the experience of that spiritual disease, that I found my universal being and had my peek into that part of my Self that is all of us. The talented writer and enlightened creator of this book that you hold in your hands has also experienced her spiritual disease.

I always suspected that cancer was my spiritual salvation. With the passage of time (and increased well being) came the faith that allowed me to give voice to that suspicion and to the deeper suspicion that the physical dis-ease that is shortening the lives of many of us and that we give many names—cancer, heart disease, diabetes—and call incurable, is nothing of the sort. But rather is this physical degeneration merely a symptom of our loss of memory, memory of our true Self, of all that went before, generations beyond counting, and of all that is yet to come. For everything that is, has been, or will be, is written on the infinite pages of the Cosmos; I know this is true for I have had my carcinogenic glimpse into that Cosmos. It is this Cosmic Memory which Maya unfolds in this book that reveals to us our sacred, spiritual nature, and allows us to proceed with what we call life; reveals to us our timeless mind and ageless body, makes us whole and harmonious...and One.

Maya Tiwari too, as she relates in this book, had her "dark passage" through the valley of cancer. Mine was at the age of twenty-nine, hers at twenty-three. That we both survived our dark journeys is not the point, but rather what happened to us along the way: abandonment of false beliefs and perceptions; acceptance of our true, that is to say our *divine*, nature; acceptance of responsibility for our disease and for our rejuvenation. Cancer was the obstacle in our lives, the celestial mountain we climbed, and through which we connected with our true self.

To deny personal responsibility for such celestial obstacles and ask for, *demand*, surgical, chemical, man-made salvation, is to deny our divine nature and miss the point entirely. What we call "incurable" is really missed opportunity: missed opportunity for the growth that is our physical rejuvenation and spiritual salvation.

The man who writes this small foreword is everyman. Not an expert, a physician or holder of a Ph.D. from any field of specialization...his expertise is nil. Certainly he is not a guru or sage or otherwise enlightened being. That he is still alive and capable of the thoughts of this humble foreword is solely because, when his false lifestyle resulted in the physical degeneration that was his celestial obstacle, he got the message. And it was divine. And it is here on these pages that you are about to read.

This book, as the person who wrote it, is like the ocean. We need only stand on the shores of our being, and the spiritual, which is to say *essential*, reward is inevitable. Stand on the beach of any ocean and gaze out at the vastness, or quietly ponder the pages of this book; you will be gently nudged towards your divine self by both experiences. The recovery of your eternal memory is up to you, but you will never again be without the tools with which to begin that journey.

So beware! To have this book in your hands is to have the oceanic presence of Maya Tiwari in your home, to have the Cosmos in your soul...remembered.

There is a universal collective that connects us all via the spiritual umbilical cord that is our true Self. This book holds the teachings that make realization of this possible for all of us—in *this* lifetime.

If there are those of you that feared the ancient tradition of Ayurveda and its secrets of healing were in danger of being lost, here is the work that lets us all sigh a collective breath of joy. For within these pages the primary healing practices, teachings and ancient scriptural knowledge of Ayurveda that has been handed down for thousands of years—from sage to sage, master to master—have been made available to us in the written record that is this book.

Welcome to a complete healing for your soul—a myriad of therapies and recipes by which to recover your vitality and joy of living and lose your disillusionment and fear of death.

Read it at your own risk, for you may lose your self in it...your false self. And find true health and happiness and eternal life.

Dirk Benedict
Bigfork, Montana
December 27, 1994

ACKNOWLEDGMENTS

My gratitude to the staff of Lotus Press, and in particular to Santosh Krinsky, my publisher; Lenny Blank, for his efforts and encouragement; Susan Tinkle for her conscientious final editing; Beverley Viljakainen, my esteemed colleague, for the line editing and exquisite refinement of the work; Jancis Salerno for the book and jacket design.

My deep appreciation to Deepak Chopra, M.D., for his kind review; Dirk Benedict, my brother of spirit, for his soulful foreword; Gladys Taylor McGarey, M.D., M.D.(H), Margaret Paul, Ph.D., and Niro Markoff Asistent for their generous review comments.

I thank the staff at New York Open Center for their kindred support; my organizers/students whose stoicity sustain the dissemination of my work around the country: Ketul, Gandharva, Aparna, Taj, Stephen, Pat, Gary, Prem Leena, Ann, Usha, Victoria, Stan, Larry and Judi.

Finally, my thanks to Leslie Hawkins, Roxanne Clement and Jeff Hollifield for assisting me with the input of the manuscript; Marnie Mikell for the final illustration of the line drawings; and Franzi Talley for the final illustration of the cover art.

AUTHOR'S INTRODUCTION

My salutation to Lord Krishna,
whose appearance is a blessing to the universe,
who is boundless joy for those who surrender to Him.
His mere glance from the corner of His eye
dries up the ocean of delusion.

—Advaita Makaranda (1.1)

The cool waters of the Ganges rush steadily over my feet. I hear God's voice in the raging thunder. The whirling sands, supported on the wings of the driven wind, take the forms of my ancestors' faces. Little do I know the true purpose of my visit to India until I stand transfixed in boundless space and infinite time. I behold the faces of my beloved people whose blood and spirit run through me. I hear the cries of my ancestors finally silenced, as the debt for their estrangement from the homeland more than a century before is paid. The first of my people to return to the sacred land of India, I am here, through the grace of my teacher, Swami Dayananda Saraswati, to receive my initiation as a Brahmacarini.

As I stand in this holy river declaring my intentions to live fully within the knowledge of the Vedas, to live in Shiva, I must never forget this moment.

Cidananda rupah, Sivo'ham. Sivo'ham.
My nature is boundless, infinite pure consciousness
I am Shiva. I am Shiva.

—Sankaracarya
Nirvana Satkam

My journey in this life began in the early fifties in a country then called British Guiana (now Guyana). My grandparents were exported from India by the British. The Indians came as indentured laborers, slightly more fortunate than the Africans who were brought by force as slaves. My people came as priests to minister the Hindu scriptures and console vast numbers of humans who were stripped of family, villages, culture, habits, and, most important, their homeland.

Like those belonging to a second generation, I grew up without knowing my grandparents. They died young, like so many others who became confused, mad, or riddled with diseases. My parents carried the heavy burden of carving a new life in a new land while maintaining the traditions left far behind across the seas. Traditional *dharmas*, never to be witnessed again in the homeland, became a cherished and sacred memory, observed with resolute devotion. I was fortunate to have had, from an early age, a teacher of colossal magnificence, my father, the proverbial jack of all trades. The youngest in his family, and blessed with rare qualities of vision, strength and devotion to his people, he crossed the invisible bridge between India and Guyana while carrying his entire family, immediate and extended, squarely on his back. His wisdom and selfless sacrifices advanced his people, and in particular his children, through multi-cultural barriers and archaic technology, into the twentieth century. Because Guyana remained fifty years behind the rest of the world technologically, we were ten-fold closer to the natural ways of *sadhana*, which, in the last few centuries in India has been translated as "religious practice," but which I have taken the liberty of reviving to what I believe would have been its original meaning: wholesome activities practiced in harmony with nature.

Eleven children, blessed by two mothers, grew up in the dear and precious lap of nature. The idyllic field of childhood play stretched from the black, salty creek waters to the stiff khaki school uniforms. Fragrant *chamelis* thickened the air; bails of Indian cotton sprawled across the merchants' tables; the virgin green rice fields danced in the *masala* flooded air; milk so white it turned blue in moonlight; skins so black they reflected the sky; these are the memories of my country. It was a vast and mysterious land layered with British noise, Indian harmonics, and African rhythm, but the smell of my people was not there. The vibrations braided into their very being were left far behind. I loved the elders with a raging passion. I huddled in their midst to sniff and smell their scent, somehow knowing that I too could not live without their innate memory.

Meanwhile, the British rule abroad was coming to an end. Guyana was one of her last adoptees. My father foresaw the inevitable fate of a fourth world country soon to gain her independence, and skillfully honed his older children, with the prowess of creative missiles, in preparation for exportation to England, the United States and Canada. In my case, I received college equivalent degrees from London University by the soft green age of fifteen. My country became independent, and the inevitable bitter racial wars began. Less fortunate than those of us who were sent abroad before the painful struggle began, my parents, the younger siblings, the aged, and the indigent were caught in the vicious cross-fire of bloody war.

As the usual atrocities of war demeaned nature, the fertile fields and prolific lands were laid waste, the crystal streams and black waters poisoned, the redwood savagely felled. Guyana, once exquisite and prosperous with her mighty rivers, reservoirs of immense riches in gold and minerals, and pre-historic species residing in the highland rain forests, remained silently weeping in shame and obscurity for two decades. Once more my people moved on and re-settled, this time in Canada.

Peerless and pressed beyond the constraints of mind and spirit, I abandoned myself to cancer at the age of twenty-three. I let my mask fall and shatter into oblivion. The light of the Divine peered through the crevices of my broken body. My expensive, false self was dying at the same time as my divine nature hunted me down. Through my five-year sojourn with cancer, I was able to cognize my karma and my purpose for being here, and re-structure a life which both honored my past and allowed my present. I was able to see my real self, beyond the pain of my people and the conflicts of my early dualistic perceptions. In fact, I discovered nature and re-acquainted myself with the poignancy and rich beauty of the simple daily sadhanas of my childhood years.

Through the cognition of my own spiritual recognizance, timeless sadhanas, and the help of one ingenious and remarkable human, Dr. James Holland, I healed into a new being. Today marks my twentieth year since I leaped from the ashes of cancer to begin my studies of the holistic principles of life.

My work with nature's sadhanas continues to grow with the knowledge I have gleaned from the Ayurvedas and Vedanta. Boundlessly poignant in their healing abilities, and vital to the culling of human divinity, the sadhanas presented in this book are adapted from the Ayurvedas. Moreover, they reflect my myriad experiences through life's fiery passages and the awakening of my deep cognitive memories.

I am not a physician, Ayurvedic or otherwise. My intentions are to share the healing secrets I have learned from practice, both in my personal life and with the many I have helped through the dark passage of cancer. Most of all, I pray to live in the wisdom of the Vedas to discover innocence, my true nature.

About the Use of Sanskrit in This Text

Sanskrit is thought to be much more than a language in that it is said to reflect cosmic sound itself. The first manifestation to emerge in the universe in the form of gravitational and vibrational fields, cosmic sound nurtures, births and sustains all other manifestations. Are we not told that the Supreme One sent the multiple forces of creation through *shabda brahman*, the word? In the form of *varnas*, pure vibration and profound silence, God's numinous energy manifests, creating the audible or imperfect sound and visible form. Using Sanskrit, therefore, is considered to be the first sadhana, wholesome practice, that, if followed, instantly reminds us of our connection, our relationship, to the One, the Whole.

The many gods of the Vedic pantheon are considered to be the seeds of the universe. From these seeds, every precise letter of the Sanskrit alphabet has been developed, portraying the various facets of the Divine Mother. Using Sanskrit, originally called Devanagari, literally, "the means of communion among the gods," is also a means of attuning to the cosmic vibration of the universe. The circumspect intonation of a word, phrase, mantra, or prayer in Sanskrit, even without knowledge of its meaning, has been found to bring clarity, prosperity, and boundless poignancy to life. The seed syllables, or combination of Sanskrit letters containing the sum total of each deity or symbol of divinity, are the most effective mantras, the most powerful being *Om*. The proper intonation of Sanskrit syllables and words in the form of mantras purifies *ojas*, our biological essence, *tejas*, our mind's subtle fire, and *akasa*, our subtle vibrational field. Each word is derived from a verbal root having an absolute meaning, without ambiguity or cultural connotation, and therefore conveys an equally absolute meaning. Wanting to share this sadhana with you, my reader, I have maintained my practice of using the Sanskrit words and names which apply to most of the therapies and medicines discussed in the book, providing whatever explanation deemed helpful along the way. May you be enhanced by this wholesome practice. *Om*.

INTRODUCTION TO AYURVEDA

The Auspicious Past

he Vedas, made up of the *Rig, Yajur, Sama,* and *Atharva* Vedas in which the ancient scriptural knowledge is found, have been handed down to us generation by generation over several thousand years of oral tradition, before finally being recorded in written form. It wasn't until about 500 B.C. that the sage Adi Sankara culled the end portions from the Vedas, called Vedanta, which reveals the knowledge that the self and the Supreme Being are one. Sankara recorded this knowledge on palm leaves, along with vast commentaries on the subject.

Rig Veda, the foundation pillar and oldest of the Vedas, contains many references to Ayurvedic principles, although Ayurveda itself was primarily developed from the Atharva Veda, the most recent of the Vedas. The mainstay of the Ayurvedic knowledge we have today is found in the two great treatises, *Charaka Samhita* and *Sushruta Samhita,* each of which first appeared at the turn of the first millenium B.C.

Charaka Samhita remains foremost, focusing on the internal body/mind medicine of Ayurveda, in which the cause of diseases and the constitution of a person are addressed first. The knowledge of Ayurvedic surgery and the details of its techniques, contained in the *Sushruta Samhita,* are lost to us today, these practices having been interrupted at the end of Buddha's life. During the medieval period, the rejuvenation and virilization therapies, known as *rasayana* and *vajikarana*, were introduced into the Ayurvedic panoply of healing practices. Around 500 B.C., Ayurveda was formed into eight branches of medicine and two primary schools of thought named after the sages Atreya and Dhanvantari. Charaka belonged to the Atreya school of Ayurveda and Sushruta to the Dhanvantari school.

Pancha karma therapy, the core of Ayurveda's healing therapies, is believed to predate even the earliest applications of Ayurveda, which is thought to have occurred some 8000 years ago. Although it has endured long periods of interruption in India, pancha karma is still practiced in many regions of the country. Central to a phenomenal system of ancient healing techniques said to have been practiced by the gods who taught the earliest seers on earth, this therapy remains the most vital link to the essential and immortal essence of human life.

The term pancha karma refers to the five principal practices used to cleanse the body of its excess bodily humors, called *doshas*. Although Charaka did not coin the term "pancha karma," he did introduce these cleansing practices as the axis around which all Ayurvedic healing therapies revolve, defining it as the one primary independent discipline to be employed in order to promote health. Charaka considered it a requisite procedure before surgical operations or the administration of any of the rejuvenation therapies. Pancha karma benefits both the healthy and unhealthy and is considered to be the most effective therapy for preventing and curing diseases, as well as for revitalizing the entire human organism.

Ayurvedic massage was developed, along with *kalari* (a form of martial arts), to enhance the welfare of the early warriors, and is still used extensively in the Kerala region of India. It is a requisite to precede pancha karma therapy. This massage is based on knowledge of the body's *marma* points, the anatomical sites where muscles, nerves, blood vessels, joints, ligaments, and bones enjoin. Recognition of marma points historically precedes and is comparable to that of the meridian points used in acupuncture. Although there are many variations of current massage practices in India, differing somewhat from classical Ayurvedic applications, the methods used are still valid in terms of their effectiveness in regaining and maintaining health.

MANDALA OF HEALING THERAPIES

Pancha karma is the core of a vast mandala of therapies. In this mandala, there are two main categories, *shodhana* and *shamana*. Shodhana refers to pancha karma's five main cleansing and elimination procedures, while shamana encompasses the supporting therapies that are the preparation and post-therapy measures for pancha karma proper. Both groups of therapies are included here as a mandala of healing practices, since both shodhana and shamana braid together to form a stupendous human synergy of potent rejuvenation and rebirth.

Existing in the body of all living organisms, the five elements congregate in a certain pattern and are known as doshas, bodily humors. The three doshas, Vata, Pitta and Kapha, are referred to respectively as the air, fire and water principles of the body. Because the human body maintains a delicate homeostasis, the process of eliminating its manifested doshas and diseases is a systematic act of cajoling, tempering, shocking, and nurturing the body. The excess doshas are never forcibly removed from the organism. In classical practice, an intricate weave of knowledge of the seasonal effects on the tissues, the precise time of the doshas' advances, the overall condition of the person, the phases of the moon, and the pertaining signs and symbols of the surrounding animals and birds all contributed to the timing and nature of the applied pancha karma treatment. Today, the minimum observation of pancha karma therapy practice involves three distinct phases —preparation, main action, and post procedures to sustain the effects of the therapy. Shodhana, the central and primary action in the mandala of treatments, is administered in the following sequence: emesis, purgation, unctuous enema (optional, depending on the person's condition), medicated decoction enema, and nasal insufflation. The timing and number of applications vary, depending on the specific condition being addressed.

Before these five *karmas*, or actions, are administered, a certain period of time is spent on the necessary preparatory actions. Two main shamana therapies are administered: a combination of *snehana* and *abhyanga*, which involve the thorough oelating and massaging of the entire body, followed by *svedana*, the inducing of sweat through fomentation. These treatments cajole and prepare bodily tissues, as well as the mind and spirit, for the central and primary course of elimination therapies.

While all of the shamana therapies may be used independently of pancha karma, pancha karma may not be performed without the preparatory and sustaining treatments of the shamana therapies. The shamana therapies are rejuvenative and strengthening in nature, whereas the shodhana processes of pancha karma are cleansing, emphasizing elimination and depletion.

Following the pancha karma treatments, a third phase of healing practices is observed. Programs of wholesome activities, diet, and Ayurvedic teas or medicines are designed for each person, in order to sustain the results of the treatments received.

The mandala group of therapies in traditional use not only restores complete health, but more importantly, enables us to enjoy a sense of rebirth. When the necessary observances of sadhanas are continued, not only as a medium for post therapy, but as an integral part of our everyday activities, we are able to touch and draw upon the potential immortality imbued in the human species.

Shamana: Supporting Therapies

*Depleted doshas may be restored by brhmana
therapy; excessive doshas may be reduced by
langhana therapy; vitiated doshas may be
eliminated by the shodhana therapies; and, while in
a state of balance, they may be maintained by the
shamana therapies.*

—Sushruta

The shamana therapies, which are often used to support the pancha karma menu of therapies, include the preparatory treatments of oil massage and fomentation treatments as well as the follow-up therapies—nourishing foods, fasting, wholesome activities, and medicinal herbs and substances, among others. Whether they are used with pancha karma or independently, they need to be administered with full awareness of the prevailing seasonal influences and the condition of the doshas in the body.

Within the shamana group, there are six distinct therapies, which fall into two categories: *langhana*, which deplete the body, and *brhmana*, which add strength and substance to the body. These terms, langhana and brhmana, not only refer to specific groups of treatments but are also the names given to two specific post pancha karma regimens. In their group context, langhana and brhmana each cover three aspects of the six shamana therapies. For instance, the langhana group encompasses *svedana*, sweat-inducing therapy, and *rukshana*, dehydration therapy, as well as the langhana regimen itself, meaning those post pancha karma or independent body depleting measures such as fasting and physical exercise. The brhmana group covers *snehana*, oelation therapy, and *stambhana*, retention therapy, as well as the brhmana regimen, those post pancha karma or independent body building measures such as the use of nourishing foods, herbs, and unctuous substances.

Langhana treatments are used primarily to reduce Kapha and Pitta conditions, and to alleviate specific conditions like blood disorders, skin diseases, extreme stagnation of malas, bodily wastes, and obesity. The characteristics of the medicines and procedures used in this form of therapy are light, hot, sharp, rough, mobile, and hard.

Langhana treatment is more a group of sadhanas than therapy. The various langhana sadhanas which safeguard against bodily excesses are: fasting; the use of herbal therapy to promote and maintain digestion; the preparation and use of wholesome foods such as the sattvic and energizing diets, discussed in Chapter Eight; wholesome exercises; and treatments performed in the open air and bright sunlight.

The second treatment of langhana therapy, called rukshana, is a process of dehydrating the body. Rukshana favors all the qualities of the medicines and procedures used in the langhana group with one exception, in that it produces a stabilizing effect on the body. Usually, a treatment in the langhana genre is mobile in nature. Although it is best suited for conditions like water retentive tissue which are more likely to need dehydration than depletion, the rukshana form of treatment may also be used for excess Pitta and Kapha conditions. Major diseases which are located in the marma points, vital junctions of the joints and muscles, are usually treated with the rukshana procedure as well.

The main and third treatment of the langhana group, called svedana, has an infinite number of procedures within it to induce profuse sweating through fomentation. According to Ayurveda, this procedure may be administered only after the body is lubricated and properly massaged. Svedana, an invigorating procedure, is specific to Vata and Kapha disorders but may also be used for some Pitta disorders.

Brhmana, the second main group of shamana therapies, provides the body with strength and substance. This group of treatments is specifically geared to major Vata disorders, such as emaciation and the diseases of old age. Many forms of injuries and addictions are treated successfully with this group of healing actions. Conditions requiring brhmana measures may be treated throughout the year, although these strengthening treatments are usually administered in the summer when human weakness tends to be at its peak.

The qualities of the medicines and procedures used in the brhmana group of therapies contrast dramatically to those used in the langhana forms of treatment. The characteristics of brhmana treatments are heavy, firm, cold, soft, oily, clear, slow, and smooth.

Brhmana treatments, also more a group of sadhanas than therapies, are tailored to relieve the many grievances of Vata, as well as to restore balance to all three doshas after the dramatic cleansing actions of pancha karma. These treatments consist of nourishing and strengthening foods such as the post pancha karma diet as well as herbal therapies to attenuate conditions such as chronic and debilitating diseases. Ayurvedic massages with aromatic and medicinal oils, sleep therapy, nurturing teas, and brews made with substances like ghee and natural sugar cane juice, are all considered brhmana treatments.

Anuvasana vasti, a medicated oil enema formulated to simultaneously remove excess Vata from the colon and enrich the tissues, is considered both a pancha karma measure as well as a snehana treatment belonging to the brhmana group. The treatment itself is described in detail in the section on pancha karma therapies.

The main treatment in the brhmana group is called snehana. The literal meaning of "snehana" is "love." In this love therapy, ample amounts of oil are used to massage the body into a blissful state. A vital form of treatment in its own right, snehana is an excellent salve for all three doshas, particularly Vata. Snehana procedures include oelation treatments to the head, such as *shirodhara*, the process of dripping oil on the forehead, and *masthiskya*, the application of paste to the head.

The second treatment within the brhmana group is called stambhana, that which allows retention in the body. Stambhana favors all the qualities of the medicines and procedures used in the brhmana group with one main exception: it facilitates dryness, whereas a brhmana form of treatment is usually unctuous. The stambhana form of treatment is specific to conditions such as severe burns from fire or alkali, poisoning, diarrhea, vomiting, and many Pitta-type disorders. Because it employs substances with dry, retentive and mostly cooling medicinal properties, stambhana is generally considered a more appropriate treatment for Pitta conditions.

When the mandala of therapies are all performed together the process takes approximately one month. A specific classical schedule (see Chapter Seven) is recommended when all five actions of pancha karma are required. Depending on the nature of the condition being treated, fewer therapies may be administered.

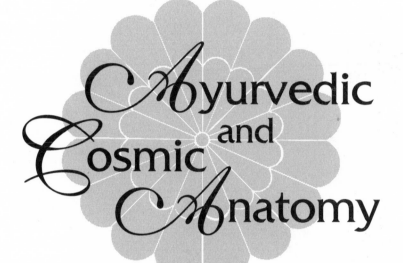

Ayurvedic and Cosmic Anatomy

OUR COSMIC BEGINNING

*T*hree primordial forces, or principles, interweaving to create the five elements—space, air, fire, water, and earth—birth the entire creation.

The principle of stillness, *tamas*, replenishes the universe and its beings and is the main principle of support within the physical universe. The principle of self-organizing activity, *rajas*, gives motility and co-ordination to the universe and human life. The principle of harmonic and cosmic intelligence, *sattva*, maintains universal and individual stasis and awareness. These three cosmic principles, called *gunas*, operating through the five elements they have created, directly interphase with human existence.

On the physical plane, tamas works closely with the physical functions of the body, summarized as bodily humors, tissues and wastes. Tamas is said to exercise the greatest influence on the body's water aspect, or *Kapha dosha*, and gives the body its ability to cogitate and to endure long periods of gestation. The tamas principle plants the natural seed of instinct in all life, permitting, for example, the vegetation to burrow beneath the snows, while the seeds throb ever so faintly in the earth—all necessary actions of stillness in order to replenish vitality and growth. Tamas' subtle force, called *ojas*, the lubricating nectar within the physical organism, imbues life with the ability to rest, to sleep, to become resolved within her Earth Mother womb.

Rajas influences the psychic plane of existence and works closely with the psychological functions of the body. On the physical level, rajas is said to exercise the most influence on the body's air aspect, *Vata dosha*. It gives us our power to transform what is being perceived externally into thoughts, concepts, visions, and dreams. Operating through the subtle forces of life-sustaining air, *prana*, this principle maintains our equanimity and influences our ability to organize what is being put into motion within this gravitational field of play.

Rajas maintains the memory of all species recorded from the beginning of time. For instance, when the bighorn sheep suspends itself high up on the overhanging cliffs of the Andes, defying gravity, it is expressing the innate structure of its species' memory preserved through billions of years only because of rajas. Also owing to rajas, the absolute chaos demonstrated by a hive of bees takes a harmoniously united form as the worker bees float in congress behind their queen. A thundering herd of elephants splash into the Ganges river and swim effortlessly, suspended across the deep waters with the delicacy of butterflies, all because of rajas' maintenance of balance within nature.

Referred to as the universe's cosmic intelligence, the third principle, sattva, permeates each and every minute cell of our being. It functions through our existential states of awareness, although it also influences the physical organism to some extent. Within the physical body, sattva is said to exercise the most influence on its fire aspect, *Pitta dosha*. Closely linked to the universal subtle fire, tejas, the sattva principle maintains the cosmic memory of the entire creation—the collective memory of the entire universe from its inception. Sattva also maintains the cognitive memory of every human—each individual's memory accumulated from the beginning of time through each rebirth until the present time—our personal wisdom, in other words. (Memories accumulated within the present life are referred to in this book as experiential memories.)

This subject will be further explored in Chapter Two. I am introducing the three phases of memory here as they comprise the core of my work in Ayurveda, and form the substratum of this presentation. Through my personal experience and Vedic studies, I have discovered the awakening of my own cognitive states, and have come to see that the three memories—cosmic, cognitive and experiential—form the epicenter of our unique human nature and, although they are not mentioned as such in Ayurveda, they do need to be understood if we are to effectively ply our remembrance of the self amid the sacred weave of nature's ways.

4

CHAPTER ONE

AYURVEDIC ANATOMY

PART ONE
Language of the Doshas

The physical, psychic and cosmic language of the body is created from the circadian rhythm of the universe set in motion some billions of years ago when the five great elements were born. Space, air, fire, water, and earth, the first material for life, are the basis of the Vedic sciences. In Ayurveda, human physiognomy is rooted in bodily humors, *doshas*, tissues, *dhatus*, and wastes, *malas*. These three principles support all of life and are more than the physical substance of our anatomy. The doshas, dhatus, and malas are the messengers of communication that interphase the external and internal nature.

When existing in the body of all living organisms, the five elements congregate in a certain pattern and are known in Sanskrit as doshas, the literal meaning of which is, "that which is quick to go out of balance." Doshas imply that the human system maintains a delicate balance or homeostasis, its dynamic elemental composition always being on the verge of disorder; all the more reason to learn how to decipher the cosmic "language" imbedded in our nature and communicated to us by the doshas, dhatus, and malas.

The doshas are a classic example of energy and matter in dynamic accord. All matter born from energy remains intricately woven within its core nature of

5

energy. The human body is an excellent demonstration of tangible matter, dhatus and malas, intimately interacting with doshas, which are more energy than matter until, that is, they manifest as diseases in the organism. In a state of balance or equilibrium, doshas are considered an energy force in that we cannot visibly detect them as they move through and support bodily function. In a state of imbalance or disequilibrium the doshas become visible as mucus, bile, wind, and physical matter. When these early signs of disorder are ignored, imbalances can quickly become full-blown diseases.

In this unique system of explaining health, air and space—both ethereal elements—form one of the three doshas called Vata. Here air exercises its power of mobility only when space is available. The elements fire and water form a second dosha called Pitta. Here the bodily water protects the heat of the body from burning through. An example of bodily fire is the acid in our stomachs, which, if leaked from the stomach, is capable of burning the organism with the force of a raging fire. Water is the buffering force that contains the body's fires. The elements water and earth congregate to form the third dosha called Kapha. Because of their mutual density, water gives earth its fluidity. Without water, earth would become stagnated and inert. Thus, the Kapha dosha enables a certain fluidity in the body without depriving it of its solid support. These three doshas co-exist in all living organisms. The degree to which each dosha exists within a person determines the individual's constitution, commonly referred to as body type.

In Ayurveda, the individual dosha is the primary consideration in diagnosis. Although there are numerous causes of diseases, such as hereditary, congenital, external, and providential factors, aggravation of the doshas is present as either a result or cause of ill health.

PHYSICAL NATURE OF THE DOSHAS

In the cosmos at large, Kapha's external nature of water and earth express themselves as the forces of cohesion, absorption, and stability. Pitta's external nature of fire expresses itself as the force of transmutation and dynamism. Vata's external nature is air, the force of mobility and exhilaration, as well as space, the field where all activities occur in dynamic containment.

Each dosha also has a primary function in the body. Vata is the moving force, Pitta is the force of assimilation, and Kapha is the force of stability. Together, they are a stupendous example of three seemingly adversarial characters in potential harmony as a result of each dosha's intricate balance of force in the body. Vata, the most dominant of the doshas, governs bodily movement, the nervous system, and the life force. Without Vata's mobility in the body, Pitta and Kapha would be rendered lame. Pitta governs enzymatic and hormonal activities, and is responsible for digestion, pigmentation, body temperature, hunger, thirst, and sight. Further, Pitta acts as a balancing force for Vata and Kapha. Kapha governs the body's structure and stability. It lubricates joints, provides moisture to the skin, heals wounds, and regulates Vata and Pitta.

Vata, Pitta, and Kapha pervade the entire body, but their primary domains are in the lower, middle, and upper body, respectively. Kapha rules the head, neck, thorax, chest, upper portion of the stomach, fat tissues, and the joints. Pitta pervades the chest, umbilical area, stomach, small intestines, sweat and lymph glands, and the blood. Vata dominates the lower body, pelvic region, colon, bladder, urinary tract, thighs, legs, arms, bones, and nervous system.

Apart from its main site, each dosha has four secondary sites located in different areas of the body. Each dosha then has five sites considered to be its centers of operation, which include the various outreach systems because of which the entire body functions. The doshas interact continuously with the external elements to replenish their energy within the body. Each of the three doshas' five sites has a specific responsibility towards the maintenance of the organism. Because the doshas also exist in the more subtle aspects of the body and universe, planes that actively affect the physical aspects, they are energetically much more influential in the maintenance of our overall health than their mere physiological expressions in the body would suggest. In fact as they manifest within the physical body, they need to be continuously discarded to prevent the body from decaying.

PHYSIO-PSYCHOLOGICAL NATURE OF THE DOSHAS

Five Airs of Vata

The five sites or centers of operation and systemic outreach through which Vata casts its influence on the entire organism are called the five airs of Vata, namely: *prana*, respiration; *udana*, throat; *samana*, stomach; *apana*, colon; and *vyana*, circulation.

Air of Respiration: Prana

Prana is the first air of the universe and of the body. Although located in the body between the diaphragm and throat, it not only pervades the region of the heart and chest, but also up into the face and brain. Prana aids in the chewing and swallowing of food and provides immediate nourishment to all vital tissues of the body. The system is constantly being rejuvenated through the natural rhythm of the breath's inhalation, exhalation, and timely retention. The activity of the colon is attuned to the respiration's rhythm, extracting prana from the digested food and diffusing it into all of the tissues in the body. When the colon is disturbed and unable to fulfill its natural ability to extract and diffuse prana, this unused prana becomes waste—a great waste, indeed.

Prana facilitates all movement in and out of the body. It moves in the region of the heart, causing it to beat; it carries food through the esophagus into the stomach. Prana sustains the heart, arteries, veins, senses, and our wisdom faculty, *buddhi*. When prana cannot function properly, our very life force is threatened. Respiratory ailments such as bronchitis and asthma result. Heart ailments and the impulse to vomit are also related to prana's imbalance. Excess Vata, which collects in the colon, joints, and other Vata locations, can lead to such conditions as painful joints and bones, arthritis, and gastritis, among others. A major cause of many diseases is the accumulation of Vata in the colon, also due to the impairment of prana.

Prana is replenished through respiration. To promote optimal health through pranic breathing, the sages devised an elaborate system of breathing exercises known as *pranayama*, which is the practice of cleansing and controlling the breath. The exercises for breath maintenance include three phases: expiration, inspiration, and retention. A fourth phase, called the silent breath, is practiced by adept yogis who have mastered the variations of the other three phases. Modern science is not yet equipped to distinguish between a yogi practicing the silent breath and someone who has physically died.

Prana: The Silent Witness

On the cosmic plane, prana is considered the first air of creation. Being the finest of the airs, it has been infused into the life of all organisms by the creator since the beginning of time, energy, and matter. Prana is referred to by the ancients as the "soul within the body," and as the cosmic breath of the Atman, the Essential Self. At our most sublime level of existence, prana is the silent witness to our journey in life. This is why it is said to sit on the throne of the heart. According to the Vedas, the heartbeat is synchronized with our breath, beating four times the speed of each normal breath. When our bodies can no longer sustain the timely rhythm of our breath, the eternal song of the heart is silenced. Broken hearts prevail when the intuitional language imbued by prana in our body is forgotten. Pranayama, the breathing practices referred to above, yoga postures and meditation, seasonal cleansing therapies such as pancha karma, and Vata-nourishing foods are all excellent ways to revitalize prana.

Air of the Throat: Udana

Udana, the second air of Vata, and prana are somewhat analogous to the sympathetic and the parasympathetic nervous systems. Udana, which means "rising air," flows upward from the umbilicus through the lung and into the throat and nose. Known as the air of ejection, it provides us with our vocal powers and clarity of sense perceptions. It also preserves our body's natural forces, such as its strength of will and capacity for effort.

Udana has the supreme task of keeping track of the number of breaths we expend. Vedic lore tells us that each person, according to his or her karma, is given a certain number of breaths at the time of conception. When this ration is used up, the person dies. Our normal breathing pace is slow and rhythmic. When our body is functioning properly, we take approximately sixteen breaths per minute. Therefore, according to the ancients, when we breathe faster or hold the breath, due to fear, anxiety, and so on, we are shortening our life.

An equally supreme task is udana's capacity to preserve memory, both experiential (memories gathered within a present lifetime) and cognitive (cumulative memories carried into all lives from the beginning of creation through all time). Impairment of udana can result in loss of memory, impaired speech, giddiness or heaviness in the head, deep-seated fears, and a shortened life span.

Udana: Keeper of Memory

At the subtle level, the creator infused, through the breath, the eternal air of udana into all living creatures, in order to track our various experiences and lives. Udana is the creator's time clock within us. Every breath we take expends karma. When the breath is long, cool, and rhythmic, we are able to increase our life span and to better serve the purpose of our journey. When the breath is shallow, rushed, and fatigued, we shorten our stay and leave the travel unfinished. The cosmic breath we received produces sound. Our voice is a reminder of our sacred origin since it expresses breath through the sound of the creator. Through wholesome and kind utterances, we are able to maintain our cognate privilege as humans. All harmonious sound produced by humans resonates with the vast and immutable consciousness. Likewise, all disharmonious noise we utter or create, whether through our own voices or mechanical devices, results in the impairment of memory, both experiential and cognitive, as well as alienation from our cosmic nature.

Udana's lesson is one of alertness and sanity. When we are able to control our sound, we protect udana. In this protection, we preserve our nature of awareness. Then we are able to hear the distant flight of a hawk, the silent crawling of the sand. We are better able to read the universal signs and to observe with reverence the sacred staff given us to walk the journey. In our own personal harmonious resonance we are able to maintain the innate link with creation, braided, as we are, to all creation through breath.

Although as separate human beings we are involved in different activities and functions, at various speeds, our cosmic nature is to remain "phase coherent" with the universe. To give an analogy: a number of pendulum clocks were mounted on the same wall by a Dutch physicist. Initially, each one ticked at its own speed, but, after a short while, they began ticking in unison. Their independent behavior became synchronized as a result of the sympathetic resonance of the collective sound waves created within the wall. The breath that ties the entire creation and all of its species together works in the same way. By becoming aware of our breath, we are essentially tuning in with, joining, the harmonic coherence of the universe.

Out of this cosmic resonance, the Vedic seers culled invaluable mantras which, when uttered repetitively and intoned properly, create a gravitational field of vibration.

Within this protective field we reverberate with all of nature. This cosmic system of sound, resonating between creator and creation, replenishes our intuitive impulses. Udana invites us to implode into the sonority of our origin where the lines between internal and external energy and matter dissolve.

The practice of silence, pranayama, yoga, wholesome activities such as the planting of herbs and foods, grinding grains and spices, seasonal cleansing of the internal body, daily cleansing of head, eyes, ears, nose, throat, Ayurvedic massage, and Vata-nourishing foods are all sadhanas to keep the udana in our body in balance.

Air of the Stomach: Samana

Samana, the third air of Vata, is located between the diaphragm and navel. It aids the movement of food through the stomach and small intestines, fans the fires of digestion by stimulating the production and activity of gastric juices and digestive enzymes and helps in the assimilation of nutrients extracted from our food. Samana is the moving force that transports these nutrients to the various tissue elements and discharges wastes into the colon. When the samana air is disturbed, it can cause mucus accumulation in the stomach, indigestion, poor as-similation, and diarrhea.

Samana: Keeper of Balance

At the subtle body level, samana represents our inner flexibility and spirit of discernment. Samana teaches us to discriminate between what is valuable and what is to be discarded as our desires for material things grow. Its lessons are rooted in our ability to balance, an apt task given its location in the mid-body. Sadhanas such as yoga, tai-chi, pranayama, Ayurvedic massage, Ayurvedic purga-tion therapy, and Vata-nourishing foods help samana to remain healthy and bal-anced.

Air of the Colon: Apana

The fourth air of Vata, apana, is located in the colon and the organs of the pelvic region. Also known as the air of elimination, apana's primary function is to relieve the body of feces, urine, flatus, semen, and menstrual waste. Its down-ward pressure maintains the fetus and the flow of its eventual birth. Apana is the most dominant of the five airs, situated as it is in Vata's primary location. Apana maintains the delayed nutrition of prana in the organism. When apana is im-paired, diseases of the bladder, anus, testicles, uterus, and obstinate urinary dis-eases, including diabetes, prevail.

Apana: Keeper of Empty

On the subtle plane, apana is our spirit of non-attachment to material posses-sions. Patanjali's yoga sutras inform us that the moral restraint of greedlessness is necessary before we can truly access our cognitive memories. True to its down-ward force of elimination, apana teaches us how to nourish ourselves, and to let go

10

of that which is in excess. Sadhanas such as seasonal cleansing of the internal body, especially Ayurvedic enema therapy, Ayurvedic massage, pranayama, warm baths, aroma therapy, and Vata-nourishing foods help to rejuvenate apana.

Air of Circulation: Vyana

Vyana is the fifth and final air of the Vata and is located in the heart. It diffuses the energy derived from food and breath throughout the entire organism including the skin. Circulatory in nature, Vyana functions in the body's circulation channels, such as the blood vessels, to transport nutritive juices and blood throughout the body. Vyana also carries sweat from the glands to the skin and is the force behind bodily expressions such as yawning and blinking. When vyana malfunctions, there is dryness of the skin and other body extremities, poor circulation, and diseases such as fever and diarrhea.

Vyana: Keeper of Charity

At the subtle level, vyana is expressed as our attention to charity and personal freedom. Teaching us to circulate in the community, to influence goodwill and charity, it gives us our inward mobility and influential nature which we are urged to express gently within activity. Sadhanas such as yoga, pranayama, body brushing, baths, aroma therapy, Ayurvedic massage, and Vata-nourishing foods rejuvenate vyana.

Five Subsidiary Airs

In addition to these five airs, Vata also has five minor subsidiary airs. *Naga* is the air which releases abdominal pressure by belching. *Kurma* controls the movement of the eyelids to protect the eyes from dust and dirt particles, light, and so on. *Krekara*, the air which causes sneezing and coughing, prevents external substances from passing up into the nasal passages. *Devadatta* controls our yawning reflex, which provides additional oxygen to a tired body. Finally, there is the air of *dhanamjaya*, which remains in the body after death, sometimes causing bloating and movement in the corpse.

Five Fires of Pitta

Pitta, formed from the elements of fire and water, also is said to reside in five sites. These sites are the centers of operation and systemic outreach through which the Pitta dosha influences the entire organism; they are: *pachaka*, stomach; *ranjaka*, blood; *sadhaka*, heart; *alochaka*, eyes; and *bhrajaka*, skin.

Fire of the Stomach: Pachaka

Pachaka is referred to in Ayurveda as the first fire of the body. It exists in the small intestine, duodenum, gall bladder, liver, and pancreas, and supports the remaining four fires, to be discussed below. Pachaka's main action is the dissolving and digesting of the food we eat. It also regulates body temperature. Once digestion has taken place, pachaka separates the food's nutritive elements from its waste elements. An imbalance in this first fire, pachaka, causes indigestion as well as a revulsion for food.

Pachaka: Keeper of the Flame

At the subtle body level, pachaka is the fire responsible for proper assimilation at the mental level. It teaches us the fine art of discrimination by enabling us to develop an alert and discerning mind. Meditation is a superb sadhana to replenish pachaka. Seasonal cleansing of the internal body, fasting, cooling baths, Ayurvedic purgation therapy, aroma therapy, and Pitta-nourishing foods appease pachaka.

Fire of the Blood: Ranjaka

True to its name, ranjaka, the second fire of Pitta, controls the formation and preservation of blood. Located in the liver, spleen, and stomach, ranjaka provides the blood with its color and oxygen. When ranjaka is impaired, bile compounds may appear in the blood and diseases such as anemia and jaundice may follow.

Ranjaka: Keeper of Passion

At its subtle level of functioning, ranjaka teaches us the spirit of invigoration and gratification. When we learn the lessons of the second fire, we are able to maintain a calm but colorful mind and tame the passions of the body. Ranjaka teaches us to play, to stimulate, satisfy, and finally to give back this invigoration to the universe. Sadhanas such as active sports, seasonal cleansing of the internal body, cooling activities, and Pitta-nourishing foods are all revitalizing to this fire.

Fire of the Heart: Sadhaka

The finest of the fires, sadhaka, the third fire, is central to the activity of Pitta. It reigns, along with prana, in the heart. In concert with udana, it governs memory and the retention and wellness of all mental functioning. When sadhaka is impaired, there may be psychic disturbances, mental disorientation, extreme emotional states, and cravings for extreme foods, drugs, and so on.

Sadhaka: Keeper of the Spirit Flame

At the subtle level, this fire is the most effective and efficient in the human body, mind, and spirit. It works within our deeper self and aids in the preservation and unfolding of our cognitive memories. Sadhaka teaches humility and cognitive truth. It allows us to cross over from the state of experiences into the fullness of our own immortality. Sadhanas such as meditation, pranayama, yoga, cleansing of both the internal and external body, studies of the sacred lore, and Pitta-nourishing foods are vital to the maintenance of excellence in the sadhaka fire.

Fire of the Eyes: Alochaka

Alochaka, the fourth fire of Pitta, exists in the pupils of the eyes. It animates sight, gives the eyes their lustre, and diffuses light and its spectrum of colors throughout the body. When the fourth fire is vitiated, there is impairment of vision and yellowness may appear in the eyes.

Alochaka: Keeper of Vision

At the subtle body level, this fire gives creative vision, hope, and alertness. It teaches consideration and accommodation of all creatures, and shows us how to accept ourselves from our very beginnings. Sadhanas such as eye exercises, painting, picnicking, strolling, sitting by a stream, seasonal cleansing of the internal body, and Pitta-nourishing foods help to maintain alochaka's equilibrium.

Fire of the Skin: Bhrajaka

The fifth fire, bhrajaka, is located in the skin, giving the skin its lustre and gleam. Bhrajaka protects the body from the depredation of the elements and facilitates the assimilation of light, wind, water, and oil through the skin. When this fire is disturbed, skin diseases such as psoriasis, eczema, and leukoderma may result.

Bhrajaka: Keeper of Beauty

At the subtle level, bhrajaka teaches cleanliness and inner luminosity. It gives us *rasa*, beauty, both internal and external. Its intention is to teach us how to share our light and influence everything in our midst with our gleam, brightness, and effervescence. Sadhanas such as cleaning and decorating our living space, daily bodily cleansing (i.e., skin brushing and anointing the body), aroma therapy, seasonal internal cleansing of the body, and Pitta-nourishing foods help to keep bhrajaka in good condition.

Five Waters of Kapha

Kapha, formed from the elements water and earth, also manifests in five doshic sites, through which centers of operation and systemic outreach it influences the entire organism. The five waters of Kapha are: *kledaka*, stomach; *avalambaka*, heart; *bodhaka*, tongue; *tarpaka*, head; and *slesaka*, joints.

Water of the Stomach: Kledaka

The first water of Kapha, kledaka, originates in the stomach. It is the cause of mucus formation in the body. Most important of the waters, kledaka's moist foamy liquid aids digestion, liquifies foods, and nourishes the remaining waters of Kapha. When this first water is aggravated, the digestion process becomes impaired, heaviness of the abdomen prevails, and nausea may also occur.

Kledaka: Keeper of Moisture

At the subtle body level, kledaka, as the keeper of moisture, teaches us the art of fluidity. We are asked to assimilate our emotions before effusing them. We can then pour oil into dryness, water into the thirsty, and fluidity into the stagnated. Only when our own nature is finely lubricated in this way can we flow into helping others. Sadhanas such as yoga, tai-chi, walking, Ayurvedic massage, Ayurvedic emesis therapy, Kapha-nourishing foods, and giving water and food to the poor, all help to maintain kledaka's balance.

Water of the Heart: Avalambaka

The second water of Kapha, avalambaka, resides in the chest and heart. It provides plasmic tissue to the heart, thereby insulating it from heat. Avalambaka also provides the limbs with their energy. When this water is disturbed, laziness and lethargy ensue. Heart originating diseases such as rheumatic fever and pains in the pericardium may also occur.

Avalambaka: Keeper of Love

At the subtle level of existence, avalambaka gives us our protective, embracing, and maternal nature. It teaches us to support the nature of Mother Earth. When we discover our own instinct for nurturing, we are then able to allow all creatures to share equally in the universe's love, light, wind, and rain. Sadhanas such as cooking, feeding the family and the poor, fasting, seasonal internal body cleansing, gardening, and Kapha-nourishing foods help us to replenish this second water of Kapha.

Water of the Tongue: Bodhaka

Bodhaka, the third water of Kapha, is the estuary which joins the five waters of the body's river. It sends water to the tongue and palate and gives the perception of taste. It registers each of the six tastes in nature and sends the appropriate impulses to the receiving tissues long before the food is ingested. Bodhaka water also liquifies food.

When this water is disturbed, crimes against the body's natural instincts are committed, due to the impairment of taste. Diseases such as obesity, bulimia, and anorexia ensue, creating, in turn, *ama*, the foul, undigested remnants of food which stick in the tissues and promote disease. Generally, a thick white coating on the tongue indicates the presence of ama in the body.

Bodhaka: Keeper of Esteem

At the subtle level of existence in the body, bodhaka guards our perceptions. It teaches us not to violate our sensory mechanisms, especially the sense of taste. It shows us how to esteem ourselves by being discerning and learning moderation. As a result, we are meant to share the knowledge of the discretionary use of our senses. Sadhanas such as fasting, seasonal body cleansing, Ayurvedic emesis

14

therapy, Ayurvedic massage, wholesome physical activities, and Kapha-nourishing foods refine our spirit of bodhaka.

Water of the Head: Tarpaka

Tarpaka, Kapha's fourth water, flows in the brain and spinal cord as cerebrospinal fluid. It soothes the sense organs and, as a result, lubricates and protects the nervous system. When this water is out of balance, the sense organs become impaired. Loss of memory and dullness of sensory perceptions are the natural result.

Tarpaka: Keeper of Peace

At the subtle level, tarpaka washes the senses clean and gives us our innate nature of calm and satisfaction. It teaches the lessons of living lightly on the earth. We are urged to use only that which is necessary to help us gain health and equilibrium. It shows us how to listen to the sacred song in the wind, rain, and light, how to cognize our essential gifts and appropriate activities, rather than craving and pursuing material possessions.

The sadhanas to maintain harmony in tarpaka are meditation, pranayama, yoga, wholesome physical exercises, daily cleansing of the body, head, eyes, ears, nose, and throat, the seasonal cleansing of the internal body, studies of the sacred lore, and Kapha-nourishing foods.

Water of the Joints: Slesaka

The fifth water of Kapha, slesaka, is located in the joints. It lubricates the joints and gives them their solidity. Slesaka's unctuous gel protects the joints from heat, and the circulation of its synovial fluid gives ease and flexibility of movement. When this water is impaired, the joints may become swollen, painful, and dysfunctional.

Slesaka: Keeper of Patience

Slesaka, meaning "that which connects," was the original Sanskrit term given to Kapha. True to its intentions, slesaka gives us the ability of connectiveness in our lives. She teaches us maternal love and gives us the power to love and to nourish. We are to learn from her to embrace even those who may not appear to be deserving of kindness. Slesaka teaches enormous cohesion and patience with all of life. The sadhanas which augment slesaka and maintain her balance are maternal activities such as nourishing oneself and others, yoga, early rising, wholesome activities, seasonal cleansing of the body, fasting, and Kapha-nourishing foods.

15

PART TWO
Dhatus: Bodily Tissues

PHYSIOLOGICAL ANATOMY

In Ayurveda, the physiological and psychological functions of the body are known to be intricately and inherently woven. Cosmic energy and universal matter are at once intertwined in our foods, thoughts, and activities. The body is sustained by prana, the life breath, and *annam*, the earth's food. Breath (oxygen-laden air) and food influence the tissues of the body and the thoughts of the mind. Both are transmuted into the cosmic essences through the physical processes of ingestion, digestion, assimilation, and evacuation. In this way, breath and food become the eternal juice for procreation, the ingredient which sprouts love and joy.

Divine transformation manifests by means of the physiological chain of events whereby bodily tissue is constantly regenerating itself. Ayurveda has identified seven constituent tissues whereby the body both lives and dies. These tissues are called dhatus. Like doshas, dhatus are formed from the five elements—space, air, fire, water, and earth. With the help of the digestive fire, the dhatus form the body's protective biological system. In other words, they nourish and defend the internal immune system. If one dhatu is defective, each successive dhatu is affected, thereby triggering a chain reaction of impairment throughout the entire tissue system.

The concentric formation of dhatus occurs through the ingestion of food substances. Infinitely well expressed by Charaka, the use of naturally healthy foods is essential to the quality of nutrients responsible for sustaining the dhatus: "The availability and consumption of a wholesome diet are imperative to promote the healthy growth of a person; likewise, indulgence in unwholesome foods promotes diseases." Equally relevant is the recognition that mental unrest or a negative disposition contaminates even the most wholesome foods once these have been ingested.

Through an enormously sophisticated process of chemical reactions, spurred by both the energy quanta of the foods and the energy vibrations of bodily tissues and mental thoughts, the nutrient called *ahara rasa* is produced. This nutrient, once absorbed into the digestive tract, is synthesized by the digestive fire to form the first of the seven tissues, *rasa dhatu*. This tissue, a milky, sticky, cold chyle

16

resembling the qualities of Kapha, is the body's plasma tissue and derives its existence from the water element. The proper conversion of the primary nutrient, ahara rasa, into plasma is dependent upon the quality of the foods, the state of mind, and the health of bodily prana. In wholesome conditions, these factors contribute to the production of plentiful rasa. In unhealthy conditions, they contribute more to the production of wastes in the form of mucus, rather than to the production of healthy plasma.

Each of the six subsequent dhatus is fed by the previous dhatu. Once rasa tissue is formed, the nutrients are refined and transported to form blood tissue, *rakta dhatu*. Again, if the nutrient quality is defective, the production of bodily waste in the form of bile is produced at the expense of healthy blood tissue. The main universal element comprising blood is fire. Not surprisingly, then, once the hemoglobin of the blood is nourished, the nutrients are further refined to provide the fuel necessary to produce muscle tissue, *mamsa dhatu*. Muscle tissue's dominant element is earth, the most matter-like element of the five elements from which the dhatus derive their form. The body's muscle tissue shares earth's nature of matter. Next in the dhatu nourishment is the fat tissue called *medas dhatu* which is pervaded by the water element.

The bone and cartilage tissue, *asthi dhatu*, which is pervaded by the elements air and space is next in the dhatu nourishment lineage. The continuously refined nutrients are then transported to the tissue comprising the body's red and white bone marrow, *majja dhatu*. The dominant element of bone marrow tissue is fire, which is reflected in this tissue's combustion/conversion/transmutation functions. Finally, the refined nutrient remaining after all these dhatus have been fed replenishes the sperm and ovum tissues, *shukra* and *artava* respectively. This last dhatu, once formed, is fed by the subtle essences of the nutrients refined through the synthesis of all of the previous dhatus. It is the subtle and pervasive essence remaining in the body before it becomes the material for procreation. If this dhatu is impinged upon, due to pollution of the nutrients, for example, the new life formed from the union of sperm and ovum is usually adversely affected in some way or other.

The condition of the dhatus is one of the main considerations during the pancha karma cleansing therapy. Certain seasons create susceptibility in the tissues, thereby making it easier to extract ama, wastes which have become imbedded in the tissues. Predisposed to positive vibrations, the dhatus respond immediately to the various stimuli exuding from herbs and other substances used in the emesis, purgation, enema, sudation, and massage therapies of pancha karma. These natural medicinal substances serve to buffer the body's internal systems, creating within the tissues a willingness to let go of the accumulation of negative forces.

PSYCHOLOGICAL ANATOMY

Kala: The Body Crystal

Dhatu transmutation in the body is a paragon and proof of the earth's dynamism occurring within us. Before the nutrients infiltrate a particular dhatu, they pass through a prismatic membrane or body crystal, called *kala*. Heated by the body's tissue fire, the nutrients are further transformed by the body crystal, which, by projecting a spectrum of vibrations, permeates the receiving tissue while it is being fed. In the same way that you can bask in the infraction of light permeating a crystal, each dhatu is bathed in a spectrum of vibrations diffusing through the kala. When the nutrients of food and mind are wholesome, the body crystal is clear and shining; when the nutrients are polluted, they cloud and may even block the crystal completely.

Essentially, while the rasa dhatu is being formed, the universal vibrations of joy and exhilaration transpire into the organism through the body crystal. This, then, is the secret that rasa carries—the cosmic joy and exhilaration infused from nature, called *prinana*. When rasa is being replenished in the body, we experience a lift in spirit as the rainbow essences of the cosmos are received into the organism. If, however, the nutrients are unwholesome, rasa dhatu exudes sadness and grief, rather than joy, and these negative emotions quickly pervade the entire organism.

As rasa feeds the blood, the joy mounts into exquisite exhilaration. The body, mind, and spirit surge forth to become boundlessly exuberant with abundant life. Kindness and the spirit of embrace imbue the organism. The secret carried in the blood tissue, then, is invigoration and life, called *jivana*. When the nutrients brought by rasa are less than wholesome, rakta dhatu, blood tissue, experiences anger, lethargy, and hopelessness, which rapidly impact adversely on both the body and mind. Rakta, in turn, feeds the muscle tissue, mamsa dhatu, which buffer and protect the internal body. The secret brought to the body by mamsa is discernment, the discernment that seals off the body from negative influences and protects it throughout its sacred journey. When mamsa receives polluted nutrients, it becomes confused and loses its ability to receive positive vibrations. Both body and mind become clouded as a result.

Mamsa, in its turn, feeds the fat tissue, medas dhatu, and every cell revels in celebration. Located in the center of the cyclical chain of dhatu nutrition, meda's secret in the body is the lavish, lubricating love called *sneha*. When sneha permeates the entire organism, there is an all-encompassing sense of esteem. Conversely, when medas is fed unhealthy nutrients, it exudes hatred and low self esteem, which in turn influences our every thought, word, and deed. Medas then feeds the bone and cartilage tissue, asthi dhatu, thereby invoking both our courage and personal wisdom. The secret that asthi whispers throughout the body-mind is that of fearless support, giving meaning and purpose to our numinous passage. It helps us to remember and stand firmly on the values intrinsic to nature. If the nutrients brought by medas are unwholesome, asthi experiences fear and indecision, which then pervade every cell of our body and mind. Asthi, in its turn, feeds the bone marrow tissue, majja dhatu, which is responsible for the body's feeling of fulfillment. Feelings of emptiness and loneliness, and all fear of death, are swept away as majja shares her passionate secret, filling the organism with rhythmic fullness. Majja's secret is called *purana*.

Majja then feeds the sperm or ovum tissue, shukra/artava, implanting wisdom in its wake. Through the precious gifts of vibrational nutrients, carried by the rasa, rakta, mamsa, medas, asthi, and majja tissues, the final and sacred transition within the body takes place. All at once, the essences of joy, invigoration, discernment, love, wisdom, support, fulfillment, and maturity implode and shukra/artava reveals the last secret carried into the organism by the dhatus—the secret of life itself. From the collective essences of all the dhatus, life-creating nectar is formed, so that when the time comes for the body to spill its nectar into the world through procreation, the cosmic cycle comes full circle to complete itself. If, however, the nutrients are polluted, the very essence of the seed of life is threatened. Depending on the severity of the impingement, physical mutation and the loss of cognitive memory in the newborn could be the result.

Ojas: The Glow of Health

Ojas is the cumulative essence remaining after the cycle of dhatu nutrition is complete. Our physical, mental, and spiritual strength is totally dependent on ojas. Our personal aura, the strength and glow we are meant to exude, is produced from an abundance of ojas, which is our best safeguard against mental and physical disease. As ojas thrives, so does the body's natural immunity. Mental clarity and cognitive memories also flourish. If, on the other hand, the body has insufficient rasa, the tissues become dry and emaciated, resulting in the depletion of ojas. Dullness of both the mental and physical fires naturally follows. Decreased ojas also fosters an increase in the ama, or wastes, produced by the body.

The Dhatus, Upadhatus, and Malas

At the end of the dhatu feeding chain, a secondary group of tissues is created, called the *upadhatu*. These tissues do not provoke a chain reaction with subsequent upadhatus, as do the dhatus themselves. Also, each primary dhatu, after having been fed, produces its own bodily waste called malas. The primary dhatus, along with their upadhatus, malas, and physical and emotional functions, are presented in the following chart.

THE PRIMARY DHATUS, THEIR UPADHATUS, MALAS, PHYSICAL AND EMOTIONAL FUNCTIONS

DHATU	UPADHATU	MALA	PHYSICAL FUNCTION	EMOTIONAL FUNCTION
Ingested foods	-----	feces urine	production of nutrient substance	joy
Rasa (plasma tissue)	breast milk, menstrual secretion	mucus	nourishment	exhilaration
Rakta (blood tissue)	blood vessels, tendons	bile	stimulation	invigoration
Mamsa (muscle tissue)	muscles, skin	ear wax, snot, navel lint, etc.	buffering the body	nurturing
Medas (fat tissue)	omentum*	sweat	lubrication	love
Asthi (bone and cartilage tissue)	teeth	body hair, beard, nails	supporting the body	courage
Majja (bone marrow tissue)	head hair	tears	filling of the bones	fullness
Shukra & Artava (repro- ductive tissue)	----	----	procreation	life

* A fold of peritoneum from another organ that supports an organ.

CHART 1A

MALAS: BODILY WASTE

In Ayurveda, the bodily wastes known as malas perform a useful function. While existing in the body in a timely way, malas are supportive of the body's nutrition by synthesizing essential elements in the dhatus as these make their way out of the body. The Sanskrit word "mala" is derived from two roots: *dharane*, which means "to sustain," and *kitta*, which means "that which must go away."

Malas are held in the body by the forces of *agni*, digestive fire, and *vayu*, bodily air. When agni and vayu are functioning properly, the dhatus are fed plentifully with the essences of foods. When they are not, the production of malas increases in the body. This excess waste, if not eliminated in a timely fashion, begins to consume live tissues, thereby causing the degeneration of life. True to the principle of natural cessation, deranged tissues that have been afflicted with excessive bodily waste cannot revert back to life; instead they are excreted from the body as malas.

The three principal malas are urine, feces, and sweat. These waste products, like the doshas and dhatus, are composed of the five elements. Secondary malas include the intestines' fatty excretions, earwax, hair (body, head, and beard), nails, tears, and menstrual discharge.

The primary waste of the body, feces, is the refuse of foods and substances excreted from the tissue cells so that they may be evacuated from the body and returned to the earth to aid in her fertility. Two daily evacuations are considered to be vital to good health. Urine, the water waste of the body, is to be passed five times a day if good health is to be maintained. An ample intake of pure water is vital to replenish the bodily fluids. Sweat is the perspiration formed to expel waste from the skin tissue.

The normal flow of the malas is obstructed whenever the doshas are increased or decreased beyond their natural state. Pancha karma, the five-fold Ayurvedic cleansing therapy, is designed to assist the body in the elimination of excess dosha and tissue waste. By bringing the primary forces of the doshas into balance, the elimination of wastes becomes an incidental result.

Vata, the dosha most often involved in the manifestation of disease, is responsible for the retention or ejection of feces, urine, bile, and other bodily excretions. When wastes such as mucus, bile, excess water, and gas remain in the body, Ayurveda strongly recommends that the cleansing therapies be administered. To balance Vata, for example, enema therapy, using herbal oils and decoctions, is prescribed and applied.

Pitta disorders are generally treated with purgation therapy, and Kapha excesses are alleviated by emesis therapy. Ayurvedic massage is frequently used to balance, stimulate, or calm all three doshas. These cleansing therapies are vital to the elimination of blockages, so that toxins, bile, mucus, and other excesses can be flushed from the body.

AMA: THE SEED OF DISEASE

When the body's digestive fire is not adequate, foods remain undigested and unabsorbed in the intestinal tract, and ama is the result. Foul-odored and sticky, ama clogs the intestines and other channels of the body, including its blood vessels. Ama obstructs the colon in its attempts to carry out one of its primary functions, extracting the vital force, or prana, from the digested foods. Ama undergoes a multitude of chemical changes, gradually creating toxins which are released into the bloodstream. Excess dosha and toxins form a sinister team as they travel with great rapidity to a weakened part of the body. Through its toxicity, the ominous ama elicits a negative immune reaction in the body's tissues until, finally, disease manifests in these organs associated with the mutated tissues.

All internal diseases begin with ama's presence in the body, and all externally-created diseases eventually produce ama. In addition to obstructing the body's channels, ama causes a deterioration in our strength and energy levels. It reduces rasa, inducing lethargy and fatigue. Equally crippling to the system is mental ama, gathered through misperception and disturbed emotions. Greed, selfishness, possessiveness, stubbornness, anger, and excessive desires become mental pollutants, also ama.

An early sign of ama in the body is a sticky coating on the tongue. In Kapha types, the coating is usually thick, sweetish, and whitish in color. Pitta types tend to have a slimy, sourish, yellowish coating and Vata types have a dryish, bitter, grayish coating. When these early symptoms occur, ama may be readily alleviated by fasting and/or the pancha karma therapies administered according to the body type and in the appropriate season.

Agni and the Six Stages of Disease

Ayurveda recognizes one main cause for and six specific stages in all diseases. The cause is rooted in the impairment of the body's main fire, called agni, the fire of digestion. Charaka tells us that, "A faulty fire leads to improper functioning of the tissue fires which, in turn, creates ama in the gastro-intestinal tract and leading to poor synthesis of tissues, which then increases the production of those malas and doshas that are harmful to the body."

Disease begins as a result of the doshas' stagnation in the body. Once a dosha (or doshas) is out of balance, it begins to accumulate as a negative force. At this early stage of disorder, the doshas express themselves through the loss of normal circulation. Vague symptoms, such as the dislike of foods containing the same qualities as the affected doshas, a general lack of lustre, tiredness and lack of clarity, prevail at this time. To restore the body's health during this initial stage of the disease process many mild rejuvenative sadhanas are practiced, including nurturing foods, herbal tonics, and Ayurvedic massage.

During the second stage of disease, the doshas extend themselves beyond

22

their normal accumulative sphere by preparing to travel in the ever ready vehicle, the mobile Vata. At this stage, the affected dosha (or doshas) gathers beyond the sites of origin and begins to spread via the blood into those bodily channels associated with the disrupted dosha. The signs of failing health are more prominent at this time when symptoms such as headaches, indigestion, nausea, constipation, and diarrhea are likely to appear. During this stage, the doshas may still be aided through the use of appropriate foods and herbs, massage therapy and wholesome activities, although pancha karma therapy now becomes necessary if the body's equanimity is to be completely restored. It is in this stage that the doshas tend to gain negative force largely because of the person's disregard for the body and also due to seasonal factors.

In the third stage of the disease process, the doshas spread to still other parts of the body and may remain dormant for some time before disease is apparent. Ayurveda suggests that pancha karma be used as the primary therapy before the doshas are expressed as fully developed diseases. In many instances, however, this therapy may prove useful even after disease becomes evident, although it requires that the practitioner be vitally cognizant of the terms of treatment and the condition of the timing and details of treatment, given the patient's condition. During this stage of disease, symptoms such as abdominal distension, burning sensation in the body, and anorexia may appear.

In the fourth and fifth stages of disease, the aggravated doshas completely relocate themselves, concentrating in specific tissues and structures of the body creating conditions for which specific features have been identified and names given. These include diabetes, heart disease, fevers, arthritis, bronchitis, cancer, and many others. The development of diseases with clinical features occurs in the fifth stage.

In the final or sixth stage, the disease may take a complex turn, for example, when an abscess passes the fifth stage of disease and bursts into a chronic ulcer. Most chronic diseases are considered by Ayurvedic practitioners sixth-stage conditions.

THE THIRTEEN CHANNELS OF CIRCULATION

The body contains numerous channels through which the dhatus, doshas, and malas circulate. Known as *srotas* in Ayurveda, these consist of both gross channels, such as the intestinal tract, lymphatic system, arteries, veins, and the genito-urinary tracts, as well as the more subtle channels, such as the capillaries. Subtle channels called *nadis* are analogous to the meridians used in acupuncture, perceived to be central channels through which the body's energies flow.

In Ayurveda, a complex system of diagnosis is employed to trace the root cause of disease. The diagnosis of all diseases is based on which of the individual doshas are compromised and which channels are obstructed. An excess of any one dosha can create a spill-over effect in the body. Thus, a disease originating from one vitiated dosha is able to travel through the channels to the site of another dosha. Dosha excesses can also create blockages in the channels, thereby obstructing their normal flow.

Men have thirteen groups of channels, and women have fifteen. Of the thirteen common groups of bodily channels, the first three are the channels through which the air (or breath), food, and water travel; these are governed by Vata, Pitta, and Kapha, respectively.

Air Channels

The body's air channels originate in the heart and the alimentary tract and conduct pranic force and vitality through the respiratory and circulatory systems. These channels become impaired by the suppression of natural bodily urges, by ingesting dry or stale food, and by excessive physical exertion. Symptoms expressed by vitiated air channels are shallow and restricted breathing, fear, anxiety, and nervous tension.

Food Channels

Food channels originate in the stomach and carry food through the digestive system. Vitiation of these channels is caused by untimely or indiscriminate eating, unhealthy foods, and low digestive fire. The symptoms of afflicted food channels are loss of appetite, indigestion, vomiting, anorexia, greed, and possessiveness.

Water Channels

Water channels originate in the palate and pancreas, and regulate the body's fluids. Obstruction of these passages is caused by excessive exposure to heat, excessive use of alcohol or other addictive substances, and ingesting very dry foods. The symptoms of vitiation are excessive thirst, dryness of lips, throat, tongue and palate, as well as selfishness and dullness.

The following seven groups of channels service each of the body's seven dhatus. Like the dhatus, the nature of these channels range from the most gross to the most subtle.

Plasma Channels

Plasma channels begin in the heart and its ten blood vessels and transport chyle, plasma, and lymphatic fluid to the plasma dhatu. Obstruction of these passages is caused by stress, grief, and excessively cold and heavy foods. The symptoms of vitiation are anorexia, drowsiness, nausea, fainting and anemia, as well as impotence, stress, and grief.

Blood Channels

Blood channels originate in the liver and spleen and transport blood (especially hemoglobin) to the blood dhatus. This group of channels is often referred to as the circulatory system. Vitiation of this system is caused by hot and oily foods, excessive exposure to the sun or fire, and exposure to radioactivity. The symptoms of affliction are skin diseases and rashes, abscesses, excessive bleeding, and inflammation of the genital organs and anus. The emotional symptoms are anger, dullness, and aggressiveness.

Muscular Channels

Muscular channels, which originate in the ligaments, tendons, and skin, supply nutrients to the muscle dhatus. Impairment of these channels is due to regular intake of heavy, greasy foods, excessive sleep, sleeping after meals, and a sedentary lifestyle. The symptoms of vitiation are usually benign tumors produced by the muscular system, tonsillitis, a swollen uvula, hemorrhoids, and swelling of the thyroid glands and adenoids. The emotional symptoms are lack of mental clarity, attachment, and nervous tension.

Fat Channels

Fat channels, commonly known as the adipose system, originate in the kidneys and the fat tissue of the abdomen; they supply fat tissue ingredients to the fat dhatus. Vitiation of this system is due to inertia, suppression of digestive activities, and excesses of fatty foods, alcohol, and other addictive substances. The symptoms of affliction are generally diabetes, urinary disorders, possessiveness, and indulgence.

Bone and Cartilage Channels

Bone and cartilage channels, commonly known as the skeletal system, begin in the hipbone and supply nutritive ingredients to the bone and cartilage dhatus. Affliction of these channels is generally caused by excessive activity, friction of the bones, and excessive intake of Vata-type foods such as excessively dry, cold or stale foods. Some symptoms of vitiation are dry, flaky nails and decaying teeth, painful joints, dry and thinning hair, and feelings of deprivation and fear.

Bone Marrow Channels

The bone marrow channels, commonly referred to as the nervous system, supply the marrow and nerve tissue nutrients to the bone marrow dhatus. In Ayurveda, the marrow is not only the matter found in the bone encasement (called white and red marrow), but is also found in the brain and spinal cord. Impairment of the bones and joints is generally caused by consumption of incompatible foods, such as the use of animal foods with milk, or hot and cold substances taken together,

25

and unwholesome activities, which, in turn, affect the bone marrow. The symptoms of a vitiated nervous system are pain in the joints, fainting, dizziness, loss of memory, blackouts, and compounded abscesses.

Ovum and Sperm Channels

The ovum and sperm channels are more subtle than the nine preceding channel groups. Originating in the testes and ovaries, these channels are ordinarily referred to as the reproductive system. They transport the semen, ovum and ojas essence to the male and female reproductive tissues. Affliction of these passages is normally the result of unwholesome activities such as excessive or suppressed sex, unnatural sex, sex at improper times, drug addictions, and abortions. The symptoms of vitiation are impotence, infertility, and defective pregnancy. The emotional symptoms are sexual indiscretion and indulgences, selfishness, and aggression.

The remaining groups of channels common to both the male and female are the body's three elimination systems.

Urinary Channels

The urinary channels begin in the kidneys and bladder and eject urine from the body. Impairment of these passages is caused by the suppression of urination. The symptoms of vitiation are generally excessive, scant, or frequent urination, as well as fears, anxieties, and nervousness.

Excretory Channels

The excretory channels, ordinarily referred to as the excretory system, originate in the colon and rectum. They evacuate feces from the body. Vitiation of these channels is caused by weak digestive fire, eating before the previous meal is digested, suppression of defecation, and ingesting disagreeable foods. The symptoms of affliction are usually diarrhea, constipation, or excessively hard stools. The emotional symptoms are attachment, dullness, and fear.

Sweat Channels

The last of the excretory channels, commonly known as the sebaceous system, originate in the fat tissue and hair follicles, and expel sweat from the body. Affliction of these channels is caused by excessive activity, heat, spicy foods, acidic foods, excessive alcohol or other addictive substances, grief, fear, and anger. The symptoms of vitiation are excess perspiration or no perspiration, rough and dry skin, burning sensation of the skin, grief, anger, aggressiveness, or dullness.

Female Channels

Two additional channels exist within the female body: the menstrual channel, which expels blood, secretions and tissue debris from the uterus, and the breast milk channel, which carries milk to the nursing mother's breasts. These two channels are both part of the plasma channel, which supply the plasma dhatus.

When the channels are blocked, their corresponding doshas become vitiated. The cleansing therapies of pancha karma restore order to the system by clearing away the obstacles so that the doshas can flow as they should.

PART THREE
The Subtle Body

THE FOURTEEN NADIS

The nadis are the body's subtle channels of energy, which operate very closely with the body's primary centers of consciousness, the *chakras*. The three principle subtle channels are *sushumna* nadi, *ida* nadi and *pingala* nadi. These three main nadis sub-divide into fourteen nadis, which in turn divide into many thousands located throughout the body.

Directly related to the para-sympathetic nervous system, the sushumna and three other nadis (ida, pingala and *varuni*) act as carriers of life's vital force, prana. Sushumna is the primary subtle energy channel of the group. This group of nadis is called *pranavaha* and deals with the body's physiological qualities. The acupuncture meridians are analogous to the pranavaha nadis. Without the life currents of prana conveyed by the pranavaha nadis, the body's para-sympathetic and sympathetic nervous systems would be rendered inoperable; without prana, the vehicle of the mind, there would be no impression of consciousness.

The *manovaha* nadis, carriers of mental energy, are directly related to the sympathetic nervous system and deal with psychological qualities. Ten nadis belong to the manovaha group, with two additional nadis, ida and pingala, shared by both the pranavaha and manovaha groups. While the para-sympathetic and sympathetic function inseparably, all mental activities being controlled by prana, they are discussed separately for purposes of understanding.

Sushumna Nadi

The sushumna nadi, located within the spinal cord, begins at the pelvic plexus and ends in the space in the cerebro-spinal axis between the two hemispheres of the brain. The seven chakras are located along the sushumna nadi from the top of the head to the base of the spine. To the left of the sushumna lies the ida nadi and to the right the pingala nadi. Ida represents the feminine principle, reflecting lunar energy; pingala represents the masculine principle, reflecting solar energy.

Ida Nadi

Ida nadi is the body's main left subtle channel, and runs from the left genitals or testicles to the left nostril. In all yogic practices, inhalation begins with the left nostril; the breath entering the left nostril stimulates ida nadi and promotes creativity, visualization, and the nurturing of the emotions, calms the nerves and silences the mind. Left nostril breathing is also said to increase longevity. In order to maintain harmony and balance, the yogic sciences advocate the use of left nostril breathing during the day, when the body is being vitalized by the sun's energy.

Gandhari and Hastajihva Nadis

The *gandhari* and *hastajihva* nadis are ida's companion nadis. Gandhari originates from the lower corner of the left eye and ends at the big toe of the left foot. Hastajihva nadi begins at the lower corner of the right eye and also ends at the big toe of the left foot. The ascending psychic energy travels, via these nadis, from the lower body to the chakra located between the eyebrows.

Pingala Nadi

The pingala nadi, the body's main right subtle channel, runs from the right genitals or testicles to the right nostril, and is activated by the breath of the right nostril. Pingala stimulates the rational, practical self. Right nostril breath promotes stamina, vigor, and vitality. Although both the body's breaths are cleansing by nature, ida cleanses the mind, and pingala revives the body's dynamic energy. Just as left nostril breathing during the day balances the aggression of solar energy, right nostril breathing is advocated during the night, when lunar energy is dominant, to activate balance and vigor in the body.

Yashasvini and Pusha Nadis

The *yashasvini* and *pusha* nadis are pingala's companion nadis. Yashasvini runs from the left ear to the big toe of the right foot, and pusha nadi runs from the right ear to the big toe of the left foot.

Alambusha Nadi

The *alambusha* nadi begins at the anus and ends in the mouth. Its function is to provide prana for the assimilation and evacuation of food and liquid, and for the assimilation of ideas and thoughts.

Kuhu Nadi

The *kuhu* nadi begins in the throat and ends in the genitals. Through tantric practices designed to master the senses, this nadi can be trained to induce the implosion and ascension of seminal and vaginal fluids.

Shankhini Nadi

The *shankhini* nadi, which originates in the throat and terminates in the anus, is located to the right of the sushumna nadi. It is activated by cleansing Vata from the colon and anus.

Saraswati Nadi

The *Saraswati* nadi, named after the Hindu goddess of wisdom, begins in the tongue and ends in the vocal cord. It is responsible for speech and the dissemination of knowledge. A companion channel to the sushumna nadi, Saraswati nadi is lunar in nature and, thus, of the feminine principle.

Pasyasvini Nadi

The *pasyasvini* nadi is located in the lobe of the right ear and connects with the cranial nerves. Traditionally, the point on the lobe was pierced with various precious metals to stimulate energy into the cranial nerves to reduce stress and certain addictive behaviors.

Varuni Nadi

The varuni nadi, one of the four pranavaha nadis referred to earlier, aids in the purification of bodily waste. This channel runs opposite and parallel to the alambusha nadi, and together they activate excretions of bodily waste. Varuni nadi originates between the throat and the left ear and ends at the anus. It works in concert with apana vayu, which circulates in the large intestinal cavities. When this nadi is disturbed, stagnation of various bodily channels ensues and Vata disorders follow.

Vishvodara Nadi

The last of the thirteen major channels, *vishvodara* nadi is located around the umbilical area, the site of the third chakra. It stimulates the adrenal glands and pancreas and also distributes prana throughout the body. Vishvodara nadi is the body's central energy stream and is often referred to as its *ki* or *chi*. All yoga and martial arts practices, especially tai chi, quigong, and pranayama, serve to strengthen this pivotal nadi.

PART FOUR
Ayurvedic Body Types

PRAKRITI

The Ayurvedic ancients provided specific guidelines to help us identify our constitutional nature. These guidelines enable us to live wisely on the earth while safeguarding our health. From the three doshas, Vata, Pitta, and Kapha, seven body types were originally identified. Our body type, which is determined at birth by genetic and karmic memory, is our constitutional nature, our *prakriti*. This prakriti is derived from the particular combinations and permutations of the five elements in the sperm and ovum that exist during conception. Once birth has made its elemental imprint, we cannot alter it without adversely affecting our balance of well being.

The human constitution, or prakriti, is comprised of all three doshas. This means that every individual has within himself or herself the dynamic forces of Vata, Pitta, and Kapha. The difference between individuals is the degree to which the three doshas interact with one another within each body type. As noted above, a person's constitution, as determined at birth by genetics, should be maintained throughout that person's lifetime, within a reasonable ebb and flow of the prakriti, which must be understood as a flowing entity, rather than static. Only our physio-psychological aspects change, influenced as they are by social, environmental, and cultural factors operating in our lives, and, as well, by our personal choices.

Although every body type's ultimate reality is one of unison, it is essential to distinguish between the doshas in order to grasp the concept of the self whose nature is both unified and whole. If this is not properly understood, individual differences will definitely be misunderstood. Essentially, the body type is merely adjectival to the endless list of attributes that make up an individual. In other words, the individual is not the body type. However, the doshas are an impressive example of apparent adversaries which, because they are also capable of functioning at a level of absolute equilibrium, need not be adversaries at all. This is worth remembering in all of our relationships, in our continuous resolution with ourselves and with each other.

31

The Seven Original Body Types

Originally, Ayurveda defined seven body types. These were Vata, Pitta, Kapha, Sama, Vata-Kapha, Vata-Pitta, and Pitta-Kapha. The first three types occur in their pure form very rarely, so seldom is it that anyone is primarily influenced by one dosha alone. Even more infrequent is the Sama dosha, also called tridosha, both names referring to the equal distribution of all three doshas, i.e., Vata, Pitta and Kapha. By far the more common are the combination body types, referred to as dual prakriti, i.e., Vata-Kapha, Vata-Pitta, and Pitta-Kapha. In more recent times, these three dual types have been expanded to include six dual types, by reversing the two doshas within each dual type and considering it a separate type, i.e., Kapha-Vata, Pitta-Vata, and Kapha-Pitta. A person who has both Vata and Pitta dominant may, therefore, be either a Vata-Pitta or Pitta-Vata type, depending on which of the two doshas is more dominant.

Note: Because so many disorders do not confine themselves to a specific body type, most of the therapies described in this book are directed to those disorders belonging to the Vata, Pitta, or Kapha dosha, rather than to a specific body type. In this way, the primary emphasis is kept on the nature of the disorder itself. Where applicable, therapies are identified by both body type and disorder. Dietary and activity recommendations are directed to both the individual therapy and body type. For the purpose of simplicity, references to body type in the therapy, formula and recipe sections are confined to three: Vata, to include Vata-Pitta, Vata-Kapha, and Vata; Pitta, to include Pitta-Vata, Pitta-Kapha, and Pitta; and Kapha, to include Kapha-Vata, Kapha-Pitta, and Kapha.

Because the body types are the basis from which all Ayurvedic diagnosis begins, they are explained here in some detail. This explanation is also intended to help you better understand your own personal constitution.

Elemental Source of Body Types

Rare Body Types

1)	Vata	air/space
2)	Pitta	fire/water
3)	Kapha	water/earth
4)	Sama	balance of all three doshas

Dual Body Types (original classification)

1)	Vata/ Pitta	air/space main; fire/water subordinate
2)	Vata/Kapha	air/space main; water/earth subordinate
3)	Pitta/Kapha	fire/water main; water/earth subordinate

Additional Dual Body Types (recognized by contemporary practitioners)

1)	Pitta/Vata	fire/water main; air/space subordinate
2)	Kapha/Vata	water/earth main; air/space subordinate
3)	Kapha/Pitta	water/earth main; fire/water subordinate

Body Type Qualities

VATA (like wind)	KAPHA (like water)	PITTA (like fire)
dry	oily	hot
cold	cool	oily
light	heavy	light
mobile	stable	intense
erratic	dense	fluid
rough	smooth	fetid
bitter	sweet	sour
astringent	sour	pungent
pungent	salty	salty

Nurturing Requirements

VATA: Nurtured by the elements fire, water, and earth

moist	sweet
heavy	salty
smooth	sour
hot	

PITTA: Nurtured by the elements water, air, space, and earth

cool	sweet
substantial	bitter
aromatic	astringent
calming	

KAPHA: Nurtured by the elements fire, air, and space

dry	pungent
warm	bitter
light	astringent
uncloying	

Determining Your Ayurvedic Body Type

Generally, everyone possesses characteristics from all three categories of body type, although one or two will usually predominate. Approach the chart below honestly. Remember that your evaluation will be colored by the qualities of your present lifestyle. Six months after making the necessary changes in your diet and daily activities and doing the cleansing sadhanas regularly, re-do the Body Type chart. The latter response will be more in keeping with your true constitutional nature.

Directions: Move horizontally across each of the sections set out in the chart below and circle the attributes that you feel most accurately reflect you. Choose at least one from each section. Ask a spouse, parent, or friend to assist you with the Emotional Characteristics portion of the assessment so that your choices will be as objective as possible. Men are advised to seek the assistance of a woman—

a spouse, friend, or mother—for both the Physical Characteristics and Emotional Characteristics sections of the chart. Then, moving down each of the three columns, count how many characteristics you circled for each body type. Whichever column yields the highest score indicates your Ayurvedic body type. For example, if your scores are 15 for Vata, 12 for Pitta and 5 for Kapha, then your Ayurvedic body type is Vata/Pitta.

BODY TYPE CHART: PHYSICAL CHARACTERISTICS

	VATA	PITTA	KAPHA
Body Frame	thin, irregular, very short or very tall	medium, proportionate, toned	heavy, broad, evenly proportioned
Weight	hard to gain, easy to lose	easy to gain, easy to lose	easy to gain, hard to lose
Skin	cold, dark and sallow, tans easily	warm, light and reddish, sunburns easily	cool, fair and oily tans easily
Hair	dry, frizzy, thin, dark	straight, fine, reddish, premature balding or graying	oily, wavy, thick, blonde, black or dark brown
Eyes	brown, gray, violet, or unusual color, small	green, hazel, light brown, almond shaped	black, blue, dark brown, big, sensual
Nails	dry, grayish, ridged	clear, well-formed, pliable	square, white, even
Appetite	irregular	intense	consistent
Evacuation	constipated, irregular, small quantity	loose, regular, large quantity	slow, regular, moderate quantity
Sweat	scanty	profuse	moderate
Stamina	poor, exertive	moderate, driven	excellent, lackadaisical
Sleep	poor, variable	moderate, light	long, deep

CHART 1B

34

BODY TYPE CHART: EMOTIONAL CHARACTERISTICS

	VATA	PITTA	KAPHA
Temperament	fearful, indecisive, nervous, perceptive	angry, intelligent, arrogant, successful	greedy, calm, stable, stubborn
Memory	learns quickly forgets quickly	learns quickly forgets slowly	learns slowly forgets slowly
Speech	erratic, talkative	decisive, articulate	slow, cautious
Spirituality	spiritually disciplined	tendency to material success	fundamentally material
Dreams	flying, fearful, erratic	fiery, violent, intense	watery, sensual, long sequences
Sexuality	cold, variable	hot, intense	warm, enduring

CHART 1C

CHAPTER TWO
COSMIC ANATOMY

PART ONE
Wisdom and Ego: Buddhi and Ahamkara

Know the self as the chariot master
The body as the chariot.
Know the faculty of wisdom (buddhi)
as the charioteer
and the mind as the reins.
The senses are the horses
and the sense objects are the arena.
So say the sages.

Katha Upanishad III (3-4)

Our cosmic anatomy functions through two main channels of information: our faculty of wisdom, called *buddhi*, and our intuitive ego, called *ahamkara*, which is also the recorder of all memories. Buddhi's main function is to provide our mind with its inner luminosity, which, in turn, directs our senses. Contemporary humans, ignorant of the numinous force of buddhi, are almost predominantly controlled by their sensory perceptions and, as a result, the mind is enslaved.

Buddhi: Light of the Mind

Both ahamkara and buddhi are aspects of our *antahkarana*, psychic instrument; however, the buddhi is far more pervasive by nature. Buddhi illumines the mind,

37

manas, which then directs the senses, *indriyas*. Without buddhi, both mind and senses are just so much inert equipment. As well as being the light of the mind and its senses, buddhi is also their life-force. Like all cosmic aspects within human anatomy, the buddhi is the potential power that enables the human to learn through knowledge, to practice through application, and to use this power as it was intended. Buddhi functions through our use of will and its associate powers of choice and self-reflection. The correct use of the trinity of buddhi, mind and senses make it possible for us to accomplish stupendous feats. Used with knowledge and reverence, the mind may enjoin the buddhi and its cognitive powers and allow us to access our entire memory through all time and space. In deep meditation, we are capable of engaging the deep breath of silence and inspiring the subtle body to travel to the far ends of the seven worlds—according to the Vedas, the earth is one of seven worlds comprising the universe. We may even travel beyond the time barrier into timelessness. At the zenith of human potential, we can dissolve all the manifestations of time-bound existence and enter the immutable, infinite space of God.

Ahamkara: Recorder of Memories

Ahamkara is commonly viewed as the ego-self or the individual expressing itself through experiences, limitations and so on; however, as part of the antahkarana, psychic instrument, it functions as the recorder of memories. Ahamkara's main function is to record the memories of our present and interphase them with cognitive memories retained from our past, as well as with the collective or cosmic memories held by the universe. These three memory functions of ahamkara occur simultaneously within each person.

Both buddhi and ahamkara are bequeathed to us from birth by the creator. These main cosmic aspects are assigned to us as instruments of navigation as we pass through each life. Ahamkara employs both the intuitive ego as well as prana, the vital force. Essentially, it is the remembering self that holds the individual memories of all lives.

The beads and the thread of a rosary provide a helpful analogy here; the thread is the ahamkara or intuitive ego, and one of the beads on it represents a present life. The rest of the beads on the thread of ahamkara are your past and future lives. The rosary as a whole, being more than the sum of its parts, holds the collective memories of all the lives of the individual passage, from inception of the first birth, through all rebirths, to the final liberation from the cycles of birth and death. The Vedas refer to liberation as *moksha*, a liberation defined in the sacred lore as the ultimate aim of each living organism, made possible only through human birth. Therefore, to be born of humankind is considered to be the most sacred and courageous accomplishment any species can achieve.

PART TWO
Three Phases of Memory

Memory is humanity's most important asset. Containing the truth of the entire universe, memory is both the inner guide for each life and the means of exchange with the universe.

We experience memory in three phases: cosmic, cognitive, and experiential. Cosmic memory, sometimes referred to as collective memory, is the complete recollection of the entire living universe from the beginning of time. Every atom and molecule of the cosmos, including the most minute cell and space within the human body, is infused with the cosmic memory of all time. The physical and emotional form and function of each species is due to this memory of the universe, referred to here as cosmic memory.

The second phase of memory, cognitive memory, is the creator's gift to the human species. Evidenced by the gods and *yogis*, this numinous ability is our least recognized feature. Totally independent of the body, mind, and senses, our cognition works only through the buddhi, our faculty of wisdom, and ahamkara, the recorder of all memory from the onset of a person's first life throughout every rebirth. I call this memory "cognitive" because it holds our past knowledge. Once we are able to invoke our cognitive memory, we may then access our higher state of personal wisdom. This memory is awakened in the human through reverent and harmonious practices given to us by nature, called sadhanas. Among the thousands of independent sadhanas given to us in this universe, the healing and cleansing sadhanas of Ayurveda's pancha karma therapies, along with its rejuvenation and virilization practices, and the maintenance and cultivation of toxic-free natural foods on earth, are the most vital sadhanas for gaining and sustaining the ultimate in terms of personal cognition. Healthy cognition within the present depends on the availability of essential information culled from foregone experiences in each of our prior existences and its retrievability in our cognitive state. The only way that we can avail ourselves of this information is through accessing our cognitive memory.

The third phase of memory, experiential memory, is based on the sum total of experiences in each of our present lives, experiences that are predominantly guided by the mind, body, and senses. As essential as experiential memory is in maintaining the complex personal interactions in everyday life, the memories we

39

experience from moment to moment are highly susceptible to inaccuracies. Experiences occurring within the span of one life have barely enough time to become assimilated within the cells and tissues of our physical organism, much less to become refined and divinized within the individual ahamkara which has been in the process of forming for billions of years—since the beginning of manifestation. As such, experiential memories are more in the nature of memory in the making, and thus cannot be solely depended upon. Nor can the mind or senses provide us with flawless memory or the infallible truth. In and of themselves, the mind and senses are considered by the Vedas to be unreliable instruments with which to gather truth and understanding about the dynamic realities of life and living.

COGNITIVE MEMORY

To die but not to perish is to be eternally present.
—Tao Te Ching

The most sublime form of universal language which the human carries is the ability of cognitive remembering. In the context of the bead and the rosary, used earlier as an analogy, cognitive memory is the whole rosary, whereas the experiential memory of each life is a single bead. Carrying the links of previous and future lives, each human bears this ineffable but seldom-used gift—cognitive memory.

Distracted by the activities of mind and senses, we are ignorant of our sacred largess. Although no moment is devoid of it, we are simply unable to draw upon it because we are unaware of its existence within us. In spite of our nescience, deep cognition often peers through unwittingly. Demeaned by names such as sixth sense, *deja vu*, gut feeling, an unusual ken, extrasensory perception, a woman's intuition, and so on, the cognitive state remains unrecognized. As long as this condition prevails, we are deprived of the very essence of our highest human ability—an ability garnered by dint of the number of lives and journeys we have endured.

Cognitive memories are those which have outlived the body of each rebirth. Real in nature, they attach themselves to the subtle body after death and are transferred to the ahamkara of the new body at the time of rebirth. The sum total of both the resolved and unresolved memories of all previous lives are carried by the ahamkara. Even future lives, yet to become memories, are held by your subtle body in the form of cosmic or universal memory which is more difficult to access. These future lives, like the present life, are determined by the imprinted record of your individual deeds from all prior lives. Since you do not use up all of your karmic account in any one life, there is always an outstanding balance in each individual karmic account waiting to be used to form future rebirths. These so-called memories of future lives yet to be lived, in the form of *samskaras*, remain in your subtle body even as you experience a present life and are not transferred into the ahamkara of the present life. Saṃskaras are the karmic impressions from all past lives carried in the subtle body, the vibrations and potential materials for all of our future lives or rebirths. In this sense, you cannot retrieve these samskaras from ahamkara; nor can you obliterate them from your subtle body. It is these karmic imprints that influence the human organism through the subtle field of cosmic vibration.

Kalidasa's eloquent remembrance, in the following verse, mimics the song of every soul:

> *How a fragment of melody or the fragrance of a*
> *flower, will evoke forgotten memories, filling the*
> *soul with sadness, as though vague remembrances*
> *from other lives are passing over the spirit!*

Honed and refined, these cognitive memories, imprints in the form of memory, have withstood the bitter test of time and rest in our deepest place of resolve. They reside within us to guide, to provide, to endorse our present and future journeys in the universe.

Cognitive memories are the residual essence of the sum total of each of our individual lives imbued with the sacred lore from the creator. They trace every existence you have experienced, all trails you have covered. Cognitive memory is our personal wisdom. More than instinct, it is our God nature. When we guide the mind and senses in their natural functions, esteem ourselves through knowing and allowing, observe the universal codes of moral behavior, dharmas, and are present in our daily sadhanas, we are able to access our cognitive ability.

Accessing Cognitive Memories

Cognition presents itself to us when the body, mind and senses are prepared as benign receptors through the continuous practice of sadhanas. The cognitive state is the simple essence of our being; when the mind and senses are allayed, cognition is readily available. In instances of extreme pain, or a near-death experience, the floodgates of cognition can swing wide open. During my cancer years, much of my cognitive memory became available to me. This was due to the fragility of the physical body and the impulses of a dying organism. When the physical body becomes exceedingly vulnerable, the subtle body prepares for its departure. Ahamkara, unable to hold its possessions, begins to relinquish its assets of memory and prana, which are then gathered up by the subtle body in preparation for its departure from the dying physical body. At the same time, the mind's attention is pulled away from its attachment to the sensory mechanism and is enveloped by the dramatic transactions between ahamkara and the subtle

41

body. In this manner, the near-death entity receives a compelling surge of cognition. However, receiving cognitive memory as a result of the physical body decaying is far from the ideal way of accessing our inner powers.

The physical body, mind, and senses were given to us as vehicles for practicing sadhanas so that we may maintain health through being available to our cognition. Through our mindfulness and presence in these practices, we are able to understand and balance our three bodies: cosmic, cognitive, and experiential. The Vedas maintain that there are no new experiences except the experience of knowing our real nature. Our cognition holds the answers to every mystery, every puzzle we create. When we do not learn the lessons from our voluminous past experiences, they appear to us as "new."

Cognitive Memory Through the Senses
Cognitive Memory Through the Six Tastes

The six tastes of nature proposed by Ayurveda are: sweet, sour, pungent, bitter, astringent and salty. Rooted in the cognitive state, the sense of taste is our primary receptor for accessing cosmic memory. We eat in order to remember all of time, from the beginning of our journey in the universe onward. Through the six tastes we can assimilate the very essence of the universe because they hold the memories of the universe from the beginning of time. They also provide the fundamental means for tapping into our own cognitive nature. For instance, when we eat a bowl of rice, its sweet, warming and nourishing taste triggers the rapture of all the memories of the sweet taste held within the universe. More than sixty percent of the natural foods of creation are sweet in nature. Similarly, when we taste a lime or grapefruit, the impulses sent deep within our bodily tissues from the sour taste awaken all the memories of sour carried in the universe from the first creation. Sour is the universe's essential taste for inspiring appetite and healthy inquiry. Because of its immense potency, it is used in small quantities.

The pungent taste carried in foods such as ginger, garlic, and peppers stimulates passion and heat in the body. The pungent taste connects us to the vast memories of the universe's passion and stimulation. The taste of bitter in our bodily system invokes constriction. It sends a jolting signal to the system that cautions it to remain light. The astringent taste, found in the tannins of barks and uncooked legumes, and which we also experience in various medicines, stimulates the system into aliveness. Both bitter and astringent tastes are used as minor tastes in our daily foods, and invoke the cosmic memories of lightness and aliveness in the body.

The salty taste cleanses bodily tissues and gives fresh potential for retrieving wisdom from the universe. Most of the universe's salt comes from water. Even the crystallized rock salt from the Sindh Mountains of Pakistan was once buried under the sea. Sea salt and water have been used for centuries in the healing therapies of India, China, and Europe. Salt and water are essential to awakening

42

and maintaining fluency of both cognitive and experiential memories. Due to its potency, salt is used as a condiment in our food, rather than a main taste. A small amount of rock salt or sea salt maintains homeostasis in the bodily water which constitutes seventy-five percent of the body's material.

The full spectrum of the six tastes originated from the water element. Without water, there can be no taste. Without taste, there is no remembering. So water serves as the most important element in the function of memory. Water-associated memories are usually the first to avail themselves to us when we begin to access our cognitive nature.

Taste, functioning through the tongue, begins in the tarpaka water of the head and stimulates expectancy in all of the body's sensory organs. For instance, long before a meal is actually served, the juices of appetite can be stimulated through the senses. This may start as far back as the field in which we saw the honey-gold grains rustling in the wind against an azure blue sky and the brilliant shafts of light from the sun. Our ears may have heard the "shoo-shoo-shoo" of the dancing crops; our eyes may have seen glimmering pieces of sun falling to the earth; our skin may have been touched ever so gently by the thin long wisps of the grain weeds, and our nose may have been flooded with the parched nutty aroma of earth and crop in spousal union. All of these cosmic experiences can invigorate our juices of appetite, when the gates of cognition open wide and the cosmic memory of the universe comes cascading in. Closer to the time of eating, bodhaka water is sent to our tongue to enliven the full spectrum of our taste and enjoyment. As evidenced by the example of the field of grains, personal participation in the sadhanas which are vital to the producing and preparing of the natural foods, is essential. By participating in this way, our sense of taste is preserved.

Contemporary humans violate their instrument of taste more than any other sense. We have developed, through the last four centuries especially, a long and hard irreverence for the bountiful foods of creation. More than taking food for granted, we have socialized it. We have succeeded in converting sacred food into poisoned fodder. In losing regard for the land, we are losing memory. The enormous poisons in the form of pesticides, fungicides, hormones, and so on, used to foster the harvest; the multi-machinery used to process, freeze, electrify, irradiate the foods; the commercial and genetic manipulation of food that distorts its very nature, all deplete the energy quanta of humanity's holiest asset on earth, natural food. The disparaging means employed to produce food, i.e. the vicious slaughtering of animals, contamination of their flesh, their milk, and their young, are all the result of humans having forgotten their own essential nature. Conversely, as a result of these atrocities, the human species is presently floating in the painful fluid of amnesia. In order to regain our human potential for cognitive living, these senseless and brutal activities must cease and the land, animals, and harvest returned to their natural resplendence.

Taste, then, as the fundamental aspect of retrieving all memory, cannot be surpassed or bypassed if we are to regain the cognition that is our great potential as a human species. The Ayurvedic seasonal cleansing therapies, when applied, are imperative sadhanas to help awaken our deepest cognitive memories through employing taste and the other senses. The food sadhanas that can help us reclaim this innate human gift of self-cognition are set out in my earlier book, *Ayurveda: A Life of Balance*.

Cognitive Memory Through the Other Four Senses

All of our senses are imbedded in our cognitive state. The sense of smell, for example, is also a vital link to self cognition. So often we experience a certain fragrance or smell which sends the mind reeling to some time in the past when perhaps a deep feeling of love, hate, or other strong emotion was experienced. During my bout with cancer, there were many incidents in which I relived past experiences from the memory recesses of both my present and past lives. In one such incident, while I was being rushed into the hospital's operating theater for the umpteenth time, I felt a deep surge of fear. The antiseptic smell of the room was very strong and the operating team was frantically trying to get a late start back on schedule. Lying on the stretcher, I observed the cacophony of noises and astringent smell and was suddenly transported back in time many, many years.

Amid the frenzy of that cold, stark, astringent space, I began to slip into a time when I was two years old and suffering from diphtheria.

I saw my father's face peering in through the tent in which I was incubated. I remembered feeling cold, wet, and uncomfortable and waiting for him to change my diaper. I longed for his visits, for the warmth of his enormous hands, the reassurance of his deep rich voice, all permeated with love . . . a love which kept me alive. Once more, I was facing the Lord of Death. Rudely, I was jolted back to the present as I was pushed under the operating lights, my arms pulled back and straddled. That frantic team had forgotten that I was still a living, breathing creature. I watched myself slip into the gray fog of anaesthesia and pull back from the far gone past the warm memory of my father's presence to keep me alive once more. Although it was an intensely difficult operation, I knew as I went under that I would come through.

Many things changed for me on that day as I saw my father's love so clearly. I suddenly understood that I had just made a second serious attempt to leave the earth because I had forgotten how much had been given to me in this birth. It was the day that I decided to leave hospitals and doctors behind. It was to be the first day of my rebirth, my new life—the day I decided to live.

There is not a single instant within any minute of life when we are not experiencing our cognitive state. Most people are simply not aware of it. We seldom encounter cognition as a "big bang." Cognition is a very subtle form of energy that permeates our entire organism, as though waiting for our recognition. If we look back carefully at our lives, we can see how often we have actually experienced this subtle and pervasive state and not known exactly what it was. For example, all our preferences, in terms of likes and dislikes, are rooted in our cognitive state. The things we like hold pleasant memories from the past, while the things we dislike hold unpleasant memories from the past.

The eyes, used more than all of the other sensory organs, are also a store-house of memories. Through seeing, we remember the entire universe. Our faculty of sight holds the greatest fascination for us. Attachment to the objects of the material world perceived by our senses occurs primarily through the sense of sight. Through sight, pleasant and unpleasant objects alike are imprinted on the mind. These impressions permeate the cellular body and are magnetically retained within the mind. One of the primary purposes of meditation is to retire the sense objects from their senses in the same way that we relieve children of their toys before they are put to bed. In this manner, the mind remains untethered, free to respond to cognitive impulses.

On my first trip to the Himalayas, I was catapulted into my cognitive state quite frequently, from both the thinness of the oxygen-deficient air and the visual beauty of the snowy peaks, the cobalt skies, and the incredible Ganges river trickling down from the mast of the highest peak. Historic site of the ancient seers and sacred lore of the Vedas, the Himalayas strip the senses of their routine experiential perceptions and hurl them face to face up against the creator and the creation.

After timeless days of journeying, I could no longer sustain my usual stamina, resorting to crawling on hands, knees, and belly before finally giving in and hiring a mule to carry me. Littering the dirt and rock corniche which winds its way to the very top of this majestic mountain, were vendors serving savories and "chai," *sadhus* smeared with ashes and practicing oblations in tiny shacks, and men and mules carrying luggage and devotees on their backs. Time was very far away, and I was light years away from the perceptions of time and space living. Saturated by the sound, sight, smell, feel, and taste of God, I was awakened to my cognition through most of that journey. Even now, I sustain it fully.

Every morning, the sun gleamed its bright heat to warm the crisp, cool air. On one particular morning, I knew I would never again be the same. The very sound of the day had a finer resonance. On this particular journey, I was accompanied by one of the *swamis* (a Vedic monk) and a fellow female student from my teacher's Ashram in Rishikesh, located in the foothills of the mountain. My female colleague had made this pilgrimage many times before. On this occasion, however, she was unhappy because she disliked the swami who was escorting us, a joyful and cherubic being, whose company I felt honored to have.

My friend's intense dislike of our companion and her constant bickering drove the swami ahead of us. Even so, I was amused by the extreme state of realities that existed on that glorious day. For me, there was at once full cognition of all the splendors of creation, literally hanging from every corner and crevice of the hills through which we journeyed, while in the other reality, the usual routine norm, I had to struggle to remain attentive. The angry exchanges of words between my friend and the swami created in me an obligation to keep the peace. Wrenching myself away from the very inhalation of majestic creation and my blissful state, I attempted to referee what had by then become a crowd-gathering event. Before I could engage their attention, the swami threw himself on his buoyant belly, in full prostration at my friend's feet, and then, with great rapidity, arose to mount his mule. In his haste, his orange *dhoti*, the cloth which wrapped his body, unfurled and flew into the hills. Suddenly, there was a stupendous vision of a rotund and almost-naked monk in full flight after his dhoti.

The path of cognition is often fettered with astounding humor. In criss-crossing between the experiential routine state of reality and the blissful state of cognition, that day I realized that living is a very humorous, if not always harmonious, process.

Yet another incident at noon that same day proved to be one of the most compelling cognitive experiences of my journey. I saw a golden eagle circling and once more was deeply absorbed in the beauty of it all. In the crevice where mother Ganga was trickling down, there was a flowering scarlet monkey plant hanging by its roots in the rock. As I peered between the rocks, I spotted a fraction of an open field. I left my friend and climbed a short distance behind the boulder to witness a most spectacular sight—a whole valley of exquisite wild flowers. The sight was so powerful that I stood transfixed in a timeless grip. As I approached the field, I saw flowers whose petals were each a different color, flowers which resembled columbines, flowers I had never seen before, yet somehow knew. I sat for a long time and then fell fast asleep, intoxicated by the powerful aroma of the field. An overwhelming dream found me being received in the court of a handsome young prince dressed in full regalia. I was not in my present body. Instead I seemed to be English or European, of a lighter coloring and a different beauty. Still, I knew that it was a dream of myself in another life.

I awoke and rejoined my party to continue the long trip to the temple of Badri Nath. The temple's presiding deities, Lord Vishnu and his goddess Lakshmi, give boons of love, money, marriage, children, and so on. It was a deeply spiritual place of pilgrimage whose natural hot springs are said to have once bathed Lord Vishnu and Lakshmi themselves. Both my friend and I were *brahmacarinis*, young aspirants of monastic life. Therefore, we would not normally pray for any of the boons Lord Vishnu and his goddess Lakshmi might offer. Nevertheless, after a bath in the invigorating springs, almost too hot to bear, I joined the others in the front row of the crowded morning *puja*. There, in full splendor, the presiding Rawal, religious head of the Hindus, who was officiating in the ceremony, threw an abundance of water on both of our heads. As his eyes locked mine, I recognized him to be the prince in the dream I had while asleep in the field of flowers. An immediate invitation was extended to my friend and me to be presented to the Rawal following the morning ceremony. As you may imagine, much ensued; and it took the wise intervention of my teacher to get me back on track.

Through the clarity of my senses, I was guided cognitively to circumstances I needed to witness once more in this life. Cognition is always awaiting our readiness to receive what is at the basis of our real nature. As I departed from that sacred place, I understood the meaning of the nearby mountain ranges, called Tien-shan, which means "celestial mountain." Such experiences, often perceived as obstacles, are the celestial mountains in our lives. My journey was yet another metaphor, except that, this time, I was finally able to take the sacred hills with me, inside of me.

During my time in India, my own connectedness to self cognition continued to increase rapidly. In part, this was due to my reasons for being there. My family left India more than a century ago, migrating with the British to what was then British Guiana. Although the tradition of a Brahmin life was maintained in my family, I always felt a part of me had been left behind in the homeland. The realities of people extracted from their cultures, especially a deeply ancient tradition such as that of India, always equate to a great deal of pain and suffering. The elders die from broken hearts long before they grow old. In our case, as in so many others, the brutal burden was borne by the first generation. My parents were of that generation. My father was a stoic man, bigger than life. He carried the entire family clan, as well as villages of broken people, on his back. Having imbibed some of the burden from him, my eventual return to India was to put to rest the pains of my people for whom India had become a country farther away than its great distance.

I was the first of my people to return. After many years in the United States, a five-year sojourn with cancer, and the death of my father, I made a dramatic choice to live my life close to nature and to immerse myself in the traditional studies of the sacred Vedas, so that I might regain my full cognitive powers as a human. In this "search of innocence," I went with my teacher, Swami Dayananda Saraswati, to India. His ashram is at the foothills of the Himalayas and on the heels of the holy Ganges river.

After my ceremonial initiation as a Brahmacarini, one who observes the monastic life of a student of the Vedas, I stood for a long time in the sacred river. All the signs on that auspicious day supported my new life. The wind raged during the previous night, swirling sand and river sky high. The turbulence continued throughout the morning of my initiation. Then suddenly, a mellow sun shone through with a stillness that resonated louder than the earlier storm. As I stood on a large rock, honed smooth by the moving waters, the faces of my ancestors, whom I had never seen in my life, flooded my cognition. They were finally at rest. All imprints of pain and longing were plucked from my bosom. The touch of the cool, smooth waters on my feet, the sound of the howling wind lashing against the water and the hillside all nurtured me in that sacred moment during which I took my vows.

47

These stories are deeply personal, my intention being to share with you the cognitive experiences received as a being of the universe. Once an experience is valid, it becomes part of our cognitive nature. As such, it belongs only to the cosmic universe. And so what I share with you belongs as much to you as it does to me. In reality, all of our cognitive occurrences belong to the universe. You may reach in and beckon this nature closer to you. It is the real nature of all people. The only requisite is that you live reverently in nature and continue to be present in the practice of the sadhanas you deem to be essential to your understanding.

Cognition in Dream

Our real nature rests in the space of the cosmic dream. The word "dream" is used here to refer to our idyllic longings, the fragments of ideas which whisper to us of our real nature, and not to the dreams which appear in your sleeping state. This word has been kept as a refuge in every language to indicate that space where we may escape to when brutal existence, that which is devoid of our cosmic guide, wages war in our mind and body. The dream space is indeed our cosmic refuge. In Sanksrit, the word for space is *akasha*, meaning that which sustains everything. Because of its profound resonance and stillness, the power of akasha is likened to pure consciousness, the absolute eternal.

The dream space is yet another way of defining the space where our cognitive memories reside. To reach for our dreams is an instinct prodded by self-cognition. In deep sleep we are able to resonate with our real nature, which is profound stillness. The dream space is the expression of the element space. It exists in a timeless state, as in deep sleep, where our physical nature is replenished through the resonance of space and we experience our cosmic nature within its essential silence.

Cognition in Deep Sleep

We experience our cognitive nature consistently for many hours at a time in the deep sleep state. When the mental and sensory fluctuations of the waking and dream states are dissolved, deep sleep remains, unafflicted by these movements, enabling us to rest totally within our cognitive nature.

The state of deep sleep transcends all of the perception-based experiences that occur in the waking state. After a sound sleep, we awake fully rejuvenated, fresh and joyous, replenished by our own pure nature. While we rest in the space of sleep, prana prevails as the silent witness, guarding ahamkara. In this state our cognition remains pervasive and sparkling, without interruption from the stimuli of the waking period. Sound, peaceful sleep is the state cited most frequently by the sages to demonstrate our real nature of self-cognition.

When we avail ourselves of this cognition, we enter deeply into the nucleus of our primal nature of inner luminosity, free of time-bound encounters. Unlike the physical, mental, and sensorial experiences, where the mind, senses, and physical organism are propelled externally to interact with their objects of perception within creation, cognition abounds only as we journey inward into our real nature of consciousness. When the physio-psychological organism tires itself by its experiential encounters, it necessarily turns into itself, through sleep or contemplation, to be re-fueled with its cosmic nature. To be one with self-cognition is to be one with the cosmic universe.

As human beings, we are capable of enjoying the complete integration of each of our component parts, i.e., mind, senses, buddhi, and ahamkara. When these parts dissolve into the pervasive oneness of our cognition, we may live harmoniously, our internal and external natures braided in such a way as to encourage self-cognition in both the sleeping and waking phases of existence. While asleep, we are helped enormously by the breaking down of universal energy into the dark phase of night. As night approaches, the physical organism requires rest. In preparation for total rest, the seers urge us to dissolve completely the activities of the waking hours. In this way, all perceptions and experiences, finished or unfinished, come to a full stop. The mind is cajoled into detaching itself from the sensory organs and leaving behind the ongoing daily agenda. When we are unable to disassociate the mind from its senses, and the senses from their sensory objects, dreams infringe upon our state of rest.

During the waking period, when the whole world alights with mobility and transformation, we are cautioned by the sages to remain especially alert in terms of activities, diet, and other aspects of daily life. In the light phase of day, ideas are created, decisions are progressed, relationships fostered, and ambition promoted. Therefore, it becomes imperative to beckon our cognitive nature and keep it close by so that we may be continuously guided in our efforts to live harmoniously and progressively, both as an individual and as a species. The waking period is a more challenging passage to manage than the time of sleep. But, through the consistent remembering of our cosmic nature and the constant practice of the sadhanas necessary to maintain both stamina and gentleness, we are able to progressively dissolve the appendages of each waking day and, in the process, resolve into our natural state of self-cognition.

Divination: A Cognitive Tool

In many rural parts of the United States, the method of divining for water is still practiced. Divination was used predominantly by the ancients and native people who understood the principle of resonance. When we declare our honest intentions to the universe, its response is invariably quick and telling. When we are clear and clean with our output, we attract the desired outcome. In divination, we become a resplendent vessel, emptying our intentions into the universe and allowing its response to guide us.

Both the Vedic seers and native shamans have culled volumes of information on the sacred meaning of all animals, birds, plants, herbs, and so on. By knowing these symbolic meanings, we can guide our intentions and outcomes. Animals are true symbols of divination. The bear, for example, when it comes to mind or is seen physically, is a messenger of stillness, a sign to go within the womb-cave of the self and allow the universe to clarify and nourish what we need in that particular space and time. White birds carry the omen of death, not necessarily a physical death, but perhaps the death of an old lifestyle or phase of life. A butterfly arrives to remind us of personal transformation, of arising from the inertia of the cocoon phase into a time of flying into our own splendid space. The eagle and hawk are both messengers of the Divine, reminding us of our spiritually attuned nature. They come only when we are ready. The owl too speaks of wisdom, but it is telling us to be wise to the self and to be alert to some form of deception currently operating in the life. A squirrel in its favorite tree, the oak, is a premonition of some preparation for the future which we may be neglecting. The turtle appears to remind us of the steadfastness we need. She is the symbol of Mother Earth and is considered to be the oldest of the earth's animal symbols. When the moose calls the moose-cow with that resounding noise from deep within its belly, which we cannot but hear, it is bellowing to us of the esteem we must have for ourselves.

In prayers, mantras, or simple words of intentions we use the affirmation of sound, which vibrates throughout both the bodily tissues and the energies of the hemisphere, causing a union of bodily and cosmic impulses. This conjunction revives the cognitive memory within us, and we feel at once a release in which hopes come alive. We may divine with a leaf, a coin, and even a grain of sand. The universe provides millions of means for us to read her and remain attuned.

Cosmic Memories Held by Animals

The Sanskrit name given to each species holds the hidden meaning of that species' purpose on earth. The goat, for instance, is named *aja*, the one who has no rebirth, inferring that the goat holds the cognitive memories of all rebirths in the universe. When we observe the goat and preserve its species, we are maintaining the knowledge of its essential memory on earth. The cow is given the same name as the sacred scriptures, *go*. This name has been further sanctified in that Lord Krishna is called *Gopala*, which means the one who protects the sacred scriptures. The cow as a species, then, holds the cognitive memory of the scriptural teachings. By protecting the cow, we may become inspired to study the scriptures, or even cognize the meaning of the sacred lore. The elephant is named *gaja*, meaning the one who holds the first knowledge of the earth's herbs and plants. The preservation of this incredible species may grant us the wisdom of its cognate knowledge of herbs and plants. This divine memory may enable us to ward off illness permanently and, in this way, reclaim our nature of immortality.

The Vedas propose that all species hold a particular form of cosmic memory and that, in the kindly and reverential preservation of each species, the memory they carry is protected. I believe that when a species becomes extinct through our exploitation and irreverence, the innate memory which that species carries is forever lost to us. As a result, we can no longer sustain within the human field of memory the particular knowledge that was held in that species' memory.

The universe provides us with trillions of clues, in the form of signs and symbols, to aid us in reclaiming our cognitive nature. Signs and symbols to guide all of our activities abound. Every creature, plant, herb and flower, even the wind, fire, water, and every grain of sand can teach us about our nature. The original people of North America understood the significance of every living thing. They cognized that every creature is imbued with a particular function of memory, and that when we regard and preserve their presence on earth in their natural, untrespassed habitat, we ensure the life of our own cognitive memories. When the ancients offered an animal as a sacrifice to mollify the gods, the act was to replace that which was somehow violated by human trespass. In the past, when people hunted animals, the chase and capture became a ceremony to inherit the innate powers of memory which that animal carried as the rites of passage borne by its species. Both ancients and natives, the most endangered of all species on our planet today, cognized the universal energy and lived only according to its permission. Contemporary humans, lacking the wisdom of such reverence, can no longer practice the chase, capture, inheritance and sacrifice of animals. They are no longer deserving of this sacred privilege. The wisdom contained in the hunt of the animal for the purpose of relinquishing its memory to the human cognition has been forgotten by the majority of the earth's people. Present day killing of animals, hunting, and sacrificial activities are devoid of intelligence—cosmic, cognitive or cellular. They are crude, violent and insouciant acts conducted by humans who have completely forgotten their own sacred nature and, therefore, that of the animals they kill.

EXPERIENTIAL MEMORY

Wisdom is allowing our intelligence faculty to illumine the mind;
Wisdom is allowing nature's primacy over all species, including humans;
Wisdom is allowing our true nature;
Wisdom is simply allowing.
—*Bri. Maya Tiwari*

As humans, we are born with senses, a mind, and a wisdom faculty, or buddhi, to use its Sanskrit word. Instead of allowing the wisdom faculty to guide our mind and in turn our senses, we use our sensory perceptions to entrap the mind, albeit unwittingly. We are not aware of our inner guide, the buddhi and the naturally boundless gifts we are made of. Every bodily tissue, each bodily humor, bodily waste, and the bodily channels serve as a means of communication within the body. Every moment we live is because of this communication, and the imprints of it all leave a history of both our learned and ignorant use of our cosmic and physical walk through time. In this manner, we become the ancestors of the future. What we learn now about our physio-cosmic nature adds to the reference of knowledge in the time ahead and to the refinement of the universe through the actions of this incredible species called humans.

The excellence of our codes of communication totally depends on memory: experiential, cognitive, and cosmic. In other words, in order to proceed progressively as a species, we must remember.

Experiential memory, memory based on the sum total of individual experiences in each life, is partially conditioned by karma, in that karma provides the circumstances or field for our encounters. Karma is the accrued result of all of the actions of all of our lives. Essentially, it can be thought of as the cosmic bank account whereby a record of our debits and credits in each life is maintained. According to the seers, karmas accrued from each person's collective births determine the circumstance of each life: birth after birth. Even genetic factors are conditioned by karma. Physiologically, each individual's characteristics at birth are caused by several factors: the doshas of the sperm and ovum at the time of permutation; the health conditions of both parents; the seasonal influences at the time of conception and throughout the pregnancy; the mother's physical, emotional, and spiritual health; the mother's diet and activity during pregnancy. These are all part of our karmic constituency. We are delivered fully stamped with the cognitive imprints from all of our previous lives, and these karmic impressions are in the form of memory.

Memory Transforms at Birth

While in the amniotic fluid of the mother's womb, the embryo sustains a heart rate of 160 beats per minute. This heightened frequency creates fluency of memory. It is said that the embryo recollects the collective memories of all of its lives while suspended in the watery domain of the womb. At the instance of birth, these memories are quenched. Emerging from the birth canal, the child is propelled into an atmosphere of oxygen and air, where the heart rate plummets to 72 beats per minute and the cognitive memories become vague. As humans, we were designed to live in an environment which necessitates the use of our mental and sensory perceptions. At the very moment of birth, all memories of previous lives are stored in ahamkara and, from here, we are meant to awaken and access

52

them by means of sadhanas. In this way, we grow into wisdom under the guidance of our cognition in each one of our present journeys.

We must understand that the cosmic intention is not for us to retrieve the experiential memories of each past life. If this were so, they would be accessible to us from the moment of birth and the process of birth through the watery domain of the womb into the oxygenated atmosphere of the earth would not have quashed our ability to recall them. Our sensitive mental and sensory faculty is barely able to hold together the present life's experiences, let alone the colossal files from all of our past lives' encounters. In actuality, all valid past lives' memories are carried in ahamkara as cognitive memories in the form of residual or essential memories of past encounters.

The present-day use of regression therapy to avail ourselves of memories of past lives is in some ways helpful in that these memories allow us to understand that our nature is not just the sum of its experiential parts within one life. In many cases, however, these therapies prove regressive if the intentions of recalling past experiences are misconstrued. A forced rush of past lives' memories may create a bombardment to the mental faculty and senses, resulting in delusions such as multiple personality complexes and mental confusion in the regressed person. Unless regression therapy is directed at providing the person with an initial introduction to his/her valid cosmic nature and then followed up with harmonious sadhanas for knowing and sustaining that nature, such therapy could prove harmful. The only known means of sustaining a truly cognitive life is through our conscious presence in the daily practice of sadhanas. The ancient sages have given us, in detail, incredible sadhanas which when practiced diligently refine the human system to the point where full cognition of the past interphases harmoniously with the present. The collation of the timelessness of the cognitive state and the time-bound phase of experiential life is the ultimate balance. The practice of sadhanas gradually prepares the human organism to integrate with its entire nature. Sadhanas cover a gamut of physical, existential, and cosmic practices, from the study of sacred lore to yoga, tai-chi, meditation, natural farming, wholesome cooking, and so on.

Valid Memory

Valid memory refers to those memories which have stood the test of time through all of our previous lives and are available to serve as our personal wisdom in present and future lives. Valid memories incurred within each life attach themselves to the subtle body at the time of death. When the tissues decay, the physical body of a person dies, and the subtle body takes flight into the creation at large. Usually, there are many unfinished agendas at the time of death which are explained in one of three ways. The first two relate to valid memory while the third explanation relates to invalid memory.

Unfinished experiences result in unresolved memories; in other words, a process has begun but the resolve or outcome has not yet been attained. All unresolved memories accompany the subtle body at the time of death if they are the result of valid experiences. A valid memory, resolved or unresolved, is automatically programmed into ahamkara while we are alive and is transferred to the subtle body when we die. These valid memories are often physical experiences, which, because they are not resolved, create intense longings in the mind. In such instances, the subtle body may not be able to mobilize its force in the direction of its cosmic origin, hovering instead around the familiar territory of its attachment. These encounters are commonly referred to as ghosts existing on the earthly plane. In most cases, the subtle body alights on its journey into creation and awaits its rebirth, according to the universal laws of karma.

The second explanation relates to the individual who has finished or properly resolved his/her encounters in the present life before dying. These finished experiences result in resolved memories and are also carried in the subtle body at death. Although resolved experiences are never lived again in future lives, they are maintained in the ahamkara of the next birth as cognitive memories of certain specific experiences. Once an experience is totally lived to its point of resolve, it is also carried in the buddhi and becomes our manifest (not potential) wisdom, wisdom that serves us in this and all the lives to come. This is why certain young people are referred to as "old souls" or as those who are "wise beyond their years."

Invalid Memories

The third possibility involves experiences that are neither resolved nor unresolved but are invalid. Even though they are carried in ahamkara during the present life, these experiences dissipate at death and are not transferred to the subtle body. False perceptions conceived by humans, it seems, endure the same finite fate as all other human inventions. Invalid experiences entertain invalid memories. As we live, we are continuously creating memories. Most experiences in life are accumulated through mental and sensory perceptions, which are not known for their accurate results. Although the invalid may prevail for only a finite period, it creates great havoc and pain for as long as it is kept alive.

It is said that, on average, seven out of ten situations are perceived incorrectly. For example, when we look at a light permeating through a crystal, we tend to attribute the spectrum of colors to the crystal, rather than to the infraction of light. The valid experience is that the crystal is clear and colorless, however, until this fact is known, the perception that the crystal is colorful will prevail, which is an invalid experience. Similarly, we may perceive the sky as blue when, in reality, it is colorless space reflecting the clouds. We may be told a truth and due to certain circumstances believe it to be untrue. The belief that we were lied to, and that the person who in actuality told the truth is a liar, is invalid experience. We may think we know someone very well and then discover that, through the superimposition of our own wishes upon the character of that person, we were blinded to the person's actual character. The sudden discovery is the real and valid experience, whereas the superimposed experience, regardless of the length of time it endures, is invalid.

Invalid experiences are usually the experiences that create the most devastating pain. This is because of three simultaneously occurring factors. At the cosmic level, we are blatantly confronted with a disconnectedness from our real nature; at the physical level, we literally have to extract the invalid conclusions from ahamkara; and at the external level, we need to retract all that was previously projected onto our friends, family, and others. The physical extraction of data from ahamkara and "losing face" to those close to you cause embarrassment to our personal ego. As necessary and painful as it is to remove the invalid information stored in memory, it is equally important to understand that a happy life can never be built on the retention of invalid memories. The cosmic realization that we need to remain connected to our cognitive nature is the positive lesson of these experiences. We can learn from it and, in the process, be comforted by the fact that even in the depths of despair, time heals all wounds.

More than being willing to change, we need to shift the very premise of our perceptions before we can actually guard against the recurrences of similar invalid experiences. Whether or not we recognize and resolve the invalid before shuffling off the mortal coil, they are, in fact, non-existent because our perceptions were inaccurate. Even though we are able to retain them in ahamkara while we are alive, in spite of their false status, they do not transfer to the subtle body when we die because the physical mind that gave them life dies with the body. Anything inaccurate or invalid cannot sustain itself indefinitely because the physical vehicle to which it is attached has a finite life. This is why, at the time of death, the dying are able to forgive grudges held for a lifetime. Before dying, a person is usually able to recognize the invalidities of all of the negative perceptions incurred during that life.

The continuous engaging of invalid perceptions indicates a lack of personal wisdom and a separation from the cognitive self. Although invalid memories are not retained in the subtle body after death, the condition of our wisdom faculty, as well as our cognitive accomplishment or lack thereof, leaves a definite imprint, a definite deposit in our karmic account, that affects our next birth.

Storing and Retrieving Memories

During the normal process of living, memories of specific experiences are constantly being stored, retrieved, composed, endorsed, and re-filed. The filing of all memory in ahamkara occurs while we are experiencing life in the physical body. Ahamkara is always being searched to locate a previous encounter which resembles a present situation. The new experience is then compared to the previously stored one and an assessment is made about its desirability or non-desirability. In this way, we are continuously reliving similar experiences, and updating the data base as we go along. For instance, the memory of eating ice cream may be filed and refiled approximately 7,200 times during one person's lifetime. Most people who eat ice cream file away the memory of a sweet and pleasurable experience.

Depending on the quality and quantity of ice cream and the frequency of use, the more valid memory feedback to be filed from this so-called pleasurable experience would be that the digestive fire may be weakened and the fire of the first tissue of the body may malfunction and in turn create more bodily waste in the form of mucus, rather than the nutrient plasma needed to feed the long chain of hungry bodily tissues. As a result, the entire organism may become listless and lethargic. Essentially, the information you file into memory is perception-based and as such, generally inaccurate. For those who are more attuned to the body and mind, the filing of the ice cream experience will have detailed the real effects of ice cream on the bodily organism, including the effects of its sweet taste.

The many invalid memories that humans maintain in ahamkara serve to clutter the files and create great confusion in the mind. As a result, clarity of the mind and enthusiasm of spirit are severely compromised.

The Role of Direct Perception in Experiential Memory

There are usually three processes which occur progressively in the experiencing and filing of memories in ahamkara: perception, conclusion, and judgment. By means of mental and sensory perception we experience a certain situation. For example, while diving we may have discovered a beautiful white bead sitting amid the flora and shells on the ocean floor. At once, the mind, having received the input from sensory perceptions, immediately jumps to a conclusion or, at the very least, entertains an assumption: the beautiful iridescent bead is a pearl. Later, having retrieved the bead and attempting to sell it, we discover that our "pearl" is a simple bauble of no monetary value. Annoyed at having allowed our hopes to build, we throw the bead away and think, "How did this useless junk get to the bottom of the ocean?" The answer, of course, is that however it got there, it certainly served as a good lesson never to jump to a conclusion or make assumptions.

Having jumped to a conclusion, the mind immediately releases the experience into ahamkara, which in turn files it away. The word "jump" is used literally here to demonstrate the leap from a potentially cognitive state (which occurs immediately after a sensory perception is received) to a state of amnesia (total forgetfulness of our cognitive nature). This process of drawing a conclusion is actually a form of mutation to our innate cognitive ability. When a perception is valid, meaning that what we see, hear, and so on, is actually real, without discoloration or mutation of the incident, the need to make a conclusion does not arise. Only when we are not certain of what we are experiencing do we push the process into the arena of conclusions. Conclusions can render potentially valid situations invalid. This occurs when a person's sense of cognition is so weak that it perceives

56

everything as false. Conclusions are almost always born from invalid, untruthful, or unreal situations.

As humans, we cannot negate the necessity of our sensory and mental mechanisms, since we exist within the physical principles of time and space. Therefore, we need to remain alert and refrain from drawing conclusions. Once this rule is observed, all perceptions are properly received into the memory files of ahamkara and stored there as valid memory impulses that can come to our service later in similar circumstances.

To return to our hypothetical discovery of the bead, the proper way to proceed would have been to leave the question of its real nature open until the appropriate verification had been made. In this way, there would be no disappointment in the knowledge that it is not a pearl. Disappointment is a product of the expectancy that arises from conclusions. As soon as we conclude that the bead is a pearl, that expectancy is filed in ahamkara. When we discover our error, we must extract that detail from ahamkara, unless we choose to compound the problem by sustaining the delusion of owning a pearl. The extraction becomes the physical emotion of disappointment. Apart from the grief and agony we spare ourselves, the universe often rewards us for not making conclusions. Chances are, that if the conclusion that the bead was a pearl had been held in check, our discovery might well have been just that.

The Role of Indirect Perception in Experiential Memory

We experience perception primarily in two ways, directly and indirectly. Direct perception, as in the example just cited, occurs when one or more of the senses are engaged directly in a particular situation. Indirect perception is when we experience a situation indirectly—through hearsay, reading about it, and so on. In instances of indirect perception, we are cautioned even more firmly to remain alert and maintain the utmost discretion, it being much easier to draw conclusions in matters that involve other than yourself. For example, if I had been told that my co-worker Harry had stolen money from our organization, and, as a result of hearing this statement, I assumed that "Harry is a thief," I have already condemned Harry. Even if Harry had been caught red-handed with the money in hand, I could not be completely certain that he had committed a theft unless I was in total cognition with myself. Better, then, to never draw a conclusion on a matter—the state of self cognition being the gentle space, brimming with the milk of human compassion, that it is. Endeavor to decipher the truth as a cognitive being, whatever the outcome. Extenuating circumstances always prevail in human life. Every human has, at some time, in some place, been overcome by feelings of hopelessness, fear, greed and so on. Knowing this maxim of human consideration, some help may be offered to Harry, if indeed Harry committed the offense. To simply refrain from drawing a conclusion about Harry will help him, since, energetically, the universe will deliver our compassionate vibrations to him.

57

The contemporary norm is not only to conclude that "Harry is a thief," but to salt the wound further with some judgment or other, such as "Harry is also a bum." Although refraining from drawing conclusions is a most arduous practice, once begun, minute by minute, it is surprising how many scores of conclusions and judgments we can retrieve daily. Even the language needed to rephrase a judgment call will often elude us, so firmly rooted in the mind are the habitual expressions of conclusion and judgment.

Most circumstances resolve themselves when we allow the natural flow of universal energy to operate on all the decisions of living. If our perceptions are accurate and conclusions are not made, we have a better than average chance of resolving even the most distasteful of incidents with grace. In this way, not only do we mature, but the offending party may grow as well. Without a conclusion, no judgment can be made.

That fount of wisdom, the Vedas, advises us never to draw a conclusion, regardless of the apparent accuracy of our perception within a given experience. Far better to allow a situation to mature in its own time so that ahamkara will not be crowded with invalid data. When our memory datum is packed with invalid conclusions, we block our divine access to our own cognitive nature. When ahamkara contains only the verifiable memories which have stood the test of time through all previous lives, we are able to remember our cognitive nature. The residue of all valid experiences are kept in order and serve to promote clarity and equanimity in the mind. The natural rhythm of our energy protects and guides us through thick and thin, dark and light.

COSMIC MEMORY

When a foal wobbles on its lanky legs moments after birth, the memory of its species, from the very first horse, is sustained. When the palm tree drops its fruit, the seed is swallowed by the earth and another palm grows to splendid heights. When a mountain goat defies gravity by hanging upside down on an overhanging ledge of a Himalayan peak, it is observing the prowess embedded in its feet through the refinement of its species over billions of years. This is the natural order of life: sustaining, refining, and emerging through the maintenance of cosmic memory.

Cosmic memories sustain the entire universe and cognitive memories sustain the journeys of all the species. Cognitive memory is imbued in every species, from the beginning of its journey through each rebirth. Cosmic memory is the collective memory of all species, matter, and energy in the entire universe refined throughout time. It is the cumulative universal experience refined from the first minutiae of manifestation through the present into the complete future. Cosmic memory is our universal nature which is forever resonating with our personal cognition. The cosmos and the body are variants of the same energy pattern. Energy and information fluctuate unceasingly between the tissues of the body and the strata of the cosmos.

Inseparable from the cosmic, cognitive memory also contains the imprints from past, present, and future. However, it is easier for us to access the cognitive past and present memories than it is to access future memories because we do not as yet have the previous attachments to the future experiences that create future memories. In this sense, it may be said that although cosmic memory directly influences our cognitive memories, we cannot access cosmic memories directly without altering our regular state of consciousness.

The Silent Breath

The silent breath, called *samadhi* in Sanskrit, is an ancient practice handed down by the Vedic seers. It is a state in which the *yogin*, one whose life is devoted to the practice of sadhanas to help attain union with God, dissolves all experiential memories of the mind and senses, as well as all stimuli from the external nature, and resonates fully within the cognitive state. After long and constant practice, and abundant grace from the Lord, the yogin is said to be able to attain the highest form of samadhi where not only the cognitive planes (which carry the totality of the past and present lives) have been conquered, but also the cosmic state which carries the totality of our past, present, and future samskaras, or karmic imprints. Only when both the state of self-cognition and the cosmic state have been fully transcended is the yogin's union with Pure Consciousness said to be complete. With this union, all potential materials and vibrations for future rebirths on all planes of existence are completely dissolved.

Timeless Nature

A timeless mind is a mind that has its attention on eternity, on the spirit, which has no beginning or ending in time. If your external reference point shifts from the ego to the spirit, which is timeless, then you break the barrier of time and start experiencing time as quantified eternity, and mortality as quantified immortality. When you start experiencing time as eternity, then, because the body and mind are inseparable, the body will become ageless. If time stands still, the biological clock stands still.

Deepak Chopra, M.D.
(Interview, *Yoga Journal*, Sept/Oct, 1993)

It takes not only immense discipline and a one-pointed focus to attain the ultimate goal of moksha (the end of the cycles of rebirth), but the complete grace of the Lord. Crossing the barriers of life into timelessness is the eventual birthright of every human being. What we need to do, however, before this can happen, is to refine our cognitive memories and make them available to ourselves. Every human, at any given stage, is capable of aspiring to and achieving absolute cognition through the practice of sadhanas. This enables us to once more evoke this cosmic language of the self which has been quashed by our human ignorance of nature. The universe provides a panoply of wholesome activities which, when practiced daily, can revive our own resplendent nature so that we are a true reflection of the immortal, the timeless.

The Vedas describe our real nature as boundless and immortal. This nature we experience while in the state of self cognition. During samadhi, our cognitive nature is awakened to the full reality of timelessness, which transcends all planes of existence including the celestial plane; and there is a complete cessation of mortality. Throughout life we fluctuate between the timeless nature of our full cognition and the time-bound existence of our experiential state. Given the composition of the physical body, mind, and senses, we are compelled to live within a time-bound reality. This does not, however, preclude us from claiming our timeless right to evoke self-cognition and instate it as our most sacred guide as we cross the time-bound straits of life.

Seasonal Influences on Ayurvedic Therapies

CHAPTER THREE

THE SIX SEASONS

PART ONE

Northern and Southern Movements of the Sun

*T*he seasons are defined according to the two directions in which the sun appears to be moving. As the earth makes its annual voyage around the sun, we also experience six distinct phases called the seasons. The northern and southern movements of the sun are created mainly by the earth's relationship to the sun and the moon. The northward movement of the sun, known as *adana* in Sanskrit, begins at the winter solstice and ends at the summer solstice. The southern movement starts at the summer solstice and ends at the winter solstice.

During the northerly phase, the sun's energy is at its strongest and sucks moisture from the earth, leaving it dry. Also the wind conjugates with the sun, adding to the harsh nature pervading the three seasons in this phase. During this half of the year, the body tends to be weakened by the sun absorbing its moisture and humidity.

The southerly phase, known as *visagra* in Sanskrit, influenced more by the moon, provides a period of cooling relief to the earth. The sun's energy begins to wane and more moisture is released into the atmosphere. During the remaining three seasons of the year, the body tends to gain strength and vitality.

THE THREE SEASONS IN THE NORTHERLY PHASE OF THE SUN

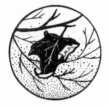

Late Winter

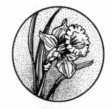

Spring

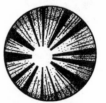

Summer

The three seasons in the northerly phase of the sun are late winter, spring, and summer. From late winter, in mid-January, the absorbing effects of the sun and wind increase progressively until their culmination in mid-June, when the sun's southward movement across the earth commences.

Due to the sun's harshness during the northerly phase, three of the six tastes—bitter, astringent and pungent—are dramatically enhanced. These three tastes share a constricting and absorbent nature which, when used in the form of food, further deplete the physical organism.

THE THREE SEASONS IN THE SOUTHERLY PHASE OF THE SUN

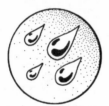

Rainy Season
(early fall)

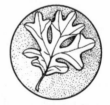

Autumn

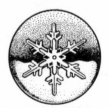

Early Winter

Contrary to the northerly phase, the sun's southward movement begins a period of reprieve for earth's inhabitants and vegetation. This phase is dominated by the quality of the moon which influences the sun's rays onto the earth. During this period, the sun and wind are also restrained by the clouds and rains, triggering a period of cooling release, which begins towards the end of summer. The stupendous powers of the sun begin to slacken as a result of the course of the earth's movement, cloud formation, and the presence of wind and rain.

The three seasons created by the southward movement of the sun are the rainy season or early fall, autumn, and early winter. From mid-June until towards the end of summer, the heat of the sun slackens progressively until its weakest culmination in mid-November, when the tri-seasonal cycle of the north phase reoccurs. The end of the southerly phase and the beginning of the northerly phase mark the most important junction of the changing seasons.

During the southerly phase, the natures of the three remaining tastes, sweet, sour, and salty are greatly enhanced. As a result, they contribute to bulk and vigor when used in the body.

AYURVEDIC CHART OF THE SIX SEASONS

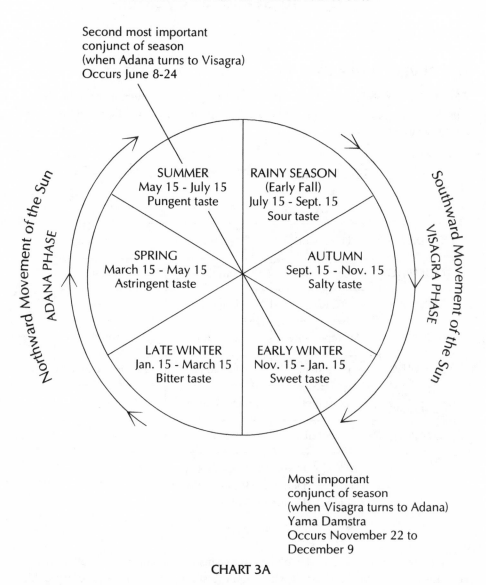

Second most important
conjunct of season
(when Adana turns to Visagra)
Occurs June 8-24

Northward Movement of the Sun
ADANA PHASE

Southward Movement of the Sun
VISAGRA PHASE

SUMMER
May 15 - July 15
Pungent taste

RAINY SEASON
(Early Fall)
July 15 - Sept. 15
Sour taste

SPRING
March 15 - May 15
Astringent taste

AUTUMN
Sept. 15 - Nov. 15
Salty taste

LATE WINTER
Jan. 15 - March 15
Bitter taste

EARLY WINTER
Nov. 15 - Jan. 15
Sweet taste

Most important
conjunct of season
(when Visagra turns to Adana)
Yama Damstra
Occurs November 22 to
December 9

CHART 3A

PART TWO
Daily and Seasonal Cycles

THE SEVEN DAILY CYCLES

The earth is a mobile force which circles the sun, just as the moon circles the earth. The daily and seasonal cycles are created by the earth's dynamic relationship to both the sun and moon.

SEVEN DAILY CYCLES OF THE DOSHAS

	VATA	PITTA	KAPHA
DAWN	Dominant	Neutral	Accumulating
MORNING	Lessening	Accumulating	Dominant
MID-DAY	Neutral	Dominant	Lessening
AFTERNOON	Accumulating	Lessening	Neutral
DUSK	Dominant	Neutral	Accumulating
EARLY EVENING	Lessening	Accumulating	Dominant
MIDNIGHT	Neutral	Dominant	Lessening

VATA: Dominant 2:00 - 6:00 am & pm
PITTA: Dominant 10:00 - 2:00 am & pm
KAPHA: Dominant 6:00 - 10:00 am & pm

CHART 3B

Each day we experience six phases of expansion and contraction, all of which are controlled by the sun. At **dawn**, when the sun is about to rise, the dry, cold, mobile aspects of Vata, gathered through the night, are prevalent. At **daybreak,**

66

the cool and heavy energy of Kapha begins to flow out of the body as we rise from rest. At **midday**, when the sun is at its peak and saps the body with its heat, Pitta prevails. In the **early afternoon**, as the sun's energy begins to wane, the dry, cold energy of Vata once more dominates. At **sunset**, when the sun has descended on the horizon, Kapha begins to pour back into the body to induce the body to rest. Finally, at **midnight**, when the sun is farthest away from the earth, Pitta once more prevails.

Controlled by the vibrational heat waves of the sun, the body's heat is at its peak at midday and midnight, the two times at which Pitta is at it height, since the bodily fire is naturally increased during these two pivotal junctions of the day. The junctions of day crossing into night, and night into day, are dominated by both Vata and Kapha.

DAILY COURSE OF THE ORGANS AND DOSHAS

TIME	DOSHA	ORGAN
11:00 am - 1:00 pm	Pitta	Heart
1:00 pm - 3:00 pm	Pitta	Small Intestine
3:00 pm - 5:00 pm	Vata	Bladder
5:00 pm - 7:00 pm	Vata/Kapha	Kidney
7:00 pm - 9:00 pm	Kapha	Pericardium
9:00 pm - 11:00 pm	Kapha/Pitta	Body Cavities
11:00 pm - 1:00 am	Pitta	Gall Bladder
1:00 am - 3:00 am	Pitta	Liver
3:00 am - 5:00 am	Vata	Lungs
5:00 am - 7:00 am	Vata	Colon
7:00 am - 9:00 am	Kapha	Stomach
9:00 am - 11:00 am	Kapha/Pitta	Spleen

CHART 3C

67

The Daily Course of the Organs and Doshas

As the earth orbits the sun, the energy fluctuations that occur directly affect the bodily organism. Each organ and dosha is susceptible to the dynamic energy transaction, which occurs naturally throughout the course of the day, a different dosha and organ being affected in a cyclical manner every two hours.

The doshas are also affected during the natural course of digestion—Vata, Pitta and Kapha each controlling a specific aspect of the process.

DOSHAS' BEHAVIOR DURING DIGESTION

	Immediately After Eating	During Digestion	Post-Digestion
VATA	Neutral	Accumulating	Dominant
PITTA	Accumulating	Dominant	Lessening
KAPHA	Dominant	Neutral	Neutral

CHART 3D

The Junctions of the Seasons

According to Ayurveda, all diseases begin at the junction that occurs before the seasons because it is at this time that the individual doshas are quick to fall out of balance. Therefore, we are urged to cross the seasonal junctions gently and with care. As you will discover in the chapter on the Ayurvedic cleansing therapies, most of the body's internal cleansing and healing take place during the seasonal junctions in an attempt to revitalize and replenish both the mind and the body. Ayurveda's unique healing system, pancha karma, was designed to facilitate this natural process. Pancha karma treatments are usually administered at the two main junctions of the six seasons. Details for transitioning from one season to the next are set out in the ancient Ayurvedic texts. These schedules have been included later in this chapter.

While passing through the full yearly cycle of the northern and southern movements of the sun, the body experiences six distinct variations at each of the six junctions of the seasons. These variations create imbalances within the doshas, which is why the seasonal junctions are deemed a vulnerable time for the body. The last seven days of the previous season and the first seven days of the ensuing season comprise the *rtusandhi*, the junctional period. It is during these days that we are advised to remain especially alert and to make the necessary adjustments in all of our activities, in our work, diet, sadhanas, and so on.

The six seasons in the year occur in early winter (November 15 to January 15); late winter (January 15 to March 15); spring (March 15 to May 15); summer (May 15

68

to July 15); the rainy season or early fall (July 15 to Sept 15); and autumn (September 15 to November 15). The Ayurvedic calendar further divides these seasons into twelve phases. In actuality, each season has an early and late phase, i.e., spring's early phase is from March 15 to April 15, and its late phase is from April 15 to May 15. The fortnight period between the early and late phases of each season is considered to be a junction point within the season. There are, then, six junctions existing within the six seasons.

There are also six main junctions which occur between each season, i.e., the fortnight which marks the ending of spring and the beginning of summer is also considered a seasonal junction. Altogether there are twelve junctions, six within the seasons, and six between the seasons. Of the twelve seasonal junctions existing, the six which occur between each season are the most crucial. The junctions serve an important purpose in Ayurvedic medicine. These are the periods when the body's cycles and doshas are most fragile.

Diseases are first rooted in the body at the time of seasonal junctions. These gaps are given serious consideration before the administering of the *shodhana* process, the therapies for eliminating bodily waste in the form of doshas.

The cleansing therapies for Vata occur twice yearly. Once within the seasonal junction of the rainy season (early fall) between July 24 and August 7, and then again between the seasonal junction of autumn and early winter. In the tropical and semi-tropical climates, this time falls between November 8 and November 20. In the temperate zone, the junction is observed as a longer period between October 20 and November 20. The reason for this extension of time in temperate climates is to facilitate the performance of the therapy before the extreme cold of winter approaches. Extending the time for therapy beyond the period of a fortnight at this time of year is also to accommodate the cleansing of both the Pitta and Vata doshas, whose elimination cycles naturally occur during this period. Kapha may also be cleansed at this time due to the excess accumulation that tends to gather because of the dampness of the previous rainy season. Thus, the end of autumn is considered a good time for tridosha cleansing and restoral.

In the tropical and semi-tropical climates, the most appropriate time to cleanse the excesses of Pitta is the fortnight between the end of autumn and the beginning of the early winter season, which is from November 8 to November 20. Although the tropics do not experience a winter season, this period of time is still referred to as early winter for the purposes of explanation.

The most ideal seasonal junction for eliminating excess Kapha is the end of late winter into spring, from March 21 to April 21. Here again, the period is extended to include two fortnights, since Kapha tends to accumulate throughout the early and late winters and so requires a longer period to thaw out. The Kapha dosha usually liquifies from the beginning to the end of the spring season and may be eliminated from the body at any time during this period. Pitta may also be cleansed at this time due to the thawing out, or liquification, of the bodily fires after the winter.

Although there are a few differences of opinion among the classical Ayurvedic scholars as to the proper timing for administering pancha karma therapy, there is a harmonious consensus on at least one point. Both Charaka and Sushruta agree that the most appropriate time to remove excess doshas from the body is at the end of their seasons of aggravation. It is at this time that the doshas are in their most liquid form and can be most easily extracted from the tissues. Thus, the beginning of the spring season is usually the best time to treat Kapha excess and the end of autumn the best time to cleanse both Vata and Pitta excesses. As mentioned earlier, Vata may also be eliminated at the central junction between the early and late phases of the rainy season. In this way, the doshas' excesses are weakened before they become rooted in the body as diseases. The cleansing therapies are not administered even in their appropriate seasons when weather conditions are extremely cold or extremely hot.

The main intent of pancha karma cleansing actions is to persuade the bodily tissues to release their waste and to help restore the natural function of both tissue and dosha. According to the Vedic seers, the bodily tissues are more willing to release ama, the foul, undigested materials stuck in the tissues, at the junction of the seasons. During this time, the body is responding to the natural influences brought on by the changing seasons, and is both vulnerable and pliable. The use of these deeply cleansing and healing therapies is intended to cajole both body and mind to let go of its excesses, toxins, and so on. In this manner, the ama is released from the willing tissues of the body and re-directed into the digestive tract, which then moves it out of the body. Any excess clogging in the mind is also removed in the process.

If, on the other hand, these treatments are administered in an unseasonal and untimely way—within the dosha's full-blown season, for example, or if they are in their first stage of building up—the body can be injured rather than helped. This is because the body is not always willing to let go of its wastes and toxins so that incorrect or untimely cleansing may actually force the ama to go even deeper into the tissues.

THE SEASONS OF NATURAL ACCUMULATION, AGGRAVATION AND ALLEVIATION

	Accumulation	Aggravation	Alleviation
VATA	Summer	Rainy season (early fall) Late winter	Autumn
PITTA	Rainy season	Autumn Rainy season (early fall)	Early winter
KAPHA	Early winter	Spring Rainy season (early fall)	Summer

CHART 3E

70

PART THREE

Seasonal Cleansing Therapies for Each Dosha

VATA: SEASONS OF AGGRAVATION

Rainy Season (Early Fall)

During the rainy season, the earth releases more gases into the atmosphere, which tends to aggravate Vata. Further aggravation is created by the dampness of the rainy season and the higher acidity in the water at that time. The rainy period comes at a time when the body, having endured the long and harsh time of the northerly phase, is at its nadir of vitality. Even though the rainy season marks the beginning of the southerly phase, a period of strengthening, the body is still too vulnerable to resist the onslaught of the rains.

Vata is the dosha that leaps out of bounds very quickly and is thus afflicted somewhat consistently throughout the year. However, it requires special help at the end of the period of major aggravation which begins in the summer and runs into and throughout the rainy season. Thus Vata's first annual cleansing period comes between the early and late phases of the rainy season.

Although Vata's main season of alleviation is the rainy season (early fall), the next appropriate cleansing period occurs at the end of autumn. In temperate climates, where there is no definitive rainy season, the vitiation of Vata still occurs at this time due to the northerly movement of the sun; therefore, the same seasonal recommendations apply.

Late Winter

Late winter is the next season in which Vata is generally alleviated. The extreme coldness of winter increases the already cold nature of Vata, and the body requires the greatest amounts of physical warmth and nourishing foods. When not amply protected or fed, the body begins to eat its own tissues, and Vata becomes aggravated as a result. Nourishing, warm foods with sour, sweet, and salty tastes are recommended to balance Vata during this time of year. Healing gems such as opal, topaz, and beryl, and aromas such as rose, mint, and jasmine may be used at this time. Ayurvedic massages, warm atmosphere and clothing, and reduced sexual activity are all deemed vital so that Vata may remain balanced throughout this season.

Although there are some cooling influences in tropical and semi-tropical climates at this time of year, the late winter cleansing programs recommended in this book do not apply.

Summer

Vata may become mildly disturbed during the summer, due to the reduction of Kapha in the body caused by the heat of the sun. If Kapha is reduced too severely, Vata suffers since Kapha provides the buffering necessary to the lean and erratic Vata character.

Vata may be nurtured at this time by light, cool, sweet, and nourishing foods, mild and gentle daily routines, decreased sexual activity, gems such as pearl, opal and amethyst, aroma therapy, gentle body rubs, and so on.

Autumn

The end of autumn is generally considered to be the time when all three doshas can be relieved of their excesses. Therefore, if Vata's condition was not alleviated during the rainy season, it may be removed through the elimination therapies at the end of the autumn season.

In an attempt to establish one particular time of year as the best time for cleansing all three doshas, practitioners in the United States, Europe, and England are applying pancha karma primarily during the autumn season and are enjoying successful results. However, we need to remain alert to the fact that we cannot expect to completely standardize this unique and dynamic practice without negatively influencing results, which, in many cases, may prove harmful to health. Also, these therapies should conform to the original uses of matter, energy, and time. Therefore, they must not be performed with equipment that requires electrical energy, nor should they be applied in an untimely manner or employ unnatural or inappropriate substances.

Ayurveda presents a vast and illuminating mandala of healing therapies. Although many of its practices have become virtually extinct, we are fortunate to have available to us still a practicing knowledge of the pancha karma and its supporting therapies. Pancha karma therapies include those treatments that cleanse and eliminate the aggravated doshas, as well as the rejuvenative and restorative sadhanas that help the tissues and doshas to regain their equanimity.

The therapies and the proper time to apply them are described below. More details are provided in the section on the actual treatments and sadhanas. These therapies may be used by all body types, according to how the doshas are behaving.

Vata Seasonal Cleansing Schedule

Climate	Season	Date
Temperate and Tropical	Junction of summer and rainy season (early fall)	July 24 to August 7
Tropical	End of autumn	November 8 to 20
Temperate	Late autumn*	October 20 to November 20

Cleansing at this time must occur before Yama Damstra (see explanation, pg. 84)

Note: Because autumn is one of the two main transitional seasons of the year (the other being spring), the cleansing time is extended to a longer period during the autumn season, rather than to just the junctional period between autumn and early winter.

Vata Seasonal Cleansing Therapies

Vasti Therapy: The Ayurvedic use of herbal decoction enemas, as well as medicated oil enemas, to clear the excess dosha from the large intestines.

Enema decoctions are derived from herbs such as comfrey, *dashamula*, *gotu kola*, and licorice. The sesame oil enema is usually administered as a separate procedure. These enemas re-direct the apana wind to its normal downward flow and soothe Vata disturbances in the body.

Pinda Sveda: The Ayurvedic use of fomentation therapy to thoroughly invigorate the body.

This therapy stimulates the vital tissues and organs, while alleviating bodily pain. Sveda therapy also awakens cellular memory and removes fear from the mind.

Abhyanga: The application of the Ayurveda system of massage, using herbal medicated oils, sesame oil, sandalwood paste, and so on.

Abhyanga is a vital Ayurvedic practice used to restore equanimity to the body's muscular system. Because this massage also stimulates the body's natural "valium," abhyanga promotes both peace of mind and strength of limb.

Shirovasti: The Ayurvedic practice of pouring medicated oil on the head and allowing it to remain for a period of time.

This therapy promotes mental clarity, stimulates cognitive and experiential memories, and completely revitalizes the body.

Shirobhayanga: The Ayurvedic application of medicated oils to the head.
Various Ayurvedic herbs such as *madhuka*, *kesare*, or *devadaru*, are boiled in sesame

oil in preparation for shirobhyanga. The head is then amply massaged with the oil, giving life and balance to the sense organs and rejuvenating the entire body.

Details on these and other healing procedures for Vata are located in Section III, Rejuvenative Sadhanas, and Section IV, Cleansing Therapies.

PITTA: SEASONS OF AGGRAVATION

Autumn

Accumulated Pitta from the rainy season becomes aggravated during the autumn season, a time when the digestive fire is already tremendously affected by the long and dry period of the previous northerly phase. Pitta is further afflicted by the extreme conditions of the rainy season that precedes autumn. As the sun begins to brighten the sky, providing the heat necessary to evaporate the moisture of the rainy season just past, it affects the vulnerable Pitta, causing both the digestion and blood systems to go awry. At this time, the liquid that Pitta has accumulated during the rainy season dampens the digestive fire, resulting in a loss of appetite.

In order for Pitta to retrieve its normal and excellent digestion, the Ayurvedic purgative therapy of *virechana* is recommended (see below). The best time of the autumn season for any form of cleansing therapy is at the tail end of Pitta's accumulation, i.e. the latter part of the season when the dosha is in its most fluent form. In tropical and semi-tropical climates, the best time is at the end of autumn.

Rainy Season

There are many Ayurvedic healing therapies that, while not part of the pancha karma or herbal therapies, may be observed during both the rainy season and throughout the autumn period. These include massage geared to Pitta types, using aromatic and cooling oils such as coconut oil combined with sandalwood essential oil; daily body brushing; altering one's activities to those that are milder and more harmonious, especially during the initial stages of doshic vulnerability; aroma therapy using oils like mint, licorice, sandalwood, jasmine, or vetiver, to calm the mind and stomach; healing gems such as pearl, coral, emerald, and crystal quartz.

Pitta Seasonal Cleansing Schedule

Climate	Season	Date
Temperate	Late autumn*	October 20 to November 20
Tropical	End of autumn	November 8 to 20

Cleansing at this time must occur before Yama Damstra (see explanation, pg. 84)

Pitta Seasonal Cleansing Therapies

Virechana Therapy: The use of Ayurvedic purgatives to clear the lower pathways of the body.

This therapy helps to purify the blood and to cleanse the stomach, sweat glands, small intestines, colon, kidneys, liver, and spleen. Substances such as psyllium husk, castor oil, senna leaves, cow's milk with ghee, flaxseed, *trivrit* and *triphala* are used to induce purgation.

Rakta Moksha: Although this form of therapy, commonly referred to as bloodletting, is seldom used in India today, and is illegal in the United States and Europe, when performed correctly it is an effective form of therapy to extract toxins from the blood.

Generally, toxins that accumulated under the skin and around the marma points (the energy junctions of the body's meridians) were eliminated through the process of blood-letting. Because Pitta manifests in the waste products of blood, many skin ailments, such as rash, eczema, and acne, are caused by toxins circulating in the blood system. The drawing of a small amount of blood from the vein relieves the blood tension created by these toxins. Internal use of certain bitter herbs, such as *neem,* dandelion leaves, burdock root, calamus root, and turmeric, may also be used to purify the blood.

Shirodhara: The use of a decoction, such as medicated ghee and buttermilk, sugarcane juice, and herbal oils on the forehead, to relieve ulcerations in the head and body and burning sensations or pain in the head.

In the traditional Ayurvedic application, the person lies down on a wide, seasoned, wooden log. A vessel called *dhara chatti,* which resembles a wide top funnel, or a *dhara patra,* a pot with a hole in the bottom, is used, through which the medicated oil is dripped rhythmically onto the center of the forehead where the third eye is located. Shirodhara is a beautiful therapy which awakens our cognitive state and lulls the entire bodily organism into a state of calmness. This therapy is used to balance all three doshas, employing those medicated oils and substances best suited to the different doshas and various ailments.

75

Details on these and other healing procedures for Pitta are located in the Rejuvenative Sadhanas (Section III) and Cleansing Therapies (Section IV).

KAPHA: SEASONS OF AGGRAVATION

Spring

Although Kapha enjoys the strongest stamina of the three doshas, she experiences her fragility in the springtime. After the long, cold, and inert periods of early and late winter, Kapha begins to thaw so that most of the semi-frozen wastes accumulated during the previous seasons liquify.

Kapha's imbalances are expressed through the feeling of lethargy, colds, tonsillitis, sore throat, lung congestion, cold body extremities, and so on. Winter changes to spring, almost at the very height of the northerly phase of the sun, when strength and vigor tend to become depleted by the sun's harshness. The thawing out of liquid waste in the body retards both the digestive fire and the body's metabolism, which is why Kapha's potential listlessness and lethargy increase. The gap before the full bloom of the spring season is the best time of year for the Kapha dosha to be thoroughly cleansed by means of both the elimination therapies and rejuvenative sadhanas. These processes relieve the excess dosha when it is in its most fluid form and not yet rooted in the body in the form of disease. Kapha then has plenty of time to mobilize during the remaining season.

Rainy Season

Kapha experiences similar difficulties during the rainy season (early fall), a time when the spring seasonal process is reversed. The end of the summer heat and the ensuing decline in strength is braced up by the damp and humid cold of the rainy season. Due to Kapha's reduced digestive fire, a feeling of listlessness may again prevail, along with Kapha's enormous inclination to hoard excesses within the body. During this period, replenishing therapies used to maintain Kapha's balance include: seasonally appropriate foods; Ayurvedic massage with *aguru* oil; inhalation therapies using aromas such as sage, eucalyptus, peppermint, and aromatic smoke; *collyrium*, various salves for the eyes; and healing gems such as emerald, lapis lazuli, ruby, and garnet.

Kapha Seasonal Cleansing Schedule

Climate	Season	Date
Temperate and Tropical	End of late winter into spring	March 21 to April 21

Note: Because spring is one of the two main transitional seasons of the year (the other being autumn), the cleansing time has been extended to a longer period during the spring season, rather than to just the junctional period between the late winter and the spring.

Kapha Seasonal Cleansing Therapies

Vamana Therapy: Vamana, also known as emesis therapy, is an ancient therapeutic method for eliminating Kapha's accumulation through the upper pathways.

For example, two glasses of salt water, or an herbal decoction, are taken in the morning. This solution aggravates Kapha and induces vomiting. The tongue is usually rubbed with the index and middle fingers to stimulate the reflex action of throwing up. Vamana releases congestion from the lungs and provides immediate relief for asthmatic and bronchial attacks. Vamana is used for serious Kapha disorders and to help with other ailments such as skin diseases, diabetes, chronic disorders of the lungs and stomach, sinusitis and tonsillitis.

Oil massage and fomentation applied to the chest on the evening before the emesis therapy are the preliminary steps taken to induce the state most conducive to this therapy.

Nasya: The nasal application of medication in both powder and liquid form.

The powdered medication is inserted into the nose through a tube and the liquid medication is applied with a dropper. The nose is the gateway to the cerebral, sensory, and motor functions of the body. Disorders associated with the movement of prana are usually corrected by nasya therapy. Kapha excess stored in the throat, nose, sinus, and head are also removed from the body as a result of nasya. Herbal powders, such as *gotu kola* and *shatavari*, as well as substances such as milk, ghee, medicated oils, ginger and garlic are used, depending on the dosha and the nature of the disorder.

PART FOUR

Relationship Between the Doshas and the Seasons

The doshas are to the body what the seasons are to the earth. Both the doshas and the seasons are created from the five elements. The elemental aspects of the seasons are in the form of galactic space, wind, sun, moon, rain, and the earth. Here, we are urged to understand the interplay between the doshas and the seasonal influences within the primacy of the five elements. The doshas are not simply the dynamic energy within the body, rather they are influenced primarily by seasonal variations. Knowledge of the seasons is germane to the balancing of the doshas. Therefore, a thorough understanding of the function of the doshas within the body necessitates an understanding of the variations within each season, the junction between seasons, and the annual rotation of the six seasons.

In many cases, the designated seasonal tastes and qualities appear to be contradictory. For this reason, the following charts are provided to assist you in coordinating your body type with its seasonal tastes and qualities.

BALANCING SEASONAL TASTES AND BODY TYPE TASTES

The apparent contradictions between the tastes and qualities beneficial to each body type, and the tastes and qualities suggested by the cyclical nature of the seasons, are to be understood in the following way: The tastes which are generally good for each body type may become heightened or prevalent in the body and external environment due to seasonal influences. For example, of the six tastes, the pungent flavor naturally predominates during the summer; although considered a generally good all-year taste for Kapha types, it needs to be used in the summer season with discretion. Similarly, the salty taste which predominates during autumn, although considered a generally excellent all-year taste for Vata types, needs to be reduced during the autumn season, even by Vata types. In the early winter, the sweet taste predominates, and although generally an excellent all-year taste for Pitta types, needs to be reduced during the early winter, even by Pitta types.

The tastes and qualities of our body, and the external environment created by the five elements, are further influenced by the dynamic inter-relationship of the earth, sun and moon. As the earth makes its annual revolution around the sun,

78

half of the year, called the northerly phase period, is heavily influenced by the effects of the sun sucking the moisturizing salves from the earth's surface. As a result of this absorbent action, the qualities and tastes dominantly produced by the earth's vegetation and atmosphere are predominately pungent, bitter, and astringent. The seasons which correspond with these tastes are late winter, spring, and summer, respectively. During these periods, our bodily tissues are then saturated with more of these three tastes than usual. Subsequently, we need to use the other three tastes—sweet, sour, and salty—and their qualities in order to promote balance within the organism.

Likewise, during the remaining half of the year, called the southerly phase, when the sun is farther away from the earth, the soothing coolness of the moon predominates. This is a period of release and relief for the earth in which the energy of the remaining three substantial tastes—sweet, sour, and salty—increases. The seasons which correspond with these tastes are early fall/rainy season, autumn, and early winter respectively. Here, we seek balance through the tastes and qualities of the more pungent, bitter, and astringent food and activities.

Each of the six tastes, when expressed in foods, contributes to life in a different and quantitative way. The sweet taste is the most dominant in the universe, comprising more than seventy percent of all foods in nature existing on the earth, due to its nurturing, building and sustaining nature. The five remaining tastes—sour, salty, pungent, bitter, and astringent—are supporting principles and are used primarily as accents and condiments to food and life. The exception here is when these tastes are naturally dominant in a particular food, e.g., the sour taste of grapefruit; the natural salt in most watery vegetables, such as zucchini and cabbage, and the pungency of ginger root, garlic, peppers, and most herbs. Bitter exists in foods like vegetable and salad greens, while as alkaloids and glycosides, it exists predominantly in herbs and medicines. The astringent principle is fundamental to medicines, as in the tannin of barks, for example. It may also be found in foods such as uncooked legumes. All six tastes form the basis, in varying degrees, for all the foods and principles of nature.

Tastes Within the Body

Ayurveda perceives the tastes as an intrinsic language permeating all of nature, present in every structure of the universe. We generally associate tastes with the obvious sensory organ of the tongue and the foods it receives. In the therapeutic aspects of Ayurvedic healing and cleansing regimens and sadhanas, taste must necessarily be viewed in its more all-encompassing light. Each taste is formed by two of the five elements combining in varying units.

The doshas and dhatus may be viewed as the bodily equivalent to the universal tastes. They function primarily through the instinct of taste. Certain tastes within the doshas and dhatus are heightened and disturbed by seasonal changes, as they are in the foods we eat. For example, the rasa dhatu, the body's plasma, lymph, and chyle tissue, consisting mostly of the water element, is in fact the body's sweet tissue. During the winter season, when the sweet taste is dominant, it is most adversarial toward the rasa dhatu. Similarly, rakta dhatu—blood, essentially—has fire as its dominant nature, and is the body's pungent tissue. During the summer, the pungent taste is considerably pronounced and directly affects the rakta dhatu. Asthi dhatu, the bone tissue of the body, pervaded by air and space, may be thought of as the body's bitter tissue. In the autumn and early winter, the bitter taste is heightened, and asthi dhatu is generally adversely affected. The nature or general quality of the doshas may also be related to taste. Vata, which is predominantly air and space, may be called the bitter dosha; Pitta, which is mostly fire and water, may be called the pungent dosha; and Kapha, predominantly water and earth, may be called the sweet dosha.

Simply put, we need to eat more of the tastes that are presently not as prevalent in the universe and in our bodies. In this way, our internal tastes are calmed and nurtured so that we are more able to flow in gentle balance with earthly nature. A chart is provided below to help you braid your personal body type requirements with the overall scheme of the earth's seasonal influences. This interphasing process will require patience and practice. After a full year's observance of the seasonal cycles and junctions, and their correspondence to your prakriti (constitutional nature), you will be better able to identify and implement the routine that best suits you, adapting it as necessary through your remaining years.

Ayurveda's presentation of the universal tastes is the basis of all sadhanas, whether they relate to our foods, activities, lifestyle, or dreams. Knowledge of the six tastes is especially relevant in Ayurveda's seasonal healing and cleansing therapies, the tastes being yet another part of the alphabet which forms the complete language of nature.

No taste is ever used exclusively of the others; a combination of all six tastes must, in some way, be present. Like the body, every form of life and atmospheric condition is a combination of all six tastes, each entity demonstrating varying degrees of the five elements imbued in the six tastes. It is essential to use all six tastes throughout the year, while emphasizing those tastes which are more vital to your health, given your individual prakriti and the requirements of the seasons.

THE TASTES OF THE SEASONS

Northerly Phase (Winter Solstice to Summer Solstice)			
Season	**Dry Tastes**	**Element Composition**	**Dosha**
Late winter	bitter	air and space	Vata
Spring	astringent	air and earth	Vata & Kapha
Summer	pungent	air and fire	Vata & Pitta
Note: the dry tastes are created by the progressive northward movement of the sun			

Southerly Phase (Summer Solstice to Winter Solstice)			
Season	**Moist Tastes**	**Element Composition**	**Dosha**
Rainy season (early fall)	sour	earth and fire	Pitta & Kapha
Autumn	salty	water and fire	Pitta
Early winter	sweet	water and earth	Kapha
Note: the moist tastes are created by the progressive southward movement of the sun			

CHART 3F

Beneficial Tastes According to Doshas

Vata: sweet, sour, salty

Pitta: sweet, bitter, astringent

Kapha: pungent, bitter, astringent

These are the general rule only and need to be altered according to the dynamic demands of each season.

SEASONAL TASTE ADJUSTMENTS

	VATA	PITTA	KAPHA
LATE WINTER	**Major:** sour, salty, unctuous **Minor:** sweet	**Major:** sweet, sour,* salty,* warm, unctuous **Minor:** bitter, astringent, cool, light	**Major:** sour,* astringent, pungent, warm, moderate unctuous **Minor:** bitter, salty, dry
SPRING	**Major:** sweet, salty, warm, moderate unctuous, alkaline **Minor:** sour, pungent	**Major:** sweet, bitter pungent,* warm **Minor:** astringent, cool, alkaline	**Major:** pungent, moderate astringent, alkaline, warm, dry **Minor:** bitter, salty
SUMMER	**Major:** sweet, sour, warm, moderate unctuous **Minor:** bitter, salty, cool, light	**Major:** sweet, bitter, cool, moderate unctuous **Minor:** astringent, light	**Major:** bitter, astringent, moderate sweet, warm, dry **Minor:** pungent, cool
RAINY SEASON (early fall) Temperate Climates	**Major:** sweet, moderate bitter,* salty, moderate unctuous, warm **Minor:** sour	**Major:** bitter, astringent, moderate salty, moderate sweet, warm, moderate unctuous **Minor:** pungent, cool	**Major:** bitter, astringent, pungent, warm, light **Minor:** salty, sour, dry
Tropical and Semitropical Climates	**Major:** sweet, salty, moderate unctuous, warm **Minor:** bitter, pungent	**Major:** sweet, bitter, salty,* warm, moderate unctuous **Minor:** astringent, pungent	**Major:** moderate salty,* pungent, bitter, warm, moderate unctuous **Minor:** astringent, dry
AUTUMN	**Major:** sweet, sour, warm, light **Minor:** salty, astringent	**Major:** sweet, bitter, astringent, cool, light **Minor:** pungent	**Major:** bitter, astringent, moderate sweet, warm, light
EARLY WINTER	**Major:** salty, bitter,* moderate sour, warm, unctuous **Minor:** pungent, sweet	**Major:** bitter, astringent, moderate pungent,* warm, moderate unctuous **Minor:** sweet	**Major:** pungent, astringent, bitter, warm, moderate unctuous **Minor:** salty

CHART 3G

82

* Vata types: If strong tendency to Vata disorders, use as minor tastes and increase the use of sweet and salty tastes during the seasons indicated.
* Pitta types: If strong tendency to Pitta disorders, use as minor tastes and increase the use of bitter, astringent and sweet tastes during the seasons indicated.
* Kapha types: If strong tendency to Kapha disorders, use as minor tastes and increase the use of pungent, bitter and astringent tastes during the seasons indicated.

Transitioning the Seasons

Although this transitioning pattern may seem tedious, it possesses great rhythm. Having practiced it once at the crossing of one season into the next, you will experience a natural ease during the next crossing. Intrinsically, we observe this pattern to some degree without realizing it. The simple act of putting away one season's clothes and bringing out the next season's reflects this rhythm. Rarely do our actions declare an abrupt end to the affairs of a particular season.

The Seasonal Junctions According to the Calendar

Late winter to spring	March 24 to April 7
Spring to summer	May 24 to June 7
Northerly to southerly phases	June 8 to June 24
Summer to rainy season (early fall)	July 24 to Aug 7
Rainy season (early fall) to autumn	September 23 to October 7
Autumn (Yama Damstra) to early winter	November 22 to December 9
Early winter to late winter	January 24 to February 7

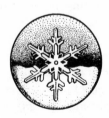

Fourteen-Day Transitional Regimen

Day	Regimen
1	1/4 of previous season's regimen and 3/4 of new season's regimen
2	full regimen of previous season and none of new regimen
3	1/4 of previous and 3/4 of new
4	1/2 of previous and 1/2 of new
5	1/4 of previous and 3/4 of new
6	1/4 of previous and 3/4 of new
7	1/2 of previous and 1/2 of new
8	1/4 of previous and 3/4 of new
9	1/2 of previous and 1/2 of new
10	1/2 of previous and 1/2 of new
11	1/4 of previous and 3/4 of new
12	1/4 of previous and 3/4 of new
13	none of previous and full regimen of new
14	1/4 of previous and 3/4 of new

Having completed this transitional regimen, remain completely within the current season's regimen until the next seasonal junction. Then repeat the above.

The Strength of Seasonal Influence

The intricate nature of the seasons is created by the course of the earth, sun, and moon, and human vitality is determined by the resulting variability. The two most important transitional periods are when the southerly and northerly phases change from one to the other. During these changes, there is a tendency toward physio-psychological vulnerabilities and stress. The period between November 22 and December 9, called Yama Damstra, when the southerly phase changes to northerly, is the most crucial of all seasonal transitions. Yama is the Lord who receives the deceased. This time holds within it an innate structure of fear and mental disturbance for a human being. To restore equilibrium in the mind and body, it is advised to observe the sadhanas of fasting, meditation, and prayers.

The period June 8 to June 24, when the northerly phase changes to southerly, is the second most important seasonal junction. Although it is not as potentially traumatic as the Yama Damstra period, it is still a vulnerable period. Sadhanas such as aroma therapy, light massage, pranayama, the careful transition of seasonal foods and so on, are vital for maintaining good physical and mental health. Since this period is preceded by another seasonal junction, occurring between May 24 and June 7, the entire month from May 24 to June 24 should be observed as a time of transition.

In review, the healthiest period of the year occurs between November and January, and the least healthy period is between May and July. The intermediate periods, February through May and August through October, are moderately balanced and healthy.

SEASONAL DO'S AND DON'TS

	DO	DON'T
LATE WINTER	sour, salty, moderate sweet, unctuous, substantial quantity of food	excess sweet, pungent, bitter, dry, cold, raw foods, meager quantity of foods
SPRING	pungent, astringent, moderate sweet, moderate salty, warm, moderate quantity of food	sour, excess sweet, bitter, too many fluids, cold
SUMMER	sweet, bitter, astringent, cool, moderate unctuous, sufficient fluid	salty, sour, pungent, hot, insufficiency of fluids
RAINY SEASON (early fall) Temperate Climates	pungent, butter, astringent, moderate salty, moderate sour, light, warm	sweet, excess sour, excess salty, cold, dry, excess unctuous
Tropical and Semitropical Climates	sour, salty, unctuous, moderate sweet, moderate unctuous, warm	pungent, bitter, astringent, excess sweet, cold, dry
AUTUMN	sweet, bitter, astringent, cool, light, non-oily	sour, salty, pungent, hot, oily, excess food, heavy foods
EARLY WINTER	salty, bitter, astringent, moderate sour, warm, moderate unctuous, moderate quantity	sweet, excess sour, excess cold, dry, excess food, raw foods

The "Seasonal Don'ts" may be used occasionally as a minor taste. See Chart 3G.

CHART 3H

Seasons and Strength

Note: S = Southerly phase; N = Northerly phase

S   Early winter, *hemanta*
    November 15 to January 15; maximum strength (peak period)
N   Late winter, *sisira*
    January 15 to March 15; maximum strength (wane period)
N   Spring, *vasanta*
    March 15 to May 15; moderate strength (wane period)
N   Summer, *grisma*
    May 15 to July 15; minimum strength (wane period)
S   Rainy season (early fall), *varsa*
    July 15 to September 15; minimum strength (peak period)
S   Autumn, *sarada*
    September 15 to November 15; moderate strength (peak period)

Strongest period of human strength—January 10 to January 24.
Weakest period of human strength—July 10 to July 24.

A Woman's Season

There is an additional season for women which happens once every month during menstruation. The beginning period of the full moon is the natural cycle for ovulation. Receiving the essence of the moon at this time, a woman's sexual impulses heighten and her vitality is once more replenished. Then, during the time of the new moon, she experiences the natural cycle of menstruation. Menstruation is caused by the sun absorbing energies from the earth, which in turn draws the menstrual waste from the body. When the cycle has not been tampered with by the use of contraceptive pills and other birth control devices, harmful foods and activities, and disruptive sexual activities, the natural ebb and flow of a woman's monthly cycle remains in harmony with the cycles of the moon.

During the full moon period, sadhanas such as aroma therapy, warm baths, the use of healing gems appropriate to each dosha, and other activities which increase the vital essences of the body may be practiced. During the period of menstruation, activities need to be reduced to the essentials so that the body experiences the least degree of intrusion. A minimum of bodily cleansing sadhanas are also advocated at this time. Quick, cool showers, or wiping down the body, is the appropriate means of bodily cleaning during menstruation. A woman should refrain from all sexual foreplay and activities, as well as from the cooking sadhanas, in order to prevent the energies of the menstrual waste from pervading the foods and so on. Considered a very fragile period for a woman, this time is to be used to rest and to allow the body to empty itself before it is renewed. Even if your cycles no longer coincide with the moon's rhythms, you may observe these sadhanas in order to eventually restore your natural cycle.

During ovulation, Pitta is most dominant, while Vata dominates the period of menstruation and Kapha the period following menstruation.

A WOMAN'S SEASON / MONTHLY MENSTRUAL CYCLE

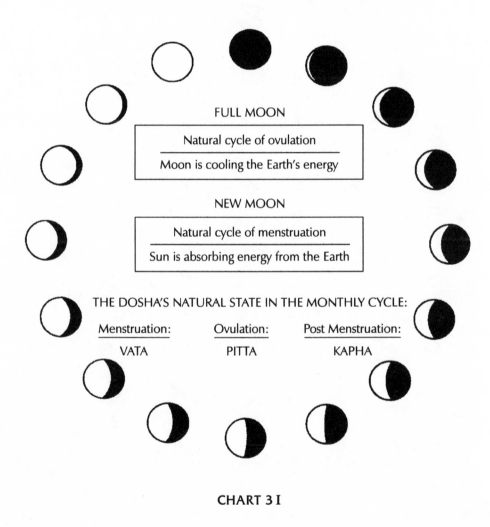

FULL MOON

| Natural cycle of ovulation |
| Moon is cooling the Earth's energy |

NEW MOON

| Natural cycle of menstruation |
| Sun is absorbing energy from the Earth |

THE DOSHA'S NATURAL STATE IN THE MONTHLY CYCLE:

| Menstruation: | Ovulation: | Post Menstruation: |
| VATA | PITTA | KAPHA |

CHART 3 I

Ayurvedic Rejuvenative Sadhanas

CHAPTER FOUR

AYURVEDIC MASSAGE THERAPY: ABHYANGA

Ayam me hasto Bhagavan
Ayam me bhagavattarah
Ayam me visvabheshajah
Ayam shivabhimarshanah

My hand is the Lord.
Boundlessly blissful is my hand.
This hand holds all healing secrets.
Which make whole with its gentle touch.

—*Rig Veda*

Abhyanga therapy is an ancient practice which predates the Vedic period. Early humans practiced life-sustaining ways of manipulating the body to produce strength, mobility, flexibility and fluent memory, memory which interlaced with the cosmos.

Vitally linked to the profound harmony of the earth, the ancients knew every movement in the cosmos to be filled with universal abhyanga. The leaves and bark of the trees are continually massaged by the wind; the rocks and pebbles are rubbed by the streams and rivers; the animals, brushed by space, wind and the forest, are forever toned by abhyanga.

91

PART ONE

The Marma Points: Charting the Course for Abhyanga

Ayurvedic massage is based on the knowledge of the marma points, the vital points of the body where structures pulsate and pain exists. Marmas, or reflex anatomical sites, are also called the junctions of prana by Sushruta. Knowledge of marma points was culled in ancient India from the Atharva Veda. During Vedic times, the knowledge of these vital points was widely used to fatally wound opponents in war, to save lives through surgery, to revitalize the body through abhyanga therapy, to strengthen the body through martial arts, and to stimulate, repair and heal these vital points through Ayurvedic acupuncture.

The body consists of thousands of marma points, with 365 essential points, 43 of which are the ones most commonly treated. Some points are more important than others, with 107 points being lethal if a blow to one of them is received.

Marma points are also defined as the junction where flesh, veins, arteries, tendons, bones and joints meet. These points are connected like a rosary by a common thread or subtle channel, nadi. Marmas are vitalized by the pranic energy carried to them via these subtle channels. Most nadis exist deep within the tissues of the body, occasionally traveling towards the body's surfaces.

Although the massage techniques given at the end of this chapter stimulate the main marmas and circulatory channels, only a cursory description and graphing of them are given. The directions given here are elementary, but are sufficient for the general application of massage and as a preliminary procedure before pancha karma.

In abhyanga therapy, a basic knowledge of marmas, nadis and the circulatory systems is important. Massage acts directly on blood, nerves, and lymph circulatory systems. The lymph system, operating through ducts, nodes and passages, does not have capillaries to carry its fluids independently as does the blood system. The lymph system's function is to supplement blood circulation. Further, the lymph system serves as a reservoir for muscles to float in. Its lymph nodes assist blood circulation by draining excess fluids from the blood stream, thus easing the labors of the heart. They also provide the body with its direct line of defense against disease. By stimulating the lymph nodes, massage therapy, especially when performed with warm oil or substances, serves to cleanse and revitalize the body.

There are three main types of massage techniques in abhyanga therapy:

active, passive and persuasive. In active massage, strong pressure is applied; in passive massage, delicate stroking is performed; in persuasive massage, the technique of pinching or kneading the small muscles between the thumb and forefinger is used. Generally, Vata and Pitta conditions are treated with a combination of active and passive massage, while Kapha conditions are treated with a combination of active and persuasive massage.

The head, face, neck, shoulders and upper chest are massaged first in abhyanga therapy; the general flow of massage then moves to the soles of the feet and continues upward towards the heart, unless a cold massage is being administered. In this event, the stroking begins on the head and continues steadily downward. Massaging the body from the soles of the feet upward activates the veins and carries the impure blood to the heart for purification. The revitalized blood is then distributed via the arteries throughout the body.

Generally, abhyanga is applied with warm substances. Occasionally, however, a cooling substance may be used for Pitta conditions. A panoply of massaging oils, aromatic oils, fragrant powders and bean and grain flour mixtures, called *ubtans*, are used to facilitate smoothness or light friction.

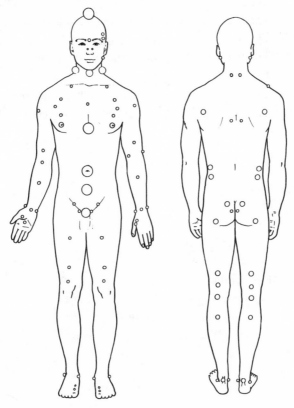

Figure 1: Main Marma Points on the Body

Forty-three Commonly Treated Marma Points

The marma points are named after their location or function in the body.

Arms and Legs:

Talahridaya	The center, or "heart," of the palm of the hand or the sole of the foot
Kshipram	Area between the thumb and forefinger on the hand or between the big toe and fore-toe on the bottom of the foot; "quickness"
Kurcha	The bundle of muscles or tendons at the base of the thumb or big toe
Kurchasira	The base of the hand or the foot; "head of kurcha"
Manibandhi	The four points around the wrist; "bracelet"
Gulpha	Ankle joint
Indravasti	Mid-forearm and mid-calf; "Indra's bladder"
Kurpara	Elbow joint
Janu	Knee joint
Ani	The lower region of the upper arm or leg
Urvi	The wide mid-region of the thigh or forearm; "wide"
Lohitaksha	The lower frontal insert of the shoulder joint and leg joint; "red eyed"
Kaksadhara	The top of the shoulder joint; "upholds the flanks"
Vitapa	The perineum, where the legs are connected to the trunk

Abdomen:

Guda	Anus
Vasti	Bladder
Nabhi	Navel

Thorax:

Hridaya	Heart
Stanamula	Root of the breast
Stanarohita	Incline (or upper region) of the breast
Apastambha	The upper side of the chest
Apalapa	Center of the upper chest; "unguarded"

Back:

Katikataruna	The center of the buttocks; "what arises from the sacrum"
Kukundara	On either side of the posterior superior iliac spine; "marking the loins"
Nitamba	The upper regions of the buttocks
Parsvasandhi	The sides of the waist; "joint of the sides"
Vrihati	The broad region of the back; "large"
Amsaphalaka	The shoulder blade
Amsa	The shoulder

Neck:

Manya	Perhaps owing to its connection with udana air which controls the voice; "honor"
Nila	From the color of the veins at the two points at the base of the neck; "dark blue"
Sira Matrika	From the arteries to the head that flow through this region; "mother of the blood vessels"
Krikatika	Two points at the back of the neck

Head:

Vidhuram	From the sensitive nature of the two points below the back of the ears; "alarm"
Phana	The side of the nostrils; "serpent's hood"
Apanga	The outer corner of the eye
Avarta	From the sensitive nature of the two points directly behind the ears; "calamity"
Sankha	The temple; "conch"
Utksepa	Above the temple; "upward"
Sthapani	Point between the eyebrows; "support"
Sringatakani	The soft palate of the mouth; "places where four roads meet"
Simanta	The skull and surrounding joints; "summit"
Adhipati	Point at the crown of head; "overlord"

PART TWO
Observances and Preparations for Abhyanga Therapy

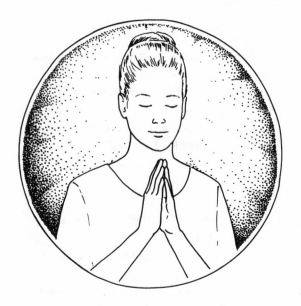

QUALITIES OF THE ABHYANGA CARE GIVER

Administer massage only while calm, clean and fresh, and free from disease. The abhyanga care giver must also be free of anger, fear and greed. Traditionally, the Ayurvedic massage therapist takes a bath and dons a fresh gown after every subject treated. At least, the hands and face are to be washed after each treatment. The hands must be warm, with the nails clipped, clean and unpolished.

As a general reminder, never administer massage during menses, or while the body is releasing toxins or discharges. (See Chapter Nine, Cleansing Ablutions for the Practitioner.)

Abhyanga Therapy Room

- Well ventilated, preferably with soft, natural light
- No harsh light (i.e., fluorescent or direct sunlight)
- No cold draft of air or wind
- Quiet with only the sounds of nature to be heard
- Dry and warm
- Natural hardwood floor, preferably
- Sparsely furnished with only abhyanga therapy necessities
- A traditional wooden massage table is preferable, approximately 6 feet long and 2 1/2 feet wide. The table may rest directly on the floor, or may be supported by legs.

Inappropriate Conditions for Care Giver and Subject During Abhyanga

- Menstrual cycles
- Bodily discharges
- Intestinal ulcers
- Fasting
- The first two hours after meals
- Full bladder
- Fear
- Loud noises/conversing with the subject during treatment

Abhyanga Procedures for Women

- During pregnancy, massage excludes the stomach and abdomen areas.
- The practitioner should be female, unless the massage is being administered by the subject's spouse.
- Only the sides of the breasts are massaged, slowly and gently.
- After delivery, a thorough massage with emphasis on the thighs, waist and abdomen is recommended. This refreshes the body, relieves pain, and renews the mother's strength. Post-partum massage also allows the waste remaining in the womb to be cleared out of the body. This massage should be performed by a midwife or a female Ayurvedic massage practitioner.

PART THREE

The Practice of Abhyanga Therapies

Benefits

Massage is the most ancient technique used for relieving pain. Still a valid and thriving art in most regions of India, and in particular Kerala, abhyanga is used to manipulate and correct dosha disorders, especially of the Vata kind; to cure orthopedic injuries; to relieve swollen tissues; and to promote regeneration of the tissues and organs, as well as the internal functioning of the body. Moreover, massage stimulates skin, muscles, veins, arteries, the circulatory systems and the nervous system. It improves the skin, strengthens the lungs, intestines and bones, and regulates the digestive system.

Massage increases bodily heat and the flow of life-supporting oxygen; it also improves circulation, causing the body to flush out its waste products more efficiently. Promoting vitality, strength, stamina and flexibility, abhyanga also improves concentration, intelligence, confidence, esteem and youthfulness.

Especially excellent for the aged and the infirm, massage therapy benefits everyone.

Necessary Aids

- Treatment gown*
- Loin cloth*
- A glass bottle containing two cups of massage oil
- A small stainless steel funnel with a 1/4 inch opening at the spout
- Two clean cotton hand towels
- A clean cotton sheet
- A comfortable upright chair for the subject to sit on during head massage

* *See Appendix D*

Abhyanga Therapy

Season: all year

Body Type: all types

Duration of Treatment

Vata: 45 minutes; early morning or early evening

Pitta: 45 minutes; early or mid-morning

Kapha: 60 minutes; early morning

Note: Subject's head should be pointing towards the east if massage is performed in the morning and towards the west if in the early evening. Full body massage treatment should not be administered after dark.

This therapy is to be administered as a preliminary measure before pancha karma or as a general body/mind rejuvenator throughout the year. As a preliminary measure before pancha karma, the massage may be shortened to forty minutes for all body types.

General Techniques

1. **Soothing rubbing movement:** Use soothing rubbing movements on the surfaces of the arms and legs.

    legs: from the sides of the feet to the groin

    arms: from the fingertips to the armpit

2. **Pinching technique:** Muscles are grasped between the forefinger and thumb, away from the bones. Apply pinching techniques only to the following areas: chest, arms, legs and back.

3. **Kneading technique:** Grasp the larger muscles with the hands and coax them into vitality. Kneading may be applied to the entire body.

4. **Pressing technique:** Press along the hard body surfaces with flat hands moving in a circular manner. Caress and compress the softer areas of the body, applying wave-like pressure while constantly moving upward.

5. **Small circular thumb movement:** Small, circular, clockwise and counter-clockwise massage movements are generally applied with the thumb to essential marma points of the body.

Order of Massage
1. Shirobhyanga
2. Padabhyanga
3. Abhyanga: Arm and Hand Massage
4. Abhyanga: Abdomen and Chest Massage
5. Abhyanga: Back Massage
6. Special Hip Massage
7. Special Belly Massage

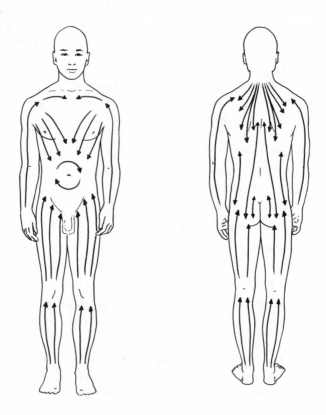

Figure 2: Directional Flow of Massage

SHIROBHYANGA: HEAD, NECK, AND SHOULDER MASSAGE
(while subject is in a sitting position)

Head Massage: First Phase

Directions
The head is the most important part of the body, carrying eight of the body's

ten sacred gates or apertures: the two openings of the nostrils, eyes, and ears, the mouth, and the most auspicious point, called *Brahma Randhra*, situated eight finger-widths from the center top of the eyebrows. The embryo receives its nutrition via the Brahma Randhra until it makes its journey from the womb. According to the Vedas, the soul departs the body from this point (also called *sushumna*, the seventh chakra) after death, and thus its name Brahma Randhra, the gate of Brahma, the creator. The remaining two gates of the body are the anus and genitalia. In abhyanga therapy, the massage always begins with the head.

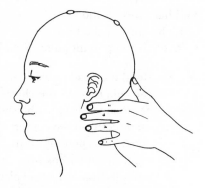

Figure 3: Three Points on Head

Benefits

Shirobhyanga increases the flow of cerebro-spinal fluid, thus strengthening the nervous system. This massage balances the pituitary and pineal glands. Eyes, lungs, heart, brain, colon, and stomach also become toned as a result. Shirobhyanga also helps to improve both experiential and cognitive memory, alertness and stability.

Ayurveda recommends that a small amount of sesame or coconut oil be placed on the summit, or soft spot, of the cranium for the first nine months of an infant's life. This measure serves to improve the child's memory, intelligence, energy and sight. A daily head massage also strengthens the nervous system and energy of the child. The same benefits may be observed by adults to varying degrees.

Oiling the Three Major Points of the Head: First Phase

Brahma Randhra: Soft spot of the head

Before commencing the massage, wash your hands thoroughly. Then, shake them and gently turn your wrists in a circular clockwise motion. Accelerate the rhythm of your hand movements until you feel a tingling sensation in your fingers. This activity allows your healing energy to flow freely.

Have the subject sit in an upright chair and take your position, standing behind the chair. Part the hair in the center and pour approximately two tablespoons of oil on the Brahma Randhra spot (Fig. 4).

- Begin by massaging the oil into both sides of the head, above the ears.
- Spread the oil over the front portion of the head, while firmly rubbing the head with both hands.

101

Shikha: Crest of the head

The crest of the head, or *shikha*, is the second most important point of the head.

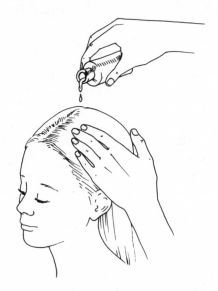

- Bend the head forward, so that the chin touches the chest. Pour approximately two tablespoons of oil directly on the center of the crest. This point is located about eight finger widths from the medulla oblongata, the place where the skull meets the neck.
- Spread the oil over the back of the head, while firmly rubbing the head with both hands.

Figure 4: Oiling the Head

Medulla oblongata: Base stem of the brain

At the center back of the head, where the skull meets the neck, is the third most important point of the head. Called the medulla oblongata, this point is pivotal to the way the brain communicates with the entire nervous system.

- Gently bend the subject's head completely forward and pour approximately one tablespoon of oil directly on the medulla oblongata point.
- Using both hands, rub the base of the skull and the back of the neck firmly to excite the fine capillaries of circulation and the nervous system.
- Finally, press both thumbs on each side of the medulla oblongata point, and hold for a minute or so.

Head Massage: Second Phase

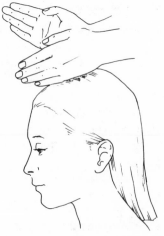

- Bring both hands together in a prayer pose. Place your clasped hands on the crest of the subject's head.
- Moving your hands in a scissor-like motion, begin to decisively pound the center line of the head, moving both hands forward while pounding the head, to the top of the forehead; then move the hands back again, remaining all the while on the center line of the head.

Figure 5: Scissor-like Motion

- As you pound towards the lower back of the head, have the subject bend his/her head forward and downward so that the chin touches the chest.
- After pounding the center line of the head, take a small amount of hair, rooted directly over the three auspicious points of the head (Brahma Randhra, shikha and medulla oblongata) and twist it (Fig. 6).
- Gently pull each one of the hair twists beginning with the Brahma Randhra point and ending with the medulla oblongata point.

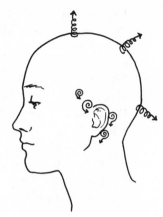

Figure 6: Twisting the Hair; Massage Points Around Ears

Head, Neck, Face and Shoulder Massage: Final Phase

- Pour approximately one tablespoon of oil into your hands and begin rubbing the neck. Use both thumbs and apply pressure along the center back line of the neck, while your fingers apply gentle pressure to the front of the neck.
- Make a fist with both hands and use the thumbs to apply gentle pressure in a subtle counter clockwise circular movement over and around the ears, with emphasis on two points behind the ears, one directly above the ear and the other behind the lobe (Fig. 6).
- Using both hands, gently stimulate the temple on both sides of the head, by subtly moving your fingers in a circular counter clockwise manner.
- Pour another tablespoon of oil into your hands and apply it to the shoulders. Massage the shoulders with broad strokes, using both hands, beginning from the center of the back and massaging your way outward toward the arms.
- Press firmly downward from the neck toward the upper back.
- While continuing to stand behind the subject, rub the subject's shoulder blades with both hands.
- By using firm downward pressure, continue to massage the upper chest.
- Guide the subject to the massage table and ask him/her to disrobe and put on the loin cloth. Cover the subject with a clean sheet and invite him/her to rest for a few minutes while you wash your hands and prepare for the full body massage.
- When you return, ask the subject to close his/her eyes and guide the subject into total relaxation.

- Pour approximately one tablespoon of oil into your hands and rub the face, beginning with the forehead and continuing to the cheeks. Use your thumbs to massage the sides of the nose, around the mouth and chin.
- Place a few drops of oil into the nostrils and quickly rub the inside of the nostrils with your index finger.
- With ease and delicacy use your thumbs to rub over the closed eyes.
- Finish the face massage by dripping two tablespoons of oil through a small funnel directly onto the third eye, the *sthapani* marma point.
- While dripping the oil, gently rock the funnel by moving it one inch from side to side over the third eye.
- Pat the excess oil from the face with a towel.

Note: Shirobhyanga may also be applied as an independent massage when *mardana,* or light pressure massage of the head, is required.

PADABHYANGA: FOOT AND LEG MASSAGE

Benefits

Padabhyanga, foot and leg massage, stimulates all the organs of the body and increases ojas and a state of deep relaxation, inducing a sense of total wellness in the entire system. Massaging the feet, one of our five organs of action, relieves insomnia, nervousness, and dryness or numbness of the feet. Massaging the legs energizes the belly, pelvis, and colon, improves circulation and fertility, and cures numbness.

Foot and Lower Leg Massage: First Phase
- Remove the covering sheet from the legs.
- Firmly shake one leg at a time by placing both hands on the back of the foot and lifting the leg slightly.
- Apply two tablespoons of oil to the sides of the right foot and rub thoroughly, massaging in a clockwise circular movement.

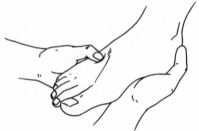

Figure 7: Foot Massage

- Place the subject's heel in your right palm and press firmly into the ankle joint with your thumb and fingers (Fig. 7).
- Using your left hand, press the tips of the toes and then pull each toe firmly. Apply oil to the toenails and rub them once more.
- Use both hands to massage the "neck" of each toe (Fig. 8).

104

- Beginning eight inches above the ankles, firmly massage the leg with both hands, gradually making your way down to the feet.
- Massage the top and bottom of the foot at the same time by holding the foot underneath with your fingers and using both thumbs to press the top of the foot.
- Repeat the same procedure on the left side, but using a counter clockwise motion, where indicated.

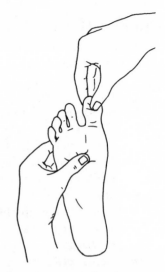

Figure 8: Massaging the Toes

Lower Leg Massage: Second Phase

- Prop the right leg up, so that the knee is bent and the sole of the right foot rests on the massage table.
- Pour two tablespoons of oil on the right leg and begin massaging from the knee downward.
- Firmly knead the muscles of the calf.
- Place your thumbs on the lower part of the knee cap and press firmly into the tendons.
- Make small circular movements with the thumb (clockwise motions on the outer leg points and counter clockwise motions on the inner leg points) on the ten essential lower leg points which follow: two points on either side of lower knee cap; two points on either side behind the knee; two points on either side of the mid-calf; two points on either side immediately below the calf; and finally, two points on either side of the leg, behind the ankle bone (Fig. 9).
- Massage the lower leg with both hands from the knee downward, ending at the ankle. Gently shake and rotate the ankle until it feels loose.
- Straighten the leg and repeat the same procedure on the left leg.

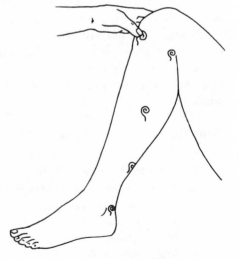

Figure 9: Lower Leg Massage

Upper Leg Massage: Third Phase

- Pour two tablespoons of oil on the upper part of the right leg.
- Using both hands, begin massaging from the top of the leg, kneading the thigh firmly (Fig. 10).
- Massage slowly downwards until you reach the knee.
- Prop the leg up slightly and continue kneading the back of the thigh.
- Gently place the leg back down and perform long rubbing strokes from the top of the leg down to the knee.
- Repeat the same procedure on the left leg.

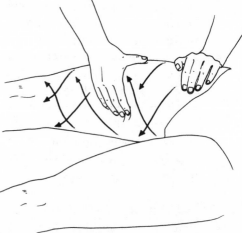

Figure 10: Upper Leg Massage

ABHYANGA: ARM AND HAND MASSAGE

Benefits

Our hands, also one of our five organs of action, energetically speaking, hold the five elements on the tips of our fingers. The earth is held in the little finger, water in the ring finger, fire in the middle finger, air in the index finger, and space is held in the thumb. Our hands are vital extensions that enable us to touch nature and refine her within ourselves.

For both the practitioner and subject, hand massage stimulates our deep cognitive memories while energizing the tissues and organs of the body. Massaging both the hands and the arms increases flexibility and refreshes the energy of the whole body.

Arm Massage: First Phase

- Pour two tablespoons of oil on the right arm and rub it in gently.
- Lift the arm and gently shake it, allowing the tension to leave.
- Starting from the shoulder, begin to massage the arm, kneading it firmly, moving downward.
- Bend the arm to flex the elbow joint. Press the nodes in the hollow of the elbow.
- Place your hands on the back of the arm and, using your thumbs, press the inner arm all the way down to the wrist.

- With small circular motions, use the thumb to massage the two essential inner and two essential outer points of the arm, clockwise on the outer arm points and counter clockwise on the inner arm points.
- Finally, place a small amount of oil in each armpit. Using your fingers, gently press into the armpit and hold for a minute or so until you feel the pulsation.

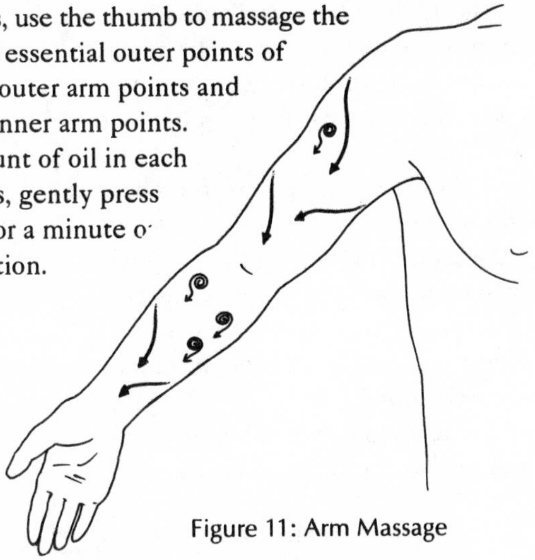

Hand Massage: Second Phase

- Rub the right hand with a small amount of oil.
- Massage the palms of the hand by pressing with your thumbs.

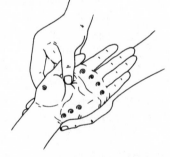

Figure 11: Arm Massage

- Use small circular clockwise movements with your thumb to stimulate the mound in the palm below each finger.
- Rub each fingernail with oil and massage each finger by gently pulling on it.
- Press each finger firmly and rotate.
- Bend the fingers backward, then forward, by extending and flexing the wrist.
- Firmly shake and rotate the wrist until it is loose and has released its tension.
- Use your thumbs and press the back of the hand, following through to the nail of each finger.
- Repeat the same procedure with the left hand, using counter clockwise motions on the mounds in the palms as indicated.

Figure 12: Palm Massage

ABHYANGA: ABDOMEN AND CHEST MASSAGE

Benefits

The navel is considered the epicenter of the body, connecting all 72,000 of its nerves. It also contains the memory of our first feeding in this life, since our first vital sustenance flowed through it from our mother.

Center of belly and body, the navel is a phenomenal base of energy. Abdominal massage helps to move stagnant energy and revitalize this basic life source.

Physically, the abdominal massage relieves constipation, tones the stomach muscles, uproots toxins from the body and induces deep feelings of wellbeing.

Abhyanga massage to the chest stimulates the heart, increases circulation, stimulates the capillaries of the blood vascular system, tones the liver and spleen, increases prana, stimulates the lungs, and dislodges mucus accumulation.

The abdomen is massaged gently; no pressure is applied to this area.

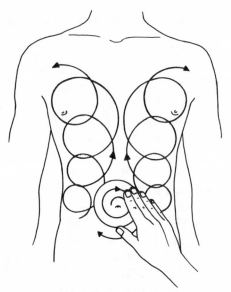

Figure 13: Chest Massage

- Pour a teaspoon of oil into the navel. Using your right hand, gently rub the area around the navel, using a clockwise motion. Begin with small movements, gradually enlarging the circles as you rub away from the navel.
- Pour two tablespoons of oil over the heart and rub evenly over the chest area.
- Place both hands over the chest and massage gently, using outward, circular strokes.
- When massaging a woman, apply no pressure on the breasts. Delicately rub around the breasts with light circular movements.
- Gently pull on the nipples of both males and females.
- Massage the rib cage with firm pressure.

ABHYANGA: BACK MASSAGE

- Have the subject lie on the stomach, placing the arms above or underneath the head.
- Pour four tablespoons of oil along the spine, starting from the base of the spine and pouring upward to the base of the neck.
- Place both hands on either side of the base of the spine and use your thumbs simultaneously to massage in small semicircular movements, with the left thumb going in a counter clockwise direction and the right thumb going in a clockwise direction.
- Gradually move upward while maintaining your semicircular thumb massage, until you have reached the base of the neck.

- Position your hands once more on either side of the base of the spine, your thumbs beside the vertebral column.
- Firmly massage the back with your fingers, moving upwards to the base of the neck.
- Knead the muscles on both sides of the spinal column, using both hands simultaneously.
- You may also quickly pinch the skin all over the back.
- Finally, rub the sides of the buttocks firmly.
- Cover the subject and let rest for fifteen minutes.

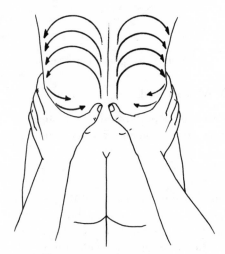

Figure 14: Back Massage

SPECIAL HIP MASSAGE

Apart from toning the muscles, massaging the hips helps improve digestive fire and the peristalsis movement of the large intestines; it also helps to tone the liver and spleen.

Directions
- Have the subject lie on the left side.
- Pour one tablespoon of oil on the right hip.
- Grip the hip firmly with both hands, your thumbs on the back of the hip and your fingers at the front (Fig. 15).
- Massage both the waist and hip areas firmly and steadily for five minutes, maintaining a general circular motion with your hands.
- Repeat the same procedure on the left hip.

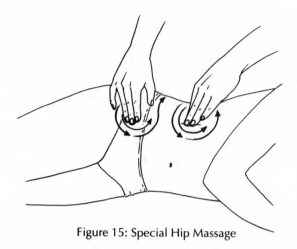

Figure 15: Special Hip Massage

SPECIAL BELLY MASSAGE

A special belly massage is performed in abhyanga therapy to tone the stomach, improve digestion, circulation and fertility, and, most significantly, to relieve constipation.

Caution

- Make certain that the subject is neither pregnant nor has an abdominal inflammatory condition such as ulcers.
- The subject should not eat for three hours before treatment.
- The subject should relieve the bladder immediately before receiving the massage.
- Discontinue the massage if the subject complains of pain in the belly.

Directions

- Have the subject lie on the back with the knees propped up, the soles of the feet resting flatly on the massage table.
- Have the subject inhale through the nostrils deeply into the abdomen and release the breath through the mouth for a few minutes.
- Rub the subject's shoulders firmly, until you feel the tension leaving the body.
- When the abdomen is completely relaxed, you may start the massage.
- Sitting on the subject's right side, pour one teaspoon of oil in the navel. Gently place both hands over the belly, covering the navel for a minute or so, in complete silence.

- Using your right fingers, gently begin to stroke the belly with a rhythmic succession of short strokes.
- Begin at the navel and move in a circular clockwise manner, creating an outward spiral until the entire belly has been stroked (Fig. 16). Maintain a delicate but firm stroking throughout the massage.
- Use the palm of your hand to continue rubbing the belly in a circular clockwise motion.
- Beginning at the lower left side of the belly, use both hands and begin to knead the muscles gently, while gradually increasing your pressure. Move upward steadily, but apply downward pressure to this area of the belly.
- Repeat the same procedure on the top of the belly and then move on to the right side of the belly, ending at the bottom.
- End the massage by pouring another teaspoon of oil into the navel. Put the middle finger of your right hand into the oiled navel and feel the pulsation of the belly for a minute or so.
- Rest both your hands over the belly for a moment. Then cover the subject with a clean sheet and let rest for ten minutes.

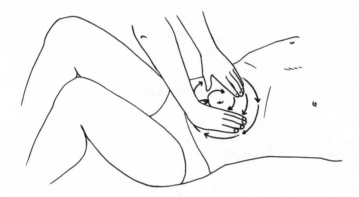

Figure 16: Special Belly Massage

Post-massage observations

- If oils were used during massage therapy, dust the body with freshly ground urad or chickpea bean powder or sandalwood powder (see formulas at the end of this chapter). Then, lightly rub the body with a towel, using downward strokes, to remove the oils and powder.
- Have the subject rest for fifteen minutes and then take a cool bath. Vata types may take a lukewarm bath.

PART FOUR
Self Application of Foot Massage

A daily foot massage, padabhyanga, is a simple and most revitalizing sadhana for maintaining good health. Padabhyanga has been practiced for millennia as a prerequisite to sound sleep, to infuse the day's activity with equanimity, and, as a more exotic activity, in the royal courts of India and China, as a prelude to sexual activities. According to Ayurveda, many marma points for the body's vital organs and sense organs are located in the soles of the feet. Padabhyanga not only invigorates and renews the entire body, but also encourages its natural "valium" to flow. A peaceful night's rest or a calm day's activity is assured after the feet are thoroughly massaged.

During the course of a day, the feet literally carry tons of the body's dynamic weight. A foot massage at the beginning or end of each day is a wonderful way to show appreciation for this valiant organ of action.

PADABHYANGA: FOOT MASSAGE

 Note: This symbol indicates therapies which may be performed at home.

Season: all year

Body Type: all types

Time of Application: early morning or before bed

Conditions

Rough or dry skin; dullness of sense organs; fatigue; insomnia; poor vision; nervous tension; lethargy

Self Massage

- Wash your hands, face, and feet and put on a fresh robe. Pour 1/4 cup of the appropriate oil into a small bowl and place it next to you.
- Sit in a comfortable posture, either on a clean mat on the floor or in an upright chair.

- Close your eyes and sit in contemplative silence for a few minutes before beginning your massage.
- After contemplation, gently lift the right leg, rest the right ankle on the knee of the left leg, and pour a small amount of oil on the right foot.

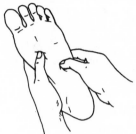

- Using both hands, clasp the foot, the thumbs resting on the bottom of the foot and the fingers resting on the top.
- Crimp the fingers and press firmly into the center top line of the foot, beginning at the ankle and moving along the foot to the middle toe. At the same time, press

Figure 17: Padabhyanga

the thumbs into the bottom of the foot, beginning at the heel and moving along the inner and outer edges of the bottom of the foot. Synchronize both hands so that they move at the same pace, the top and bottom of the foot being massaged simultaneously.
- Continue this procedure for five minutes, always starting from the heel and working the fingers and thumbs towards the toes, repeating the process until the entire outer surface of the foot has been thoroughly massaged.
- Release the foot and move to the toes. Beginning with the big toe, press on both sides of the nail, using the thumb and index finger of your left hand. Gently pull the toe and then firmly massage the under side, starting from the root. Rubbing this point stimulates the brain and helps the sight.

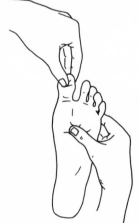

- After a time, proceed to the index toe and repeat the same procedure. This toe releases energy to the lungs.
- Continue in this way, toe by toe. The meridian for the large intestine flows through the middle toe; massaging it helps to tone the colon. The fourth toe is the location of the kidney meridian; massaging it helps to

Figure 18: Toe Massage

increase the flow of vital energy to the kidneys. The little toe houses the heart meridian; massaging this toe stimulates the heart and enables its beat to remain slow and rhythmic.

- The entire massage may be repeated once more. Before changing feet, press your thumb firmly into the four marma points indicated on the bottom of the foot (Fig. 19).
- Reverse the position of the legs and repeat the entire procedure on the left foot.

After massaging both feet, gently rub off any remaining oil with a dry towel. Wash your hands and observe a brief meditation. Prepare to greet the day with joy or succumb to a peaceful night's rest.

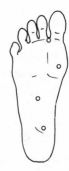

Figure 19: Marma Points of the Foot

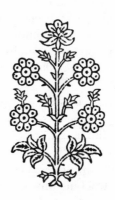

PART FIVE
Abhyanga Formulas

ABHYANGA OIL PREPARATIONS

Oils are used in both abhyanga massage and snehana therapies to soothe and stabilize the body; they also act as a carrier for the nourishing herbs and substances added to the oils. Oils regulate the doshas of the female genital organs and provide the body with heat. They tone the skin and bodily tissues. Oils usually alleviate Vata disorders, stabilize Pitta disorders and aggravate Kapha.

A wide variety of Ayurvedic oils is used for massaging each part of the human body. Sesame oil is used as the dominant base for most rubbing oils due to its warm, nutritive and penetrating qualities. See Appendix A for extensive lists of massage oils.

Formulas for Ayurvedic Herbal Oils

Herbal Oil Decoction

4 c water
1 c oil
1/4 c herb

Bring water to boil in a stainless steel pot. Add oil and herbs, cover and simmer on low heat for 4 to 6 hours, or until all the water has evaporated. Allow herbal oil to cool, then pour oil through a tea strainer into a glass jar. Cover and store in a cool place.

Herbal Oil Infusion

1 c oil
1/4 c herb

Bring oil to boil in a stainless pot. Add herbs and remove from heat. Cover and let steep for 10 hours. Pour oil through a tea strainer into a clean glass jar. Cover and store in a cool place.

Fresh Herbal Oil Sun Decoction

1/4 c fresh herbs

1 c oil

Lightly mince the fresh herbs and place them in a clean glass container with the oil. Cover with a piece of cotton gauze and secure with a rubber band. Allow the jar to sit in the sunlight between the hours of 10:00 a.m. and 3:00 p.m. for 25 days. Be careful not to expose the jar to extreme cold, rain or moonlight. At the end of the infusion period, strain into a clean glass jar. Cover securely with a proper lid and store in a cool place.

Combining Oils

Generally, Ayurveda does not combine the base oils. Instead, oils are either added to herbs and other substances or are used singularly. Essential oils are added in minute quantity to primary rubbing oils for accent. When adding essential oil to a base oil, use ten drops of essential oil to one fluid ounce of base oil.

Combining Oils with Juices and Gels

The blending of oils, herbs and aromas is a fine art intrinsic to the Ayurvedic rejuvenative practices. For example, the fresh juices of herbal roots, such as ginger and garlic, or the fresh herbal juice extracted from mint and cilantro, may be combined with warm or cool oil. The proportion is usually one part juice to two parts oil. When a gel, such as aloe vera, or gum resins, such as asafoetida or pine gum, are added to oil, the procedure is slightly different. For a gel substance, the ratio is one part gel to three parts warm or cool oil. A hard gum resin is grated to a powder, added to the warm oil, and let sit for a few hours before using. When the gum resin is soft, it is added to the oil and the mixture is simmered over low heat for 15 minutes. Generally, ten pinches of gum powder or ten drops of soft gum resin are added to one fluid ounce of base oil.

When fresh juices or gels are combined with oils, the preparation should be made fresh before each application to avoid spoilage.

Warming Massage Oils

Generally, Ayurveda recommends warming the oils used for abhyanga. In certain instances when Pitta conditions are being treated, the oils may be used at room temperature. It is best to warm the oils in a double boiler, unless the oils are diluted with water. Never use electrical stoves or electrical heating devices to warm massage oils. Electrical energy disrupts the energy quanta of the oils, which in turn send chaotic vibrations through the skin when the oils are applied. Gas stoves, or other heating devices which produce an open flame, are best for heating the oils and substances used in abhyanga.

Massage Oil Containers

In ancient times, various metal, glass, ceramic and earthenware were used as conductors of energy for massage oils. The materials used to make the containers influenced the energy of the various oils they contained. For instance, gold, bronze, or brass containers were used to carry the oils used for Vata and Kapha disorders, while silver, pewter, or platinum containers were used to hold the oils used for Pitta conditions. Generally, earthenware and ceramic containers were used to maintain warmth and impart humility to the oil, which in turn transferred that vibration to the patient to whom the oil was applied. Glass containers of various colors were also used to contain the oils, since each color carries its own unique healing vibration. Moreover, the transparency of a glass container allowed the oil it contained to be influenced by the energies of the sun or the moon, when the numinous vibrations of solar or lunar energies were necessary to the healing of the person for whom the oil was intended.

Likewise, appropriate gems were placed in oils intended for massage, and special mantras were recited, in order to produce the desired results after the oils were administered.

You, too, may continue the use of these ancient and luminous procedures as you practice these timeless sadhanas of healing.

Abhyanga Oil Formulas

Base oils

The following base oils or lubricants may be used alone or as a base for the appropriate herbs or essential oils best suited for each type.

Vata: dark or light sesame, ghee, jojoba, avocado, walnut, almond

Pitta: light sesame, coconut, sunflower, canola, ghee

Kapha: light sesame, canola, corn, walnut, almond

Essential oils

The following are a few examples of the essential oils which may be added to the appropriate base oils for each type. Use ten drops of essential oil to one fluid ounce of base oil. Add the essential oil after the base oil is removed from heat, if the base oil is to be heated.

Vata: jasmine, rose, sandalwood, cardamom, yellow champa, nutmeg, cinnamon, lavender, frankincense, saffron, lilac, vetiver

Pitta: sandalwood, jasmine, fennel, coriander, lavender, peppermint, lemon, lime, saffron, orange, lilac, rose

Kapha: sage, myrrh, patchouli, allspice, eucalyptus,
cardamom, cinnamon, yellow champa,
lemon, lime, neroli, geranium

Herbs used in oil infusion and decoctions

The following are a few examples of the herbs which may be used in oil
infusion or decoction for abhyanga.

Vata: ashwagandha, bala, bhringaraja, gotu kola, licorice,
cloves, comfrey, calamus root, ginger, ginseng

Pitta: neem, mahabala, amalaki, gotu kola, gokshura,
shatavari, bhringaraja, peppermint, fennel, licorice

Kapha: bhringaraja, gotu kola, bibhitaki, haritaki, gokshura,
neem, wild ginger, rosemary, sage, horseradish

Ubtans

Fresh ground flours, *ubtans*, from a myriad of beans, and occasionally grains,
have been used even before Vedic times to enliven the skin tissue, stimulate the
body and make it glow. Ubtan is an inexpensive and irreplaceable final measure
to abhyanga or preliminary process before baths.

Ancient cultures used the earth's sacred grains and legumes not only to cleanse
the body, enhance its physical prowess and nourish it, but also to clean the dishes
and living space as well. Inherently astringent in nature, the ground legumes
combined with certain antiseptic herbal powders become a powerful all-round
cleanser.

Application of Ubtans

To remove excess oils from the body after massage therapy, and preserve
moisture in the skin, apply an ample amount of finely ground powder on the body
with long upward strokes.

Remove the powders by using firm downward strokes until the body is cleared
of both excess oil and powder. A lukewarm bath may be taken afterwards.

Ubtan Preparations
Season: all year
Body Type: all types

> 8 parts legume flour
> 1 part oil
> 1/16 part herbal powder

Note: Occasionally, grain flour may be used instead of legume flour (see legume and grain grinding directions below).

Note: See "Base oils" for each type in abhyanga formulas above.

Legume Flours

Vata:	chickpea, mung, urad, brown lentil, brown rice, wheat and oat
Pitta:	chickpea, aduki, soya, urad, barley, wheat and millet
Kapha:	aduki, chickpea, mung, red lentil, corn, millet and barley

Herbal Powders

Vata:	ashwagandha, bhringaraja, bala, haritaki, vidari, ginseng, jasmine, rose, ginger, walnut, rose hips, sandalwood, star anise, licorice, cloves, cinnamon, cardamom
Pitta:	bhringaraja, shatavari, musta, neem, gokshura, turmeric, raspberry, red clover, rose, jasmine, white oak, wintergreen, strawberry leaves, lemon grass, hibiscus, coriander, fennel
Kapha:	bhringaraja, neem, musta, ajwan, ashwagandha, bibhitaki, turmeric, strawberry leaves, sage, rosemary, peppermint, wild ginger, lemon balm, cloves, cinnamon, cardamom, birch

Grinding Legumes/Grains

Use a hand food grinder to grind enough legumes or grains for a fortnight's use. (See grain grinding technique in Appendix E.) The beans or grains may be ground to a fine flour for dusting excess oils from the body or to a coarse grainy texture for bodily cleansing needs. These flours, coarsely ground, may be used for cleansing the face as well.

PART SIX

Preliminary Fomentation Treatment

Fomentation therapy, also called *svedana*, is performed to aggravate the fat tissue, thereby forcing excess sweat out of the body. Used as a preliminary treatment before pancha karma, fomentation helps to liquify and uproot the aggrieved doshas, rendering them ready for expulsion from the body. The primary therapies in pancha karma, namely emesis, purgation and/or enema treatments, complete the process of ejecting the fluid and uprooted excess doshas from the system.

Fomentation treatment also helps to relieve bodily stiffness, heaviness and coldness. Although sweat therapy is used to evacuate the excesses of all three doshas, it is generally used to relieve Vata and Kapha disorders. Because of the production of sweat, the channels of the body are cleansed, thereby regulating Vata. Vata is further assuaged by the soothing action on the joints caused by the heat during fomentation.

Due to the regulated production of sweat in the body during fomentation, Kapha is also relieved in that it is reduced, along with conditions such as excess weight, lethargy, loss of appetite and low digestive fires.

Because of Pitta's natural bodily heat, only mild forms of fomentation treatments are recommended. (See Chapter Six for the various forms of svedana therapies.)

For preliminary fomentation treatment before pancha karma, a steam room, heated by hot rocks or bricks sprinkled occasionally with water to facilitate steam, is preferred. An enclosed steam room or wooden box, traditionally called baspa sveda, heated by a gas generator, will also suffice. Avoid electrically charged steam rooms or boxes. If a steam room or box is not available to you, the simple sudation applications which follow may be used.

FOMENTATION TREATMENT

Time of Application
> Vata and Kapha: 30 minutes
> Pitta: 15 minutes

Note:

1. Fomentation therapy is to be applied after abhyanga therapy and before pancha karma.

2. The conditions and restrictions set out in Chapter Six are to be adhered to here as well.

Ginger Compress

Ginger compress may be applied to the body and limbs, but not to the head. Use two extra-large, heavy stainless steel pots filled with ginger water. One pot of ginger decoction is kept simmering over low heat while the other pot of decoction is in use. Follow directions for Ginger Compress given below, adjusting the amounts to 4 gallons of water and 2 cups grated ginger, and applying a towel compress to the whole body.

Note: See list of Ayurvedic herbs used in svedana and common sweat-producing herbs in Appendix A. These may be used in the decoction in combinations of three to seven different herbs, depending on the intensity of heat required for fomentation.

Ginger Compress - Treatment for Kidneys
1 gal water
1 handful of grated fresh ginger

Bring water to boil in a large stainless steel pot. Place the grated ginger in a small, clean cotton pouch, secured by a draw string. Using your stronger hand, firmly squeeze the pouch so that the ginger juice seeps through the bag and into the boiling water. Then drop the ginger pouch into the pot of boiling water. Cover and let simmer on low heat for thirty minutes. Donning protective mitts, remove the pot from heat and carefully carry it to the treatment room; let sit for five minutes before uncovering.

Directions

Hold the ends of a towel with both hands, and dip the slack of the towel into the pot with the hot ginger water, without letting the water touch the ends you are holding. Twist the towel to relieve any excess water into the pot. Cover the pot to retain the heat of the water. Firmly shake the towel loose to release some heat. First test the temperature of the towel by gently placing it on the subject's back for a brief moment. Check with the subject to make certain the heat is bearable before applying the compress.

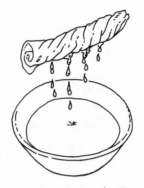

Figure 20: Wringing the Towel

Fold the towel and apply directly over the kidney area on the lower back. Use your hands and apply firm pressure over the towel. When the temperature of the towel turns lukewarm, remove it and repeat the dipping and wringing procedures in the hot water.

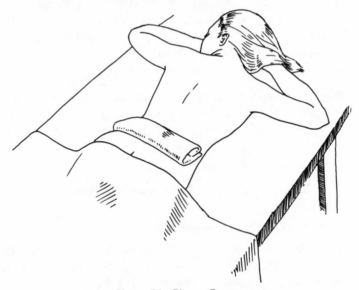

Figure 21: Ginger Compress

Repeat application of the hot towel on the subject's back approximately five times or until ginger water loses its heat.

Pre- and Post-procedures

Rub an ample amount of warm sesame oil on the back of the subject directly before treatment and directly after treatment.

Nadi Sveda for the Whole Body

Nadi sveda may be used to foment the entire body, instead of just a localized part, as explained in Chapter Six, Part Three.

Alter the treatment to accommodate the whole body, excluding the head, observing all of the rules which apply to nadi sveda.

CHAPTER FIVE
AYURVEDIC LOVE THERAPY: SNEHANA

The entire body is made up of unctuous
substances and all of life depends upon them.
—*Sushruta*

The meaning of the Sanskrit word *sneha* conveys stupendous love and immense tenderness, the essential spirit imbued in human nature. Snehana therapy is meant to invoke these deeply imbedded codes of our nature and re-awaken our cognitive memories.

The main emphasis of this therapy is on oelating, anointing, lubricating, and caressing both the internal and external body. The outpouring of caring energy from the practitioner into the person, along with the inpouring of oily substances, aids the body/mind/spirit to bend, stretch, and remember its cognitive nature. The most loving of sadhanas, external snehana is a holy alliance of nine intrinsic qualities carried by Ayurvedic herbs and substances deeply into the tissues through the skin. These nine qualities are wetness, strength, invigoration, tenderness, mending, fluidity, accommodation, restfulness, and cognition. Together they form a symphony of synergy to force the negative elements from the body and lubricate the passages of memory. Snehana re-opens the channels through which information and energy flow. As a result, we are able to freely access ahamkara, and sustain a fine balance between our experiential activities and cognitive memories. Without snehana, life can be truly loveless and cold.

In Ayurveda, snehana therapy may be used for both internal and external lubrication. Snehana is administered externally as the first preparatory therapy before pancha karma treatments begin. It may also be used as an independent therapy to alleviate Vata, Pitta, and Kapha disorders. Both internal and external snehana treatments are used effectively to cure Vata disorders.

External snehana is applied in twelve main ways. Many snehana therapies involve both massage and oelation. Anointing the entire body with oils or ghee, *abhyanga*, is also used as an independent treatment and is an extensive art of massage in itself, as discussed in Chapter Four.

A special therapeutic form of oil massage for nervous disorders as well as a dry form of massage for Kapha disorders such as rheumatoid arthritis, is called *udvartana*. In this massage, firm pressure is applied with a consistent flow of upward strokes. This therapy is also used for dissolving excess fat. Generally, udvartana is only performed with the supervision of an Ayurvedic physician. Due to its complexities, this therapy is not discussed in this book.

The process of plastering the body with medicated substances is called *lepa*. There are various forms of lepa therapy which are used extensively in both snehana and svedana therapies. The technique of shampooing the body, placing emphasis on the back, with oils and water is called *samvahana*. This process is used to rejuvenate the skin, muscle, and blood. It is a refreshing, yet soporific treatment for all body types. *Parisheka*, considered both a snehana and svedana process, involves the use of a complex formula containing several Ayurvedic herbs prepared in an affusion and used to massage the entire body. Parisheka treatment, described in detail in the svedana section, closely resembles the samvahana treatment and may be used to yield the same results.

As discussed in the preceding chapter, the anointing of oil on the feet is a traditional form of massage which has been practiced for more than five thousand years. This massage is called *padaghata* or *padabhyanga*. The anointing of the head shares equal importance with the massaging of the feet. There are many forms of head massage in Ayurveda, the most prominent being *shiro tarpana*, the application of oil to the head; *shirobhyanga*, the anointing of the head with oil; *shirovasti*, an elaborate procedure that applies oil to the shaven head; and *shirodhara*, the process of dripping a medicated decoction onto the forehead for a certain length of time. Padabhyanga and shirobhyanga massages are also described in greater detail in the abhyanga section.

Ayurveda employs a most wholesome therapy for maintaining excellence in the oral cavity. The procedure called *kavalagraha* is performed by maintaining a liquid decoction in the mouth for a short period of time. This therapy refreshes the sense organs, especially the senses of taste, smell, and sight. A similar decoction is used to massage the ears by dripping fluid into the ear channels; this process is called *karna purana*. Herbal decoctions are also used to revive the eyes, the washes known by *akshitarpana*.

126

One remaining procedure in the external snehana group of therapies is called *pichu*, the process whereby a piece of cloth is soaked in medicated oil and kept on the forehead.

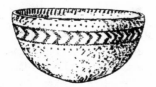

PART ONE
Observances Before Snehana Therapy

Like all Ayurvedic rejuvenative practices, snehana therapy is used only during the appropriate seasons and for certain specific conditions. The therapy should always be performed in a clean, warm, light, well ventilated room, free from dust and humidity. When thus applied, the benefits are enormous. Snehana improves the digestive fire, removes excess fat, warms the body, embraces the mind, induces sleep, adds smoothness to the skin and flexibility to the limbs. It promotes timely evacuation of bodily wastes, and brings clarity and brilliance to the mind and senses.

A healing diet of light, warm rice gruel and mild bean soups is usually taken during the course of snehana treatments and for the same period of time following treatment. To assuage any fears or anxieties the patient may have prior to treatment, a linctus prepared with brown sugar, Sucanat, jaggery or honey, is given, along with a light breakfast.

Three additional pre-snehana steps involving the head are also observed. These measures are taken to clear any obstructions remaining within the channels, as well as to quiet the stomach. A mild laxative such as castor root tea along with ginger tea is served. Gargling with triphala decoction follows. Finally, a mild nasya treatment with diluted ginger juice is administered.

Conditions for which Snehana Therapy is Appropriate
- As a preliminary treatment before pancha karma therapy
- As an independent rejuvenative therapy for all types
- For Vata disorders, such as dryness of skin, nervousness, loss of memory, insomnia, and mental stress
- For the weak, exhausted, anemic, and impotent
- For the aged and children
- For alcohol and drug addictions
- For conjunctivitis and cataracts
- After strenuous physical activities and long journeys
- As a seasonal rejuvenating routine

When seasonal and other required conditions are not adhered to, snehana may cause adverse conditions such as headaches, fainting, tiredness, body stiffness, confusion, burning sensations, constipation, weak digestion, indigestion, jaundice, and nausea.

Cleansing ablutions are to be observed by both the practitioner and the patient prior to beginning therapy (see Chapter Nine). A schedule of calming diet and activities is maintained during snehana therapy and for a period of time thereafter. Details on the healing diet and activities are presented in Chapters Eight and Nine.

Preliminary oil massage and fomentation treatments are to be administered on the subject prior to the following snehana therapies (see Chapter Four). The appropriate massaging oils for each body type are also mentioned in Chapter Four.

Inappropriate Conditions for Snehana Therapy

- Obesity and high Kapha disorders, unless a snehana therapy such as *udvartana* is prescribed and supervised by an Ayurvedic physician
- If there is impairment of digestive fire, weak or excessive indigestion, abdominal and metabolic disorders
- During nauseous or anorexic conditions
- Directly after pancha karma therapy—emesis, purgation, enema, and nasal insufflation
- During pregnancy or directly after delivery
- While intoxicated
- If there is poison in the body
- If there is aversion to foods and unctuous substances
- During menstruation period
- If there is extensive weakness and emaciation of the body
- During feverish conditions

Seasonal Snehana Guidelines for Each Dosha

Pitta disorders:	autumn:	mid-morning
	early evening:	summer
Vata disorders :	autumn:	mid-morning
	summer:	early evening
	early rainy season: (July 15 to August 15)	early evening
	late spring: (April 15 to May 15)	mid-morning or early evening
Kapha disorders:	late spring: (April 15 to May 15)	mid-morning
	early winter:	mid-day
	late winter:	mid-day

Improper Times and Seasons for Snehana

- As a general rule, snehana should not be performed during early spring—March 15 to April 15—especially for Kapha body types, because of the preponderance of Kapha in the universe at this time of year.
- Snehana should not be performed during the daylight hours of summer. This causes further vitiation of both Vata and Pitta.
- Snehana should not be performed during the dark hours (evening) of winter. This causes vitiation of Kapha.
- Snehana should not be administered in the rainy season, except for Vata disorders.

Characteristics of Substances for Snehana Therapy

In snehana therapy, Ayurveda uses an extensive pharmacopeia to mollify the tissues and encourage the emotions of love and tenderness in the human mind. Specific herbs, powders, roots, oils, and liquids such as milk, ghee and sesame oil are used in this therapy because they comprise the nine sacred characteristics which are required in the application of snehana. These nine qualities are unctuous, heavy, cold (although the warm quality is also used externally), soft, fluid, viscous, mobile, and/or slow, and subtle. All substances used in snehana are predominantly of the water element.

The unctuous property provides wetness and softness to the body. The heavy character adds strength while breaking down waste matter either in the skin during external snehana or in the tissues during internal snehana. The cold property used in substances taken internally promotes astringency and invigoration in the tissues, which in turn, produces clarity and self-cognition; it also alleviates burning and thirst sensations in the body. The cold attribute dominant in the herbs which medicate the various snehana oils used externally gives sharpness and lightness to the oils and promotes stimulation as well as substance absorption into the skin.

The soft quality of substances used in snehana therapy alleviates burning or inflamed conditions of the skin or internal tissues. It also promotes softness and tenderness in the body. The fluid quality serves mainly as a vehicle for carrying all the other properties deeply into the tissues or skin. This quality is essential for the body/mind/spirit to sustain the happiness and moistness essential to being alive. The liquid quality, when taken internally, carries the unctuous substance throughout the body and liquifies the excess doshas in preparation for their removal through the elimination processes of pancha karma therapy.

The viscous quality acts as a revitalizing tonic to the body. It helps to mend broken skin, internal fractures, slows digestion, and rests the body. The quality of mobility initiates the movement of substances in the body and allows them to become fluid or liquid. This quality advances Vata in the skin or body and promotes the timely evacuation of the bodily wastes. The slow quality of substances used in snehana therapy keeps the mobile factor in check. This action slows the movement of unctuous substances as they travel through the skin into the tissues, allowing ample opportunity for the substance's interaction with the excess doshas, dhatus, and malas. The slow characteristic subdues the aggravated doshas and gives sneha, love and affection, to the dhatus.

The subtle property of snehana substances is defined as atomic, fine, and penetrating. Called *suksma* in Sanskrit, there is no exact translation in English. This property is a principle of the subtle bodily fire known as tejas. It pierces through the body's most minute atomic particles, while keeping them knitted together, and operates through the subtle bodily channels, which are not visible to the naked eye. Its principle function within a substance is to produce combustion and promote metabolism. It carries the essences for lustre, color, and radiance to the body. The body's finest essence of tejas, carried by the subtle property of ingredients, sparks cellular memory which in turn ignites self-cognition.

PART TWO

Application of Snehana Therapies

LEPA: SNEHANA PLASTERS AND POULTICES

Snehana applications employ much more than medicated oils and unctions to the body. The application of a medicinal plaster or poultice on the body, called lepa therapy, has been used from the beginning of time to alleviate inflammatory swellings. In Ayurveda, these are applied in three main ways. A thin, cold layer of plaster, called *pralepa*, may be applied to the body to restore blood disorders and reduce Pitta vitiation. A thick or thin, warm or cold plaster known as *pradeha* may be applied to the body to reduce Vata and Kapha disorders. This type of plaster, which is usually non-absorbent, is used to facilitate the healing of bodily injuries and to reduce swellings, thus relieving pain. The third process, called *alepanam*, involves the application of an astringent plaster and is used for ulcers and other inflammatory conditions. The details of this latter process are set out below.

Alepanam - Topical Application of Medicinal Plaster

> **Season:** all year
>
> **Body Types:** all types
>
> **Time of Application:** morning or afternoon
>
> **Conditions**
> Ulcerated swellings, hard inflamed masses
>
> **Benefits**
> This procedure arrests localized hemorrhaging, softens masses and ulcerated swellings, extracts putrefied flesh from the body, and stops the formation of pus. Alepanam application also reduces pain and burning sensation of the skin and blood, cleanses the skin and subdues the aggravated doshas.
>
> **Necessary Aids**
> • Sterilized stainless steel bowl containing the plaster
> • Sterilized stainless steel bowl containing warm water

- Sterilized stainless steel bowl containing witch hazel solution (pg. 203)
- 2 pieces of sterilized cotton gauze
- 2 hot damp sterilized hand towels
- Sterilized stainless steel spatula
- Pair of sterilized rubber gloves

Note: See sterilizing procedures in Appendix E.

Directions

When an alepanam plaster is prescribed for ulcerated swellings so as to soften a mass and/or withdraw the putrefied flesh from its cavity, it should be administered once daily for thirty minutes, until the formation of pus ceases and the putrefied mass is completely drawn out.

This process may be used for any affected area of the body, except the eyes. The posture of the subject during treatment is determined by the location of the swelling.

- Allow the person to sit or lie down on a wooden table covered with a clean sheet.
- Gently massage the head of the person to ensure comfort during treatment.
- Wash your hands in the witch hazel solution and put on the sterilized gloves.
- Clean the affected area with a piece of sanitary cotton cloth soaked in the witch hazel solution.
- Apply the plaster immediately after mixing it with a stainless steel spatula.
- Use continuous upward strokes to apply the plaster, starting from below the swelling and finishing 6 inches above it.
- The final thickness of plaster should be an even half-inch, amply covering the swollen area.

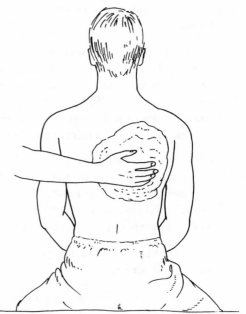

Figure 22: Alepanam Topical Poultice

133

- Allow the plaster to remain for thirty minutes, or until it begins to harden.
- Use a cool, damp hand towel to remove the plaster by applying gentle downward strokes.
- Clean the area first with a clean piece of cotton gauze soaked in witch hazel, and then with the clean, damp hand towel.
- Allow the person to rest for a short while afterwards.

Alepanam Formulas

Season: all year
Body Type: all types

> 1/2 lb aduki beans
> 1/2 c water
> 1/4 c dried wild cherry bark
> 1 tbs bhringaraja powder
> 2 fl oz witch hazel
> 20 drops white oak essential oil
> 10 drops uva ursi essential oil

Note: This amount of plaster will cover the surface area of the average female chest.

With a hand-operated food grinder, grind the beans to a medium-fine powder. In a medium-size stainless steel pot, bring the water to a boil and add the wild cherry bark. Cover and simmer on medium heat for 15 minutes, or until half the water has evaporated. Use a small colander to strain the liquid, while retaining the decoction in a medium-size stainless steel bowl. Add the bhringaraja powder to the hot bark tea.

Cover the bowl and allow it to sit for ten minutes. Mix in the ground aduki, white oak and uva ursi oils, and the witch hazel until the plaster becomes a smooth, soft paste, making it easy to spread and to adhere to the affected area of the body. Cover the bowl with a clean wet towel while you prepare the subject to receive the plaster.

Use a freshly made batch of plaster for each application. Never re-use old or used plaster.

Note: Use the sterilizing procedures in Appendix E for this formula and its application.

Lepa: Medicinal Plaster

A special application of lepa to relieve bodily aches and pains is used in Ayurveda. This application may be used on all body types and throughout the year. It is especially suitable therapy for athletes as well as Vata types. This plastering procedure may also be used for the entire body in order to restore the doshas to normalcy, and as a complete rejuvenation to the body.

Season: all year

Body Type: all types

Time of Application: morning

Conditions

Muscular spasms; bodily stiffness; prickling bodily pains; backache; oedema

Benefits

In addition to relieving the above conditions, this therapy also has the effect of revitalizing bodily tissue, restoring the doshas' equilibrium, and calming the mind.

Necessary Aids

- Bowl with plaster
- Bowl with warm water
- Small bowl of aromatic massage oil
- Covering sheet
- 2 clean hand towels

Application For Backaches

- Allow the person to remove all clothing and to recline flat on the stomach on wooden table covered with a clean cotton sheet.
- Use a separate clean cotton sheet to cover the area of the body which is not being treated.
- Administer a gentle massage of the head, using a small amount of the medicated oil.
- Continue by gently anointing the entire area which will receive plaster application (in this example, the whole back will be treated).
- Massage the back by applying gentle pressure with your hands from the nape of the neck down the center of the spine to the mid-back.
- With the fingers of both hands fully spread, begin to massage simultaneously both sides of the upper back. Allow the thumbs to remain almost parallel to the spine and move your hands gradually towards the direction of the subject's upper arms.

135

- Then move to the mid-back and gently massage the center back in both upwards and downwards strokes.
- Finally, move to the torso area and beginning from the crest of the buttocks and ending at the mid-back gently massage the area in both upward and downward strokes.
- Pull the sheet to cover the person's back for a few minutes while you wash your hands and prepare for the plaster application.
- Keep your plaster bowl within reach, pull back the sheet to expose the back and begin to apply the warm plaster from the crest of the buttocks going upwards towards the nape of the neck.
- The plaster should be evenly spread by upward strokes across the back. Apply the plaster on the complete back, covering all exposed skin. Cover the lower half of the back first and then the upper part of the back (Fig. 23).
- Allow the plaster to remain on the back for approximately thirty minutes, until it is about to become hard.
- Immediately remove the plaster from the back by using a clean damp hand towel.

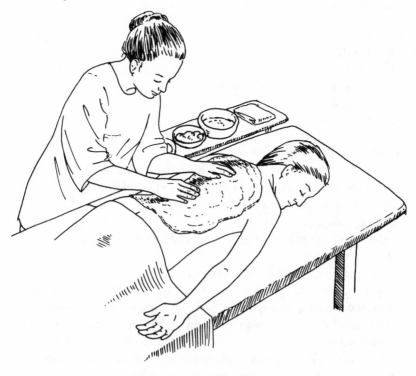

Figure 23: Lepa Application

- Use downwards strokes to remove the plaster.
- Clean off the remnants of the plaster with another clean, damp hand towel.
- Use an atomizer containing warm water and aromatic oils to gently spray the back.
- Pull the sheet to cover the back and allow the person to rest for a short while.

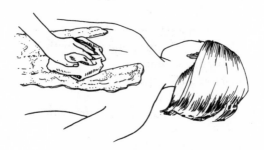

Figure 24: Lepa Removal

Lepa Plaster

2 lbs whole mung beans
2 oz minced fresh ginger
1/4 c certified raw cream
1/4 c ghee
1/4 c sesame oil
1/4 c mustard oil
1 c water

Note: The amount of this plaster will cover a surface area the size of the average male back.

Use a hand-operated food grinder and grind the mung beans to a medium fine powder. In a small stainless saucepan bring the water to a boil and add ginger. Cover pan and simmer for 15 minutes on medium-low heat, or until half the water has evaporated. Strain through a tea strainer. In a medium-size stainless bowl combine the cream, ghee and oils with the tea. Add the mung powder and work into a smooth, soft paste which is easy to spread and which will stick onto the affected area of the body. Cover the bowl with a clean warm damp towel, while preparing the subject for the application. The plaster should be applied warm.

Use a freshly made batch of plaster for every application. Never re-use or refrigerate old or used plaster.

Aromatic Oil

Vata: Combine 3 tablespoons sesame oil with 10 drops
          rose or jasmine essential oil.

Pitta: Combine 1 tablespoon sesame oil, 1 tablespoon
          ghee with 10 drops sandalwood essential oil.

Kapha: Combine 1 tablespoon sesame oil, 1 tablespoon
          sunflower oil with 5 drops eucalyptus essential oil.

Aromatic Mist

Vata: Combine 1/2 cup spring water with 10 drops rose
          or jasmine essential oil.

Pitta: Combine 1/2 cup spring water with 10 drops
          sandalwood oil.

Kapha: Combine 1/2 cup spring water with 10 drops
          eucalyptus oil.

Pour fragrant water into an atomizer or a small spray bottle with a fine spray cap. Refer to Appendix A for the complete variety of oils which may be used for each body type.

PART THREE
Snehana Therapies for the Head

There are scores of snehana therapies used in Ayurveda for the treatment of the head, since it is considered to be the most important part of the human body. The head contains four of the five sensory organs of the body and seven of the nine bodily apertures through which we interact with the external universe. On the very top of the head is the sacred shrine called *sahasrara chakra*, through which the soul is said to enter the body at birth and leave after death.

Five of Ayurveda's gentlest and most nurturing treatments for the head are as follows: shiro tarpana, the maintenance of oil on the head; shirodhara, the process by which oil or medicated liquid is methodically dripped onto the forehead from a specially designed pot hung directly above the forehead; pichu, a procedure in which a piece of cotton cloth is soaked with medicated oil and placed on the head; shirovasti, an elaborate procedure whereby the head is shaved and a tall, leather cap is fitted onto it; and, finally, a simpler yet effective process, called masthiskya, similar to shirovasti but without the oiling cap, in which a paste is applied directly onto the head.

These therapies are effective for conditions such as heart disease, insomnia, mental disorders, exhaustion, migraines, weakness of bodily joints, facial paralysis, blood disorders, eye diseases, baldness and premature graying, dandruff, scalp sores, and inflammation of the head.

Shearing the Head

In both masthiskya and shirovasti snehana therapies, the head of the subject is shaved prior to treatment. Shearing the head has been a Vedic tradition from the beginning of time, the sages and yogis observing the sadhana of timely head shaving on the eve of the full moon. True to the spirit of Vedic tradition, these actions are rooted in the wisdom of living and reverence for nature. In Ayurveda, the hair is considered a secondary vital tissue of the body. It is related to the Kapha dosha and is a direct result of both the tissue of bone marrow and the central nervous system of the body. Thus the timely removal of the hair stimulates the central nervous system, renews the bone marrow tissue, and allows the entire bodily system of Kapha to revive. As soon as Kapha is rejuvenated, the other doshas generally fall into harmony.

139

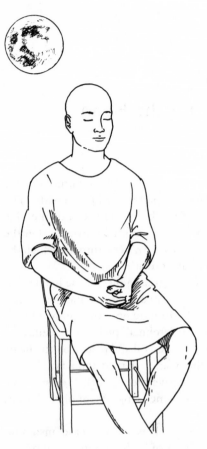

Figure 25: Shearing the Head

Because shearing the hair also renews both body/mind and spirit, the sages and yogis of yore consciously exfoliated their worn tissues for new ones, while shedding their attachment to the physical body, preferring instead to embrace their immortal and timeless self. Symbolizing self-sacrifice, the removal of the hair is a definite means of illuminating the spirit.

During my own lifetime, I have been graced with two invitations to shear my head. During my cancer years, I intuitively felt that the removal of my hair would somehow lighten my burdens. Acting on this intuition, I kept my head naked for three years and, as a result, began to grow into an abiding luminosity of my own being. A more recent invitation was extended to me when I took the vows of brahmacarani. Once more, I witnessed the burdens of material life being lifted from my spirit by the removal of my hair. I felt the wind brushing against my head and I began to remember my cognitive being once more.

Because the hair also carries the experiences of our lives and is intimately braided with ahamkara, its removal means that much more than hair is cast off. Providing the hair is removed during the proper circumstances, it becomes easier to view our timeless spirit of innocence, so often shrouded by this profuse mane.

As with the removal of all appendages bestowed on us, there is a proper time and place to do so. However, unless we live as yogis, sages, and poets, the maintenance of hair is vital to the necessary vanities of daily living. All the more necessary is the observation of daily living sadhanas, including timely and temporary removal of our ego in the form of hair.

Over the years, I have seen many cancer subjects through their dark passages. Among the sadhanas I have encouraged them to practice is the temporary shearing of their heads, which has proven to be an important part of allowing the self to find its true esteem. A naked head makes it easier to face the pure and unadorned spirit of our self so that we may come to terms with its truth and esteem it for what it truly is. A major disease is not, however, a prerequisite for the observation of this simple sadhana. In the snehana therapies of shirovasti and masthiskya, for example, the head is necessarily sheared.

Traditionally, a specific length of treatment determined by each dosha's disorder is recognized as essential in pancha karma and its preparatory practices. The Ayurvedic sages determined that by fine-tuning the timing of the treatments specifically geared to the Vata, Pitta or Kapha conditions, the disorder of each dosha can be more effectively alleviated. True to Vedic wisdom, they further cognised that by maintaining a decisive time ratio of 2:3:4: for disorders born of Kapha, Pitta and Vata respectively, each dosha responded more efficiently. This length of time is especially important when treatments are being administered to the head. For instance, Vata disorders are treated for exactly 53 minutes, Pitta disorders for exactly 42 minutes, and Kapha disorders for exactly 31 minutes. Although current practices have altered the time for each dosha's treatment to 60 minutes, 45 minutes and 30 minutes, respectively, the original timing for the head therapies is recommended, keeping in mind that more alertness will be required on the part of the practitioner.

MASTHISKYA - MEDICINAL PASTE ON THE HEAD

Season: all year

Body Type: all types

Time of Application: morning; 7:00 a.m. - 10:00 a.m.

Duration of Treatment: seven consecutive days

Vata disorders:	53 minutes
Pitta disorders:	42 minutes
Kapha disorders:	31 minutes

Conditions

Vata and Kapha disorders: facial paralysis; loss of sensation in skin; insomnia; dryness of nasal passages, mouth, and throat; heart disease; diseases of the head (including tumors); exhaustion; headache; urinary disorders; fear and anxiety; loss of bodily lustre; weakness of the joints; anorexia

Pitta disorders: pharyngitis; eye diseases (including cataract); head sores and inflammation; premature graying; blood disorders; jaundice

Note: For serious conditions (e.g., facial paralysis, heart disease, severe eye diseases, tumors, inflammation of the head, severe urinary disorders such as diabetes, emaciation, and anorexia), a 14-day treatment for 45 minutes each day between 7:00 and 10:00 a.m. is recommended.

Benefits

In addition to relieving the conditions listed above, this treatment has the added effect of revitalizing the whole body, relieving exhaustion and balancing the doshas. It also restores prana in the heart, makes the face gentle and flexible, strengthens the ojas and bodily joints and restores a healthy appetite in the subject.

Necessary Aids

- Medium stainless steel bowl containing the paste
- Small pottery bowl containing the massaging oil
- Hot damp towel to cover the bowl of paste (if the paste is applied cold, use a cold damp towel to cover it)
- Clean cotton covering sheet
- Clean cotton treatment gown*
- 2 warm damp hand towels
- Warm, dry hand towel
- Clean cotton cloth, 24 inches square, to wrap the head afterwards
- Atomizer or a spray bottle with a fine mist cap, containing the aromatic water
- Clock which shows the minutes

See Appendix D

Note: A small portable double boiler is a good asset for the treatment room. Among other uses, it will keep massaging oils warm while the plaster is being applied.

For best results from masthiskya therapy, the preliminary procedures of ab-hyanga (oil massage) and fomentation treatment (to induce sweat) are suggested. If these preliminary measures are observed, they should be performed in the early morning, followed by masthiskya therapy in the late afternoon.

Masthiskya Directions

- Arrange to have the subject's head shaved on the evening preceding treatment. This should be done just before the full moon.
- Have the subject disrobe, take a bath, and put on a clean treatment gown.
- Have the subject lie on his/her back on the treatment table which has been covered with a clean cotton sheet.
- Cover the subject's body with a clean sheet, leaving the face and head exposed.
- Using the appropriate oil, according to each body type, gently massage the subject's face, neck, and head.

- Before applying the paste to the head, have the subject move the head to the very edge of the treatment table.
- Apply the paste thickly over the head with your hands, beginning with the forehead, working your way to the top of the head, and then around the back of the head.
- Once the head is fully covered with the paste to approximately 1/2-inch thickness, encourage the subject to rest while you remove the bowl of paste and wash your hands.
- After the prescribed length of treatment has passed, use a clean cotton hand towel to remove the paste from the head.
- Follow up this initial cleaning procedure, using a clean damp hand towel to wipe off all the remaining paste.
- Applying a small amount of the rubbing oil to your hands, briskly anoint the subject's head for a few minutes.
- Using the atomizer, spray a fine mist of warm aromatic water over the head.
- Gently pat the mist from the head with a clean, dry cotton hand towel.
- Have the subject rest for a short while before rising.
- Before the subject leaves, wrap the head with a clean piece of cloth to prevent exposure to the elements.
- Advise the subject to avoid exposure to excessive cold, heat, and/or dampness and to keep the head covered when outdoors. This procedure is to be observed throughout the treatment period and for one week thereafter.

Masthiskya Formulas

Season: all year

Body Type: all types

Takra Dhara (amalaki buttermilk)

Note: In addition to its use for all body types, this formula is also used internally for Vata types.

> 1 c certified raw whole milk
> 2 c water
> 1 c amalaki powder

Combine the milk and water and pour into a heavy, stainless steel, medium-size pot. Place over medium-low heat until the mixture is warm—approximately 108°F. Remove from heat and mix in the amalaki powder with a wooden spoon, stirring well until all the powder is blended with the milk. Pour into a 12-inch tall stainless steel bucket. Use a large, clean cotton terry cloth towel to cover the bucket, wrapping the excess toweling around the bucket, and securing it with a 3-foot length of twine. Store the bucket in a room where the temperature is between 75° to 80° for 12 hours, or until the herbal milk turns into a thick cream with the consistency of buttermilk. The portion of the mixture, referred to as buttermilk, used as masthiskya paste for the head should be measured out before the remaining buttermilk is refrigerated. The refrigerated portion may be taken with meals by Vata types, being very effective for reducing Vata disorders.

Warm Herbal Paste

1/2 c amalaki buttermilk
4 tbs sandalwood powder
2 tbs lotus powder
1 tbs bamboo powder
1 tbs musta powder
2 tbs hot water

Pour the buttermilk into a medium-size stainless steel bowl. Add the four powders and the water, blending thoroughly with a wooden spoon to a smooth paste. Cover the paste with a hot, damp towel. Apply the warm paste immediately after it is made. Make a fresh batch of paste for every application.

Note: For Pitta conditions, allow the paste to cool entirely before applying.

Massaging Oils

Vata and Kapha disorders
    Warm 1/4 cup of sesame oil and keep it covered in a small pottery bowl to help maintain the heat.
Pitta disorders
    Warm together 2 tablespoons each of sesame oil and ghee; allow to cool completely. Pour into a small pottery bowl and cover to maintain the coolness.

Aromatic Mist

Vata, Pitta, and Kapha disorders

Warm 1/2 cup of water and add 10 drops of the essential oils recommended for Vata (see glossary of essential oils, Appendix A). Pour the water into an atomizer or a small spray bottle with a fine mist spray cap.

Note: Use cool water for Pitta conditions.

SHIROVASTI - MEDICINAL PASTE AND OIL ON THE HEAD

Shirovasti, another snehana treatment for the head, involves the use of both paste and oil while the subject is in a sitting position. After the head is shaved, the lepa plaster is the first remedy to be applied. Then, warm oil, retained by a leather cap on the head, is poured directly over the plaster.

Shirovasti is performed only after the preliminary processes of oil massage and fomentation therapy, and, if necessary, vasti therapy is administered. Shirovasti is generally performed for seven consecutive days, the preliminary procedures being done in the early morning and shirovasti in the late afternoon.

Although this therapy is similar to masthiskya, and may be used for the same menu of diseases, it is generally used for severe conditions such as facial paralysis, heart diseases and tumors of the head.

Body Type: all types

Season: use seasonal guidelines

Temperate and Tropical Schedule

Vata disorders:	July 22 to August 7
	October 20 to November 20
Pitta disorders:	October 20 to November 20
Kapha disorders:	March 21 to April 21

Time of Application: 3:00 to 4:00 p.m., on the day after the full moon.

Duration of Treatment: seven consecutive days

Vata disorders:	53 minutes
Pitta disorders:	42 minutes
Kapha disorders:	31 minutes

Note: The preliminary procedure of abhyanga is to be performed between 7:00 a.m. to 9:00 a.m., followed by fomentation therapy. The subject then is to rest. Shirovasti is to be administered between 3:00 p.m. and 4:00 p.m.

Conditions

Vata disorders: facial paralysis; eye diseases (including cataract); heart disease/chest pains; diseases of the head (including tumors); insomnia; loss of sensation in skin; dryness of nasal passages, mouth, and throat; urinary disorders (including diabetes); grayish coating on the tongue; migraine; weakness of the joints; mental and physical exhaustion

Pitta disorders: indigestion; pharyngitis; conjunctivitis; burning sensation of skin and shoulders; excess sweating; blood disorders; hemorrhaging; jaundice; herpes; yellowish coating on tongue; greenish, yellowish coloring of urine and feces

Kapha disorders: anorexia; loss of appetite (revulsion for food); heaviness of body; excessive sleep; weak digestion; white coating on the tongue; mucus; indigestion; obesity

Benefits

In addition to alleviating the conditions listed above, this treatment has the added benefit of rejuvenating the whole body, relieving exhaustion and restoring lustre to the skin. It also relieves mental stress, restores prana in the heart, balances the doshas and increases ojas of body and mind.

Necessary Aids

- Medium-size stainless steel bowl containing the plaster
- Hot damp towel to cover the bowl
- Medium-size pottery bowl filled with warm sesame oil, covered to keep the oil warm
- Smaller pottery bowl, also for warm sesame oil
- Clean cotton covering sheet
- Clean cotton treatment gown*
- 2 warm damp hand towels
- Warm dry hand towel
- 2 pieces of cotton gauze wrapping, 48 inches long by 4 inches wide and 36 inches long by 4 inches wide
- Pair of scissors
- Atomizer or spray bottle with a fine mist cap, containing the aromatic water
- Leather cap* to hold the oil on the head
- Clock that records the minutes
- Clean cotton cloth, 24 inches square, to wrap the head after treatment

See Appendix D

Note:

1. Along with the usual treatment table or chair and work table, the treatment room should also have a sink, a small chair placed next to the sink, a stainless steel bucket under the sink, and a washing table next to the sink. The sink used in hair salons, having a curved front rim to cradle the head and neck, is recommended for the shirovasti treatment room.

2. A small portable double boiler, to keep the oil warm while the plaster is being applied, is also recommended for the treatment room. The cleaning towels for removing the plaster and oil from the subject's head, as well as the small bowl of sesame oil and the aromatic mist (in the atomizer), need to be placed on this table.

Shirovasti Directions

After the preliminary procedures of abhyanga and fomentation have been performed and a period of rest has been observed, the subject is ready for shirovasti therapy.

- Advise the subject to have his/her head shaved the evening before treatment. This should be done just before the full moon.
- Have the subject disrobe and put on a clean treatment gown.
- Place the shirovasti cap to dry under direct sunlight and remove when the leather is dry, but still supple.
- Burn a small piece of dried sage in an earthen pot and allow it to smoke. Hold the leather cap over the smoke for a few minutes to remove whatever energies may have been retained from its previous use. Never re-use the cap without thoroughly cleaning it, using the methods given here.
- Have the subject sit on the comfortable upright chair provided for treatment.
- Stand directly behind the subject and apply a small amount of the sesame oil onto the head. Gently anoint the head for a few minutes.
- Use your hands and apply the lepa plaster (see recipe information below) directly on the subject's head. Beginning from the center back of the head, plaster the entire outline of the head, excluding the ears, neck, and forehead. Then plaster the top of the head, making sure that the head is completely covered with the plaster, evenly spread and approximately 1/2 inch thick.
- Quickly wash the paste from your hands, dry them, and return to the subject.
- Using a 48-inch by 4-inch piece of cotton gauze, and beginning from the nape below the center back of the head, carefully wrap the head in a clockwise direction, retaining the plaster under the gauze

until the entire head is covered. Tuck the
end of the gauze securely beneath the
head wrapping, ensuring that the wrapping is secure.

- Place the shirovasti cap over the bandaged
head, without catching the ears.
- Using the 36-inch by 4-inch piece of
cotton gauze, firmly wrap the bottom of
the cap around the head to prevent the
oil, which will be poured into the cap,
from leaking out. In this way, the oil is
retained on the plastered head for the
duration of the treatment. Leave the first
4 inches of gauze hanging over the
forehead.

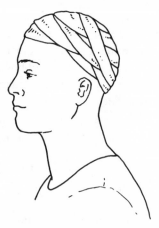

Figure 26: Bandaging Head

- After securely wrapping the bottom of the cap to the head, take the
end piece of gauze and tie it to the piece of gauze hanging over the
forehead using a tight knot.
- Pour one cup of oil into the cap (Fig. 27).
- Invite the subject to close his/her eyes and to rest quietly in the
sitting position.
- Ensuring that the subject is totally comfortable, allow the oil to remain on the head
for the prescribed length of time,
depending on each dosha's
condition.
- Before removing the oil cap
and the bandaged plaster
from the subject's head,
make sure that the clean-
ing aids you will need are
in order.
- Place the chair by the
sink with its back toward
the sink. The chair
should be low enough to
allow the subject to bend
the head backwards
directly over the sink.
- Guide the subject from
the therapy area to this
chair.

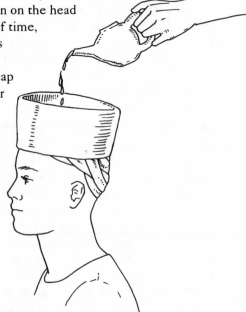

Figure 27: Shirovasti Cap on Head

148

- Assist the subject to slip down slightly into the chair so that the back of the neck is comfortably cradled on the rim of the sink.
- Snip off the knot of the bandage with a pair of scissors, while carefully removing the oil cap and emptying it in the sink.
- Remove the cap from the sink and place it in the bucket underneath the sink.
- Loosen the head bandage and remove it so that most of the plaster on the head comes away with it.
- Using the warm damp hand towel, wipe the remaining plaster from the head, as well as from behind the ears and neck.
- After the head is completely clean, ask the subject to sit up. Using the atomizer, spray the head with the aromatic mist.
- Gently pat the mist off and anoint the head briskly with a few drops of sesame oil.
- Guide the subject to a comfortable place where he/she may rest for a little while before leaving.
- Before the subject leaves, wrap the head with the clean piece of cloth prepared for this purpose so that undue exposure to the elements might be prevented. (See Appendix D for head wrapping procedures.)
- Advise the subject to avoid exposure to excessive cold, heat, or dampness, and to keep the head covered when outdoors.

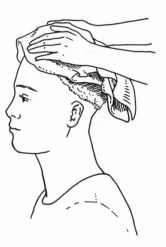

Figure 28: Removal of Paste & Oil

This procedure is to be observed throughout the period of treatment and for the week following treatment.

Shirovasti Formulas

Plaster

Prepare the lepa plaster from the recipe on pg. 137. Place the plaster in a medium-size stainless steel bowl and cover it with a warm, damp cotton towel.

Note: When administering shirovasti, the plaster is applied while still warm for Vata and Kapha disorders, and at room temperature for Pitta disorders.

Warm Sesame Oil

Vata and Kapha disorders:

Pour 1 cup of sesame oil into a small stainless steel saucepan and warm over low heat for 10 minutes. Pour the oil directly into a pottery bowl and cover it securely to help the oil maintain its heat.

Cool Ghee-Sesame Oil

Pitta disorders:

Pour 1/2 cup of sesame oil into a small stainless steel saucepan and warm over low heat for 10 minutes. Remove from heat and add 1/2 cup of pure ghee. Let the ghee melt in the oil and cool the mixture to room temperature.

Aromatic Mist

Vata, Pitta, and Kapha disorders:

Warm 1/2 cup of water in a small pan. Add 10 drops of sandalwood essential oil. Pour into an atomizer or small spray bottle with a fine mist spray cap. This aromatic mist is used in the final procedure of shirovasti.

SHIRODHARA - DRIPPING OIL ON THE FOREHEAD

Shirodhara is a titillating form of snehana treatment, whereby the oil or therapeutic substance methodically drips along a coarse thread onto the forehead. A metal or clay vessel, the dhara patra, is suspended directly above the forehead. The oil or other fluid is poured into the pot, then seeps through a hole in the bottom of the pot and slides down a 4-inch-long thread, half of which hangs through the hole. The drops of oil from the thread drip directly onto the subject's third eye, or center of the forehead.

This therapy, as all pancha karma treatments, requires two well-trained, disciplined attendants working together with clockwork precision, consistency, and speed. These qualifications are vital, for example, to achieving the precision timing needing to be maintained between the actions of pouring the oil onto the subject's forehead and sustaining the slight rocking motion of the oil vessel itself.

An ancient technique, shirodhara is meant to be maintained at a certain rhythmic speed while awakening the third eye. Vast and miraculous healing occurs when this technique is performed to perfection. The rhythm of the oil trickling onto the third eye, which is the seat of our cognitive vision, evokes deep cognitive memories. Through the arousal of these memories, bodily tissues are transformed and good health is restored.

Before shirodhara is administered, the preliminary procedure of abhyanga massage is performed. A soporific treat, shirodhara soothes and invigorates the senses as well as the mind. A total state of wellness is induced in the process.

Shirodhara

Season: all year

Body Type: all types

Time of Application: 7:00 to 10:00 a.m.

Duration of Treatment:

Vata disorders:	53 minutes
Pitta disorders:	42 minutes
Kapha disorders:	31 minutes

Conditions

General: All afflictions of the head and sense organs

Vata disorders: prickling pain in the head; loss of hair; loss of hearing; fatigue and mental exhaustion; grayish coating on the tongue; insomnia; headache; dryness of face and scalp; constipation

Pitta disorders: burning sensation in head and body; ulcerated or inflammatory conditions of the head; pharyngitis; conjunctivitis; excess sweating; dimness of vision; blood disorders; hemorrhaging; jaundice; herpes; yellowish coating on the tongue; greenish or yellowish coloring of urine and feces

Kapha disorders: excessive sleep; heaviness of body; indigestion; mucus; obesity; weak digestion; white coating on the tongue; white urine and feces; loss of appetite; repulsion for food; anorexia

Benefits

In addition to relieving the disorders listed above, this treatment has the added effect of awakening the third eye, invigorating the body and mind, and stimulating cognitive memories.

Necessary Aids

- Small stainless steel bucket containing the warm oil or liquid substance, kept covered until treatment begins
- Makeshift double boiler (large pot, half filled with boiling water, in which the oil bucket is placed) to maintain the oil's warmth
- Small stainless steel cup for dipping the oil
- Dhara patra,* or a separatory funnel with ring and stand (available through chemistry equipment suppliers)
- Clean cotton treatment gown*
- Clean cotton covering sheet
- 2 clean cotton hand towels
- Clean cotton cloth 12 inches square, folded in three to create a blindfold for protecting the subject's eyes during treatment
- Clean cotton cloth, 24 inches square, to wrap the head and forehead after treatment
- Utility sink in close proximity to the shirodhara treatment room where the dhara patra may be washed
- 2 high chairs for the attendants to sit on while administering this therapy
- Step ladder to hang up and take down the dhara patra

* *See Appendix D*

Shirodhara Directions

- Administer abhyanga in the very early morning immediately before shirodhara is to be performed.
- After abhyanga, have the subject sit up and put on a clean treatment gown.
- Have the subject lie down on the treatment table on his/her back. Pull the covering cloth up to the neck.
- Place the folded piece of cloth over the eyes to protect them from oil or liquid seepage. Ensure that the dhara patra has been hung from the ceiling and suspended directly above where the subject's forehead will be.
- Have your treatment assistant sit in a high chair on the left side of the subject and pour the oil or liquid substance slowly into the dhara patra, while you hold the suspended vessel to keep it still.

152

- Sit in a high chair on the right side looking over the dhara patra.
- As your assistant steadily pours the oil into the dhara patra, gently rock the vessel back and forth with a slight movement of the hand, an inch or so in either direction, so that the oil trickles along the center vertical line of the subject's forehead.

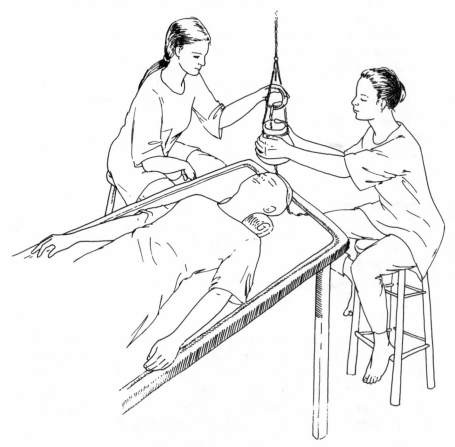

Figure 29: Shirodhara Application

- Make sure that the dripping of the oil is consistent and is maintained throughout the treatment and that a rhythmic and precise rocking of the dhara patra is maintained.
- Maintain this procedure for the length of time prescribed for each dosha's disorder.
- At the end of the treatment time, two actions occur simultaneously: while you hold the vessel in place, your assistant stops pouring the

153

oil and quickly removes the vessel from its hanging position into the sink.

- Have the subject remain lying down, undisturbed, for another five minutes.
- Using a dry clean cotton towel, gently pat the excess oil off the subject's forehead without removing all of it.
- Remove the soaked cloth from the eyes and gently pat any oil away from the eyes.
- Again, have the subject rest for a short period of time.
- Before the subject departs, wrap his/her head and forehead.*
- Advise the subject to avoid exposure to excess cold, heat, or dampness, and to keep the head and forehead covered when outdoors. This procedure is maintained throughout the treatment period and for a week thereafter.

* *See Appendix D*

Shirodhara Formulas: Oils

Season: all year

Dashamula Oil

Body Type: Vata disorders

    16 c water

    1 c dashamula powder

    4 c sesame oil

Pour the oil and water into a large stainless steel saucepan and bring to a boil over medium heat. Add the powder, cover and simmer on low heat for approximately 4 hours, or until all the water has evaporated. Cool the oil, then strain it through a fine sieve into the stainless steel bucket. Cover the bucket until the treatment begins. Place the bucket in a large half filled pot of boiling water to keep the oil warm during treatment.

Warm Sesame Oil

Body Type: Vata and Kapha disorders

Pour 4 cups of sesame oil (3 cups for Kapha disorders) into a medium-size stainless steel saucepan and warm over low heat for 10 minutes. Remove from the heat and pour into the stainless steel bucket. Cover the bucket until the treatment begins. Place the bucket in a large half-filled pot of boiling water to keep the oil warm during treatment.

Sesame Oil and Ghee

Body Type: Pitta disorders

    2 c sesame oil

    1 1/2 c pure ghee

Pour the oil into a medium-size stainless steel saucepan and warm over low heat for 10 minutes; remove from the heat. Melt the ghee by adding it to the warm oil. Leaving the saucepan uncovered, cool the mixture to room temperature. Then pour into the stainless steel bucket. Cover and take directly to the treatment room.

Licorice Oil

Body Type: Pitta disorders

    12 c water

    3 c sesame oil

    3/4 c licorice powder

Pour the oil and water into a large stainless steel saucepan and bring to a boil over medium heat. Mix in the powder, then cover and simmer over low heat for approximately 4 hours, or until all the water has evaporated. Let cool and strain through a fine sieve into the bucket. When the oil has cooled to room temperature, cover the bucket and take it to the treatment room.

Other Shirodhara Substances

Season: all year

Body Type: all types

Conditions

Urinary disorders, heart disease, indigestion, anorexia, diseases of the eye and ear, premature graying and balding, headache, insomnia, exhaustion, weakness of the joints, fear and anxiety. A total restorative for all three doshas.

Takra Dhara (medicated buttermilk)

Note: See recipe under masthiskya therapy.

Use freshly made takra dhara and apply at a temperature of 75° to 80° F.

Milk and Musta Cream

16 c water

4 c milk

1 c musta powder

2 c takra dhara (medicated buttermilk)

Pour the milk and water into a large stainless steel saucepan and bring to a boil over medium heat. Add the powder. Cover and simmer over low heat for approximately 4 hours, or until the liquid has reduced to one fifth of its initial volume (approximately 4 cups). Add the takra dhara, blending thoroughly into a warm cream. Pour this medicated cream into the stainless steel bucket. Cover and place in a large half-filled pot of hot water to keep warm during treatment. Apply this cream at a temperature of 75° to 80° F.

PICHU - OELATION OF THE FOREHEAD

Pichu is a snehana process whereby a piece of cotton cloth, which has been soaked in a specific oil, is kept on the forehead for a period of time. Pichu is the simplest of the snehana procedures and may be performed frequently as a treatment at home to help balance the doshas and bring calmness to the body and mind.

Season: all year

Body Type: all types

Time of Application: morning and early evening

Conditions and Appropriate Oils

stiffness in eye muscles	- padmaka oil
dryness or sores on scalp	- padmaka or kaseesadi oil
inflammation of head or face	- padmaka or kaseesadi oil
vaginal bleeding	- padmaka oil
hemorrhoids	- kaseesadi oil

Benefits

Relieves pain and stiffness in the eyes, moisturizes the scalp, reduces inflammation of the head and face, and is excellent for nose bleeds. Moreover, pichu application relieves vaginal bleeding and hemorrhoids.

Necessary Aids

- Pottery bowl, 6-inch diameter by 3 inches deep, one-quarter filled with oil
- Clean cotton cloth, 12 inches square
- Clean cotton hand towel

Pichu Oils

Pour 1/4 cup of either padmaka or kaseesadi oil into a small stainless steel saucepan and warm over low heat for 5 minutes. Then pour into the pottery bowl. Fold the clean piece of cotton cloth so that it forms three even layers of cloth. Holding the cloth at either end, dip the middle eight inches of cloth into the warm oil, soaking it thoroughly. Let the ends hang over the sides of the bowl so that they remain dry. Place the bowl so that it is within easy reach during your treatment.

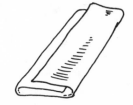

Figure 30: Folding the Cloth

Pichu Directions

- Wash the hair a few hours before pichu treatment is to be administered.
- Assemble the oil, cloth, and a clean hand towel onto a clean towel spread out on the floor.
- Place a clean mat along side your treatment items and lie down on it.

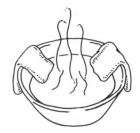

Figure 31: Soaking the Cloth

- Observe a 10-minute meditation, inviting all the thoughts and stressful details of your life to subside from the mind.
- Take naturally deep and relaxing breaths through the nose during this 10-minute meditation time.
- Then soak the cloth in the oil and place it across the forehead, from ear to ear.
- Using both hands, press down gently on the cloth.
- Use the hand towel to wipe any excess oil from your hands and face.
- Close your eyes and rest quietly for 30 minutes.

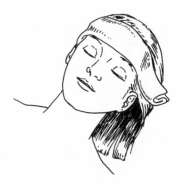

Figure 32: Pichu Cloth on Forehead

- Sit up very slowly, removing the cloth from the forehead.
- Using the hand towel, gently pat away any excess oil from the forehead.
- Clean your oil utensil and wash the oil-soaked cloth thoroughly by hand.
- Rest for 30 minutes and maintain a peaceful attitude for the rest of the day.

Note: This treatment may be applied twice daily for seven days.

PART FOUR

Routine Cleansing of the Senses

The snehana therapies for eyes, nose, and mouth are becoming a lost art in contemporary living. As simple as they are rejuvenative, the routine observance of these procedures enhances the senses and maintains clarity, freshness, invigoration, and joy in our lives. The sense organs are our only apparent means of communication with the external world. By maintaining them in excellent health, we are better equipped to use the innate cognitive abilities that braid us with the universe and our own sacred journeys from the beginning of time. It is impossible for diseases to take hold if the sensory organs are kept in excellent health.

KAVALAGRAHA - GARGLING TREATMENT

There are two main Ayurvedic gargling procedures: *kavalagraha,* in which a comfortable amount of fluid is retained in the mouth for gargling purposes, and *gandusa,* in which the mouth is completely filled with fluid thereby rendering gargling impossible.

During both procedures, it is advised to sit upright and to clear the mind of stressful thoughts. Gargling stimulates and soothes the sense organs, freshens the breath, and invigorates the mind. This sadhana is recommended to be done every morning after brushing the teeth.

Kavalagraha & Gandusa

Season: all year

Body Type: all types

Time of Application: early morning

Conditions

Bad breath; dryness of face; dullness of senses; exhaustion; anorexia; loss of taste; impaired sight; sore throat; all Kapha-related disorders

Benefits

In addition to alleviating the conditions listed above, this treatment has the effect of drawing out excess doshas through the eyes, ears, nose, and mouth.

Note: Special gargling fluids are used to restore each dosha to normalcy. Heat-producing unctuous fluids are used for Vata disorders. For Pitta, sweet, cooling, pungent, and salty fluids are prescribed; to restore Kapha, heat-producing and drying fluids are used.

Gargling Directions

- Prepare your gargling fluid and place it on the sink, along with a clean cotton hand towel.
- Clear the mind of stressful thoughts by sitting in contemplation for a short while before gargling.
- Sit on an upright chair, with your back comfortably erect.
- Fill your mouth two-thirds full with the gargling fluid. Retain for 60 seconds (Fig. 33).
- Release the fluid from your mouth, then refill the mouth with the same quantity of fluid and retain it for two minutes. Then release again.
- Finally, pour another measure of decoction into the mouth. Lean the head slightly backwards and gargle the fluid in the throat. Then release from the mouth (Fig. 34).

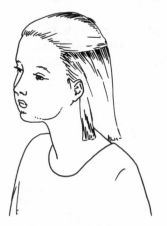
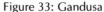
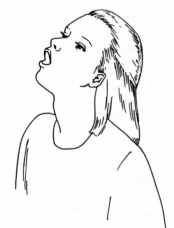

Figure 33: Gandusa   Figure 34: Kavalagraha

For serious conditions such as anorexia and loss of taste, follow the above procedure, increasing oral retention time to two minutes, or until the eyes and nose begin to ooze. Then release the fluid from the mouth.

160

Gargling Tonics

Season: all year

Eucalyptus Gargling Tea

Body Type: Vata

    1/2 c water

    1 tsp caraway seeds

    2 tsp sesame oil

    2 drops eucalyptus essential oil

Bring the water to a boil in a small stainless steel pot. Add the caraway seeds, cover and simmer on medium heat for 3 minutes. Remove from heat and steep for 3 more minutes. Using a tea stainer, strain the seeds, retaining the tea in a large cup. Finally, add the oils. The gargling tea should be used when tepid, but not too warm, so that retaining it in the mouth is comfortable.

Ashwagandha Gargling Brew

Body Type: Vata

    1/4 c milk

    1/4 tsp ashwagandha powder

    1 tsp sesame oil

    2 drops cinnamon essential oil

Warm the milk and sesame oil in a small stainless steel pot over low heat for 3 minutes. Add the powder and essential oil and then remove from heat. Cover and steep for 5 minutes. The brew should be tepid, but not too warm, so that retaining it in the mouth is comfortable.

Fennel Gargling Tea

Body Type: Pitta

    1/2 c water

    1 tsp fennel seeds

    1/4 tsp turmeric powder

    1/2 tsp brown sugar

Bring the water to a boil in a small stainless steel pot. Add the fennel seeds and simmer over low heat for 5 minutes, or until half the water has evaporated. Remove from heat and strain through a tea strainer, retaining the tea in a large cup. Add turmeric powder and brown sugar. Stir and let cool for 10 minutes.

Peppermint Gargling Brew

Body Type: Pitta

    1/4 c milk

    1/4 c water

    1 tsp dried peppermint leaves

    1/4 tsp shatavari powder

    2 drops essential oil of blackberry

Combine the milk and water in a small stainless steel pot and bring it to a boil over low heat. Add the peppermint leaves and shatavari powder. Remove from heat, cover, and steep for 10 minutes. Strain the leaves through a tea strainer and retain the milk brew in a large cup. Add the essential oil to the brew. Stir and check the temperature to make sure it is cool enough before using.

Eucalyptus and Honey Gargling Tea

Body Type: Kapha

    1/2 c water

    1/4 tsp guggulu powder

    1/4 tsp coarse black pepper

    2 drops eucalyptus essential oil

    1/2 tsp honey

Bring the water to a boil in a small stainless steel pot. Add the guggulu and black pepper. Cover and simmer on low heat for 5 minutes, or until half the water has evaporated. Remove from heat. Using a fine tea strainer, separate the pepper grains from the liquid, retaining the tea in a large cup. Add the essential oil and honey; let cool to a comfortable temperature before using.

Neem and Cardamom Gargling Tea

Body Type: Kapha

    1/2 c water

    1 tsp green cardamom pods

    1/4 tsp neem powder

Bring water to a boil in a small stainless steel pot. Add the pods, cover, and simmer on low heat for 5 minutes, or until half the water has evaporated. Remove from the heat, add the neem powder, cover again, and steep for 5 minutes. Use a tea stainer to separate the pods, retaining the liquid in a large cup. Cool to a comfortable temperature before using.

Salt Water Gargle

Body Type: all types

   1/2 c water

   1 tsp rock salt or sea salt

   1/4 tsp turmeric powder

Bring the water to a boil; then dissolve the salt and powder in it. Remove from heat, cover, and steep for 5 minutes. Use when the temperature is comfortable enough to retain in the mouth.

Licorice Gargle

Body Type: all types

   1/2 c water

   1/4 tsp licorice powder

   1 tsp sesame oil

   2 drops licorice essential oil

Bring water to a boil; add the powder and oils. Remove from heat and cover, steeping and cooling for 15 minutes before using.

Note: A strong licorice tea may also be used as a regular gargling tonic; use 1 teaspoon of licorice powder to 1/2 cup of water.

Honey and Turmeric Gargle

An excellent gargle for children.

Body Type: all types

   1/2 c warm water

   1 tsp honey

   1/2 tsp turmeric powder

Dilute the honey in warm water and add turmeric powder. This gargle is especially beneficial for sore throat and hoarseness due to honey's astringent property.

Triphala Gargle

Body Type: all types

   1/2 c warm water

   1/2 tsp triphala powder

Dilute the triphala powder in hot water. Cover and allow the infusion to sit for 10 minutes, before using as a gargling solution.

AKSHITARPANA - CLEANSING THE EYES

Akshitarpana is the process of keeping fluids and/or unctuous substances in the eyes. This therapy improves the sight, heals stiffness, pain and roughness around the eyes. It strengthens the eyes and protects them against the sun's sharp rays. Akshitarpana is also very helpful for serious eye disorders, such as glaucoma, ulcerated cornea, or inflamed lesions surrounding the eyes.

Akshitarpana

Season: use seasonal snehana guidelines

Body Type: all types

Time of Application: early morning

Duration of Treatment: 14 days

Conditions

Loss of vision/blurred vision; eye injuries; pain in the eyes; darkness around eyes; paleness around eyes; roughness around eyes; loss of lachrymal secretion; excess lachrymal secretion; hemorrhaging of the eyes; glaucoma; ulcerated cornea; inflammation in the eyes

Benefits

In addition to relieving the conditions listed above, this treatment aids gradual improvement of serious eye diseases, and has the added benefit of bringing about clarity of mind.

Necessary Aids

- Clean cotton covering sheet
- Clean cotton treatment gown
- 2 clean cotton cloths, 12 inches square
- Clean damp cotton hand towel
- Cotton bandage for the eyes, 24 inches long and 8 inches wide
- Large cup with triphala decoction, for the preliminary eye-wash and gargling procedures
- Small stainless steel bowl containing the masha (urad bean) paste, covered with a damp cloth
- Small double boiler to keep the medicated ghee warm
- Small covered pottery tea pot, containing the medicated ghee
- Clean wooden surface on a utility table to lay out the masha paste
- Utility sink for washing up

Directions

For best results, this procedure should be done after the preliminary therapies of emesis, purgation, and enema have been administered. Akshitarpana is a delicate therapy and requires a certain length of time to thoroughly cleanse the doshas, as well as the eyes. As with the pancha karma therapies, this treatment should only be performed under the supervision of an Ayurvedic physician or by trained pancha karma attendants. Early morning sunlight filtering into a well ventilated room are also standard requirements for this therapy. The treatment table should be covered with a clean cotton sheet. All the necessary substances and utensils should be conveniently located before the subject arrives.

Akshitarpana is administered in the early morning, after the necessary ablutions are performed by both the attendants and the subject.

Treatment

First day:

- Have the subject disrobe and put on the clean treatment gown.
- Assist the subject with the preliminary eye wash and oral gargling before beginning akshitarpana procedures (see details below).
- Have the subject lie comfortably on his/her back.
- Spread the cotton sheet over the subject, leaving the face and head exposed.
- Gently rub his/her face with a clean face towel and apply a thin film of sesame oil over it.
- Using your thumbs, gently massage around the closed eyes.
- Take a handful of the masha paste and divide it into four walnut size lumps.
- Take two lumps and place them on the clean surface of the utility table. Flatten each lump with the heel of your hand, and then shape it into rectangular flat biscuit-like dough, approximately 1 1/2 inches wide, 4 inches long and 1/2 inch thick.
- Repeat this process with the two remaining lumps. After all four rectangular pieces are made, carefully pick one up and curve it into

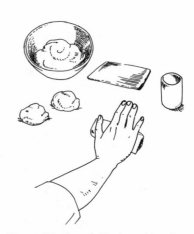

Figure 35: Dough-Tank Making for Akshitarpana

165

a wide ring the shape of a napkin ring holder, approximately 2 inches in diameter and 1 1/2 inches in height.

- Place the index and middle finger through the ring and firmly press the two ends of the ring together by pressing the two fingers against the thumb. This paste ring construction is called a tank.
- Gently place each paste tank over the subject's eyes.
- Encourage the subject to rest for another 10 minutes until the paste tank dries.
- While the subject's eyes are closed, pour the warm medicated ghee into each tank until the eyelid is completely covered (Fig. 36). Approximately one tablespoon of ghee is poured into each tank.

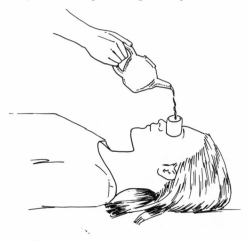

Figure 36: Pouring Ghee on the Eyes

- After 2 minutes, ask the subject to slowly begin to open the eyes and to blink slowly and repeatedly without too much effort.
- Continue this process for 5 minutes.
- Then, gently remove the tanks, one at a time, wiping off the medicated ghee with a clean cotton cloth. Ask the subject to keep the eyes closed during this cleaning procedure.
- Using the clean damp hand towel, wipe the excess ghee from the face and place the cotton bandage over the eyes.

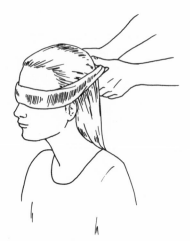

Figure 37: Protecting the Eyes

166

- Have the subject rest for 20 minutes before rising. The eyes must not be exposed to light or cold for five hours after treatment, and then only to filtered or dim light.

Note: Since the subject is to be sent home with bandaged eyes, he or she must be accompanied.

Treatment

Second and third days: Repeat the above procedures, increasing the time of medicated ghee application to 6 minutes.

Third to seventh day: Repeat the above procedures, increasing the medicated ghee application by one additional minute every day, up to 10 minutes.

The treatment schedule, then, is as follows:

Day 1	- 5 minutes	Day 8	- 9 minutes
Day 2	- 6 minutes	Day 9	- 9 minutes
Day 3	- 7 minutes	Day 10	- 8 minutes
Day 4	- 8 minutes	Day 11	- 7 minutes
Day 5	- 9 minutes	Day 12	- 6 minutes
Day 6	- 10 minutes	Day 13	- 5 minutes
Day 7	- 10 minutes	Day 14	- 5 minutes

Akshitarpana - Home Care for the Eyes

Season: all year

Body Type: all types

Time of Application: early morning or before bed

Necessary Aids
- Eye-glass (small container for washing the eyes)
- Sink
- Clean cotton hand towel

Preliminary Eyewash Procedure
- After cleansing the oral cavity and face, pour the triphala tonic into the eye glass.
- Close your eyes, lean forward slightly over the sink, and quickly cup the right eye with the liquid filled eye glass. Keep the hand towel close by to wipe off any fluids that may leak out onto the face.
- After cupping the eye with the eye glass, quickly lean the head backwards and begin to blink into the fluids for approximately 15 to 20 seconds.
- Then lean forward over the sink, release the eye glass, and wipe off the excess liquid.
- Repeat the same procedure for the left eye.

Preliminary Gargling Procedure
Refer to kavalagraha (gargling) instruction given above. Use the same triphala tonic for this preliminary gargling procedure and immediately before the akshitarpana treatment.

Akshitarpana Formulas

Season: all year

Body Type: all types

Triphala Eye Tonic

1 c water

1 tsp triphala powder

Boil water in a small stainless steel saucepan. Add the powder. Cover and simmer over medium heat for 5 minutes, or until half the water has evaporated. Remove from heat and cool. Using a fine strainer, strain the decoction, separating the sediments from the liquid.

Note: Used for preliminary eyewash and gargling procedures. This decoction and procedure may be used on a daily basis by all types to maintain clarity and coolness of sight.

Masha Paste

Yield: 2 "tanks":

2 oz whole urad beans

2 oz pearl barley

1/4 c water

Grind the urad beans and the barley in a hand food grinder to a coarse powder. Place in a small stainless steel bowl and add the water very gradually, while kneading into a firm paste dough. Be careful not to make the paste too watery or too soft. The consistency must enable you to build the miniature "tanks" used around the eyes to hold the medicated ghee, as described above. Prior to constructing the tanks, rub a few drops of sesame oil into the hands to make handling the paste easier.

Tikta Ghrita (bitter herbs and ghee)

Like all medicated ghees, *tikta ghrita* is prepared by knowledgeable, well-trained Ayurvedic pharmacologists. Medicated ghees are available from domestic sources, some of whom are listed in Appendix G. The word "tikta" refers to a particular blend of bitter Ayurvedic herbs, generally used to reduce excess Pitta and Kapha. "Ghrita" is the Sanskrit word for ghee. Ghee-making is a necessary sadhana, the method for which is described in Appendix F.

To prepare warm tikta ghrita for akshitarpana therapy, place two tablespoons of tikta ghrita in a small earthenware pot. Bring the water to a boil in a small stainless steel saucepan. Remove from heat and place the tea pot with the ghee into the boiling water. Cover the saucepan and take it into the treatment room. A double boiler may also be used for this purpose.

KARNA PURANA - OILING THE EARS

Karna purana is the process in which warm oil or medicated liquid is poured into the ears. This treatment is usually performed annually during either the autumn or the late spring season. Specific problems for which karna purana is administered include excess ear wax, earache, headache, neck pain and jaw pain. This treatment is also used for most Vata disorders relating to bodily aches and pains.

Season: all year

Body Type: all types

Conditions
Earache; nervous disorders; pain in the jaw, neck, head; loss of hearing; excess earwax; ringing sensation in the ear

Benefits
In addition to alleviating the conditions listed above, this treatment improves hearing and stimulates the sense organs. It also calms the mind and helps to balance Vata disorders.

Necessary Aids
- Clean piece of cotton cloth
- Ear dropper
- Small bowl containing the oil or other medicated liquid

Karna Purana Directions
- Clear the mind of stressful thoughts by sitting in contemplation for a short while.
- Place the container of oil or other liquid in the ear dropper, and a clean piece of cotton cloth within easy reach.
- Spread a mat on the clean floor and lie down.
- Turn onto your left side and assume the fetal position, the head slightly downward.
- Using your right hand, fill the ear dropper with the oil.
- Squeeze approximately ten drops (about 1/2-dropper tube) into the right ear. Give the drops time to trickle down the channel of the ear.
- Gently tug on the lobe of your left ear in a downward motion.

- Rest in the same position for 5 minutes.
- Cover the ear with the cotton cloth and gently turn onto your right side, once more assuming the fetal position.
- Repeat the ear drop procedure in the left ear, remembering to tug gently on the ear lobe to enable the oil to flow freely into the ear channel.
- Rest on your right side for 5 minutes. Remove the piece of cloth from the left ear and use a clean piece of it to mop up any excess oil or liquid from the entrance of the left ear.
- Lie comfortably on your back for a short while before rising.
- The head should not be exposed to extreme cold for a few hours after treatment.

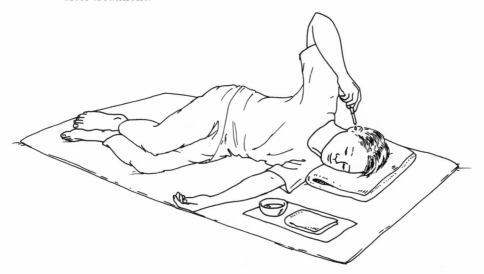

Figure 38: Oiling the Ears

Karna Purana Formulas

Season: all year

Body Type: all types

Masha Ear Tonic

Conditions

Nervous disorders; excess earwax; loss of hearing

Ingredients

    1 tbs masha oil (sesame oil may be substituted)

In a small container, warm the oil on low heat for approximately two minutes. Remove from heat and cool slightly. Ensure that the temperature of the oil is comfortable before using.

Note: For ringing in the ears or pain in the head, jaw, or ear, substitute nirgundi or bilva oil for the masha oil in this formula.

Garlic-Clove Ear Tonic

A general tonic for all ear disorders.

    1 1/2 tbs sesame oil

    1 clove garlic (peeled and slightly crushed)

In a small stainless steel container, warm the garlic in the oil on low heat for 4 minutes. Remove from heat, cover, and let sit for 5 minutes, or until the oil has cooled to a comfortable temperature for use in the ears. Remove the garlic and pour the oil into a small bowl.

Note: 5 clove buds may be substituted for the garlic. All body types may use both oils. Usually, however, Vata and Kapha types fare better with garlic oil, while Pitta types respond more favorably to the clove oil.

PART FIVE

Nasya Therapy: Nasal Insufflation

Nasya therapy, one of the five main actions of pancha karma, is also an independent snehana treatment. Generally, nasya is administered as the final therapy in pancha karma. Nasya therapy benefits all three doshas and is especially effective for Vata and Kapha disorders. Excess doshas that have accumulated in the throat, nose, sinus, and head are removed as a result of this therapy, by insufflating substances into the nasal passages.

There are several forms of nasya therapy, some of which may also be used as a daily sadhana for cleansing the pathways of the mind. Because the nose is the direct entrance to the brain and to our cognitive functions, the life force of prana enters the body through the nose. Prana controls the vital cerebral, sensory, and motor functions of the body. Nasya therapy gives immediate relief to most disorders relating to these functions.

Ayurveda relies primarily on five nasya procedures. *Navana nasya* is used for mild conditions of the head and face; it is also administered to strengthen the sensory organs. Navana nasya comprises two parts: the administering of unctuous substances through the nasal channels as a palliative measure for many disorders and the use of highly pungent decoctions or powders to induce the elimination of excess doshas from the body. Both processes may be used on a regular basis to maintain excellent health.

The second nasya procedure employed by Ayurveda is called *avapedanasya*. Here, a soft, astringent paste is introduced into the nasal passages to alleviate conditions such as hemorrhaging and bronchial disorders, poisonous snake bites, and many types of phobias.

The third nasya procedure, *dhmapana*, inserts medicated powders into the nasal channels through a straw or tube. This therapy is generally used for severe mental disorders, such as insanity and epilepsy, and for removing the effects of poison from the body.

The fourth nasya procedure, *dhoma nasya*, is the inhalation of medicated vapors made from herbs which are boiled in a decoction. This therapy is generally used for Kapha conditions such as colds, flu and congestion.

Finally, the introduction of medicated oils into the nasal passages, known as *marsha nasya*, is used to treat the disorders of children and the elderly, as well as those suffering from emaciation and extreme fragility. Depending on the strength

173

of the medicated oils, this therapy may also be used on a routine basis to ensure the maintenance of good health.

Nasya therapy stimulates the brain by creating a healthy shock to the cranial system. Nasal insufflation affects the tarpaka water of the head, resulting in the easing of cranial conditions such as hemicrania, coryza, headache, lockjaw, facial paralysis, neuralgia, cervical spondylitis, torticollis, and so on. Except for the daily or occasional use of nasya home treatments described below, this therapy, when performed as part of pancha karma, should be administered only by trained pancha karma attendants.

Navana Nasya

Season: all year
Body Type: all types
Seasonal Guidelines

Spring, autumn, winter:	morning
Summer:	mid-day
Rainy season, Vata types only:	dawn

Time of Application

Pitta types:	12:00 to 12:30 p.m.
Vata types:	3:00 to 4:00 p.m.
Kapha types:	8:00 to 10:00 a.m.

Conditions

Headache; gum disease; earache; dryness of face; premature wrinkling; facial disorders; jaundice; sinusitis

Benefits

In addition to relieving the conditions listed above, this treatment has the added benefits of giving strength to head, face, neck, shoulders, and chest, and improving rhythmic breathing. It also stimulates the brain, tones the sight, relieves fear and anxiety, and improves sleep.

Conditions during which navana nasya should not be administered

- During childhood and old age
- During pregnancy or after giving birth

- After sexual intercourse
- During fevers
- Directly after bathing
- Directly after meals or drinking alcohol
- During internal bleeding or menstruation
- Chronic insomnia
- Chronic sinusitis

Necessary Aids
- Small pottery bowl for the nasya substance
- Small pottery bowl for the massaging oil
- Eye dropper, to introduce the drops into the nasal passages
- Clean, wet, hot towel
- Clean cotton cloth

Directions
- Place the bowls with the nasya substance and the massaging oil, along with the already filled eye dropper, the clean cotton cloth, and the wet towel, within easy reach.
- Clear the mind of stressful thoughts by sitting in contemplation for a short while before the treatment.
- Wash the face and hands, then lie down on a mat on a clean floor or on a clean firm bed.
- Use a roll pillow (see sketch below) to prop the neck up while reclining the head as far back as is comfortable. The openings of the nasal passages should be facing the ceiling.
- Pour a small amount of oil into both hands and rub the entire face. Then concentrate on massaging the area around the eyes and nose.
- With both thumbs, press the sides of the nose and the areas of the sinuses.
- Crimp the fingers and gently press the cavity directly below the eyes, and then above the eyes. Both hands working simultaneously.
- With the heels of the palms, gently press the closed eyes.
- Take a few deep breaths through the nostrils and release the hands.
- Using whichever hand is most comfortable, pick up the eye dropper and squeeze 8 drops of liquid or 4 pinches of powder into the right nostril (see Increasing the Dosage below).
- There will be an immediate sensation, or "hit," to the top of the head, similar to that experienced immediately after eating raw horseradish. This treatment usually causes the eyes to water and sometimes the nose, due to the release of emotional excesses. Wipe off the discharge with the clean cloth.

- Allow a few minutes to regroup before applying the substance to the left nostril.
- Repeat the same procedure, using the same amount of liquid or powder substance.
- Rest for a few minutes before getting up.
- As a daily measure and/or a final step, wash the hands and place a few drops of sesame oil on the little finger. Insert into each nostril, turning the finger around inside each nostril to gently lubricate the nasal passages.

Note: Do not expose the head to extreme cold for a few hours after treatment.

Increasing the Dosage

The initial dosage is increased by one drop of liquid or 1/2 pinch of powder each day for the next six days. This procedure is repeated every week. For example:

Day	Drops		Pinches
1	8	or	4 pinches
2	9	or	4 1/2 pinches
3	10	or	5 pinches
4	11	or	5 1/2 pinches
5	12	or	6 pinches
6	13	or	6 1/2 pinches
7	14	or	7 pinches

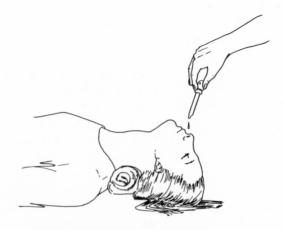

Figure 39: Navana Nasya

176

Nasal Oils and Decoctions

Season: all year

Body Type: all types

Time of Application

Vata types:	between 3:00 and 4:00 p.m.
Pitta types:	between 12:00 and 12:30 p.m.
Kapha types:	between 8:00 and 10:00 a.m.

Anu Taila (oil)

Anu taila may be used regularly to maintain mental clarity and balance.

Pour enough oil into a small bowl for your daily nasya treatment. Fill the eye dropper with the prescribed amount of oil before introducing it into the nostrils.

Sesame-Ginger Oil

Season: all year

Body Type: Vata and Kapha

Conditions

Nervous disorders, loss of memory, mental dullness, head colds, anxiety, fear, dryness of face, headache, earache, sinusitis, pain in the face, loss of smell

Ingredients

> 1 tbs sesame oil or 1 tbs ghee
> 1/2" piece of fresh, plump ginger

Warm the oil or ghee in a small stainless steel pan. Remove from heat and pour into a small bowl. Peel the ginger and mince it with a fine grater. Gather the grated ginger in the palm of your hand, make a tight fist, and squeeze the ginger juice into the oil. Cover the bowl and let sit for 30 minutes. Make sure there are no remnants of ginger in the oil before using. Fill the eye dropper before lying down to administer the oil.

Prepare only the amount of oil decoction needed for each day's use. Never re-use or refrigerate nasya substances.

Ginger Decoction

Season: all year

Body Type: Vata and Kapha

Conditions

Headache, sinusitis, colds, flu, nervous disorders, anxiety, fear, restlessness, weakness of vision, pain in the neck, shoulders, or chest

Ingredients

>1 tsp minced fresh ginger or 1/2 tsp minced
>horseradish root
>4 tbs water

Place the minced ginger or horseradish in the center of a clean cotton handkerchief or in a small cotton pouch. Gather together the ends of the handkerchief and squeeze the juice from the minced root with your hand through the cloth into a small pottery bowl. Add the water. Before using the decoction, make sure that there are no root remnants left in it. Fill your eye dropper before lying down to administer. Prepare only the amount of liquid needed for each day's use. Never re-use or refrigerate nasya decoctions.

Hot Pepper Decoction

Season: winter/late spring

Body Type: Kapha

Conditions

Congestion and mucus, bronchial disorders, colds and flu, excess nasal and oral secretions

Ingredients

>4 dried red hot chilies or 1/2 tsp coarse black pepper
>3 tbs water

Boil the water in a small stainless steel saucepan and add the chilies. Cover and simmer on low heat for 10 minutes. Remove from heat and cool for 15 minutes. Strain the peppers through a tea strainer and retain the liquid. Fill the eye-dropper with sufficient pepper water before you lie down. Prepare only the amount of decoction needed for your specific use. Never re-use or refrigerate nasya decoctions.

Nasya Powders

Traditionally, *virecan churna* and *nasika churna* are the powders used for nasal insufflation. Other powders used are calamus root, gotu kola, ginger, garlic, black pepper, and cayenne.

A nasya treatment involving powdered substances is better administered by an attending person. A straw or tube, 8 inches in length and 1/4 inch in diameter, is used to introduce the powders into the nasal channels. The appropriate amount of powder is poured into the straw via a tiny funnel, corking one end of the straw with the thumb to prevent the powder from falling through. Traditionally, the nasya attendant administers the therapy by inserting one end of the straw into the subject's nasal passage and then carefully blowing the powder into the nose.

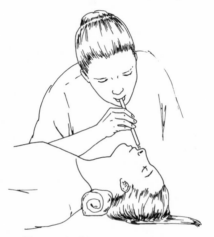

Figure 40: Dhmapana Nasya

If you are self-administering powdered substances, sit in an upright chair with your head tipped backward, propped against the back of the chair. Use a pre-filled eye dropper to introduce the powders into your nasal passage, or place the exact amount of powdered substances in a bowl and use a straw to inhale it deeply into the nasal channel.

Nasya Juices

The warmed juices of fresh asparagus root, aloe vera, and gotu kola are used to alleviate Pitta disorders such as loss of hair, ringing in the ears, anger, jealousy, and excess heat in the head. Warm milk or medicated milk decoctions are also used for Pitta disorders. This form of treatment provides sedative relief to excess Pitta.

To prepare a juice or milk decoction, two teaspoons of juice are warmed slightly in a small stainless steel pan. Optionally, a half teaspoon of ghee may be added to the warm mixture. The decoction is then put in an eye dropper ready to use.

179

CHAPTER SIX
AYURVEDIC FOMENTATION THERAPY: SVEDANA

*S*vedana therapy is a rudimentary form of nature's meditation, wherein all living things are mollified, massaged, and stimulated by the wind, rain, light and earth. The very stillness of nature is instinct with a vast immutable rhythm, as in the whispering of the wind across a desert, the trickling, shimmering raindrops on the leaves of the trees in a forest, the gurgling of the deep water as it invigorates the earth while passing through her.

When the elephants and their calves dig into the sand and breathe the minerals from the earth, they are observing nasya therapy. When the piglets dip into the mud, gleefully coating their little bodies, they are performing svedana and snehana therapies. When the fleeting wind brushes the leaves and water caresses our skin, all of nature is participating in cosmic abhyanga. Similarly, all Ayurvedic rejuvenation therapies mimic the essential rhythms, salves, sound and touch inherent in nature.

Svedana therapy, the topic of this chapter, is designed to induce sweating, which occurs through the skin, by way of the hair follicles, and through the fat tissues of the body. As a result, the body's fiery content increases, stimulating agni, which then facilitates the rounding up and expulsion of ama from the system.

Appetite and taste are both enhanced as bodily ama is expelled. Svedana therapy also works with the water that regulates all bodily waters. This regulating water, kledaka, is continuously cleansed as sweat is eliminated through the skin. Sweat is one of the waste materials produced by the body's fat tissues.

Ayurveda considers bodily wastes to be nourishing to the organism as they make their way towards the body's exit points. Once evacuated from the body, they naturally serve to nurture the earth so that it may sustain vegetation and other forms of life. In many Ayurvedic therapies, the dung of the cow and other animals is used to incinerate the rejuvenative powdered remedies, called *bhamsa,* that contain precious stones and metals such as pearl, gold and silver. Still more fundamental uses of bodily wastes are practiced by the yogins who drink their first urine in the early morning to stimulate the entire organism. Urine is the residual liquid waste generated from the foods that have already nourished the tissue chain. Introducing this latent waste material is medicinal to the system since it resonates with familiarity in the body from which it was so recently eliminated. Rather than being a putrid waste, urine may serve as an essence residue to the organism. Of course the yogins who reabsorb their urine also observe a wholesome diet and way of life, both of which are reverent to nature; therefore, their residual waste has the same excellent qualities as do their food and tissue condition.

Since sweat is a response to heat, the svedana therapies are performed to aggravate the fat tissue and thereby force excess sweat out of the system. Svedana, like snehana, is both a preparatory procedure for pancha karma and an independent form of treatment. In pancha karma, svedana is applied after snehana and before vamana, or emesis therapy, is performed. Svedana liquefies the aggravated doshas, which generally become ungrounded by the preceding snehana therapy, thus rendering them ready for expulsion from the body. The remaining therapies in pancha karma, namely emesis, purgation and/or enema therapies complete the process of ejecting the fluid and uprooted, excess doshas from the system.

Svedana therapy involves various forms of sudation treatment, which help to relieve bodily stiffness, heaviness and coldness. Although these treatments are used to eliminate excesses of all three doshas, they are best suited to Vata and Kapha disorders. Svedana is excellent for conditions such as the loss of appetite, bodily toxins, rheumatism, arthritis, heaviness in the body, and low digestive fire.

Due to the production of sweat, the channels of the body are cleansed, thereby regulating Vata. As a result, bodily wastes—urine, feces, flatus, and sweat—are efficiently eliminated. Vata is further relieved because of svedana's soothing action on the joints. Due to the regulated production of sweat in the body during svedana, Kapha is also relieved in that it is reduced, along with conditions such as excess sleep, lethargy, and excess weight.

There are thirteen classic forms of svedana therapies and within these are scores of variations. The thirteen therapies are: *sankara, prasthara, nadi, parisheka, avagahana, jentaka, kuti, ashmaghna, bhu, kumbhika, karshu, kupa* and *holaka*. These thirteen therapies are classified into three main groups: the wet therapies, sankara, prasthara, parisheka, and kumbhika; the dry, sauna-type therapies, jentaka, karshu, kuti, bhu, kupa, holaka, and ashmaghna; and, finally, the therapies specific to a certain part of the body, nadi and avagahana.

The sankara form of therapy, also known as *upanaha*, is performed with a large ball, known as a bolus or pinda. The size of an orange, the bolus contains medicated paste wrapped in cloth and is rubbed firmly over the body to produce fomentation. Upanaha is a generic term indicating the use of a poultice. The term is also used when a particular limb or part of the body is bandaged with a poultice application. The sankara or upanaha method of therapy includes a variety of treatment such as *pinda, bandhana, sthambana, anna lepa* and *paca kizhi*. Pinda sveda, the most commonly used bolus form of therapy, is a process by which a poultice of rice, milk and herbs is made and wrapped into a large ball covered with cloth. After a detailed procedure that involves massaging the body with oil and applying a paste to the head, the subject assumes various sitting and reclining positions while being rubbed with the warm boluses. Generally, two attendants, one on each side, apply the boluses simultaneously. Many poultices are used, depending on the nature of the disease.

In prasthara sveda, a poultice bed containing heating grains and herbs or spices and wrapped in silk or woolen cloth, is used to generate the fomentation.

In nadi sveda, a long, curved, perforated tube attached to a pitcher of hot herbal decoction is used to steam various parts of the body. The perforations on the tube are generally covered with leaves that are nurturing to Vata. In parisheka sveda, a pitcher with holes on the bottom fitted with bamboo tubes is used to shower warm decoctions generally made from Vata alleviating roots.

Jentaka sveda was performed even before Buddha's time. This form of sudation is performed in a specifically designed circular lodge, which is surrounded by water. In the heart of the sweat lodge is a circular oven built of clay with large apertures around it into which wood is placed. Jentaka sveda is as intense a sudation method as it is ancient and is rarely practiced today, even in India, due to the enormous technicalities involved in the construction of the lodge.

Ashmaghna sveda is the process by which a large slab of stone is heated by burning various herbs on its surface. After the fire ashes are removed, water is sprinkled on the stone to cool it down to a bearable temperature. Silk or woolen cloth is then spread over the stone's surface. The subject, wrapped in cotton or covered with animal hide, then reclines on the stone for a period of time.

In karshu sveda, an elongated pit is dug in the earth, and a fire is made from certain woods and herbs. When the fire becomes smoke free, a sleeping cot heavily covered with animal hide and cotton blankets is placed over the smoldering pit of embers. The subject, totally clothed in cotton apparel, then lies on the cot.

In kuti sveda, a round sweat lodge is built with thick walls and no windows. The inner walls of the lodge are plastered with various herbs and cow dung and/or mud. Traditionally, the sveda cot is covered with animal hides, cotton blankets and kusha grass and placed in the center of the room, surrounded by burning furnaces. The subject lies on the cot fully clothed.

In bhu sveda, an area is cleared on the earth, sheltered from the air, and certain herbs and wood are burned there. The ashes of the fire are then removed, and the earth is sprinkled with water, then covered with animal hides or woolen blankets. The subject, also heavily covered in woolen blankets, lies on the covered, heated earth for sudation.

In kumbhika sveda, a sleeping cot is placed over a pitcher of hot decoction which is half buried in the earth. Hot iron balls are thrown into the decoction to maintain a steaming temperature. The cot is covered with a thin silk or cotton sheet, and the subject wears thick and loose clothing.

Kupa sveda, similar to karshu sveda, involves lying on a covered cot over a smoldering pit of smokeless flames. In kupa sveda, the pit is heaped with the dried dung of elephants, camels, horses, and cows, instead of wood and herbs, and is then ignited.

In holaka sveda, the dung of elephants, horses, cows, and camels is burnt directly on a six foot surface of the earth. A cot covered with thin cotton sheets is placed directly over the smokeless ashes. The subject, loosely clothed in cotton, lies on the cot and receives sudation.

Avagahana sveda, also ancient, is generally used to treat conditions of the lower body, such as hemorrhoids. A tub of warm herbal decoction is prepared, and the subject sits in it. Before treatment, medicated oil is applied topically to the problem area, the subject then sitting in the warm decoction until perspiration is induced.

Soft, Wet, and Dry Effects of Svedana Treatment

There are three main ways in which svedana treatments may be applied. By decreasing the applied pressure and heat intensity, as well as the potency of the medicated substances and herbs used, a wet or dry treatment may be altered to become a soft or mild svedana. Generally, a soft sveda is used for conditions that require delicate handling, i.e. Pitta disorders, where the digestive fire is vulnerable, and conditions germane to the elderly or the extremely weakened. Soft sveda is also used for disorders that occur in excessively cold weather.

The naturally wet svedana, such as the treatments which use poultice or steam, are generally recommended for Vata disorders. Depending on the nature of the condition, a wet therapy may be altered to become either soft or sharp. Svedana performed with dry heat, such as the sauna type therapies like bhu and jentaka, are mostly used to alleviate Kapha conditions. Treatments used for Kapha disorders are generally sharp and strong, but, once again, depending on the nature of the disorder, may be altered to become mild or soft.

The therapy recommended for each dosha, and the various disorders the therapies address, are indicated before the description of each therapy.

The Ten Natural Living Forms of Sudation

The process of svedana occurs naturally within certain human activities. These activities are:

- Physical exercise or activity
- Being in a warm room
- Wearing heavy or warm clothing
- Hunger
- Excessive use of alcohol or drugs
- Fear
- Anger or rage
- Application of poultices or medicinal properties to the body
- Intense sports, i.e., wrestling, physical sparring, running, jumping
- Exposure to the sun

Like all Ayurvedic rejuvenative treatments, svedana may only be performed at certain times and for specific conditions.

PART ONE

Observances Before Svedana Therapy

Appropriate Conditions for Svedana Therapy

- As a preliminary treatment before pancha karma.
- As an independent rejuvenative therapy for all types, but mostly for Vata and Kapha disorders.
- For Vata disorders such as arthritis, paraplegia, dryness of skin, nervousness, earache, loss of memory, insomnia, mental stress, stiffness of joints and constipation.
- Kapha disorders such as colds, cough, phlegmatic disorders, rheumatoid arthritis, headaches, water retention, anemia, obesity, heaviness of body, lethargy and anorexia.
- For bilious disorders.
- While observing celibacy during and for a short while before and after treatment.
- While the body is fairly strong.
- While refraining from cold drinks, cold foods, cold baths and exposure to cold, during and for a short while before and after therapy. Cool fluids and unctuous foods may be taken before treatment during the summer season.
- While the subject's head is pointing towards the east, if treatment begins in the morning, or towards the west if treatment is given in the late afternoon or early evening.

When svedana is applied during improper seasons or for inappropriate conditions, it causes adverse conditions such as headaches, fainting, tiredness, weakness and wasting of the body, burning sensations or coldness in the limbs, indigestion, diarrhea or constipation, jaundice, bilious disorders and nausea.

A schedule of calming diet and activities is maintained during svedana therapy and for a period of time thereafter. Details on the healing diet and activities are presented in Chapters Eight and Nine. Cleansing ablutions are also observed by both the practitioner and the patient prior to beginning therapy (see Chapter Nine).

Preliminary oil massage and fomentation treatments are to be administered on the subject prior to the following svedana therapies. For details on massage and appropriate massaging oils for each type, see Chapter Four.

Inappropriate Conditions for Svedana Therapy

- Pregnancy, or directly after giving birth
- Menstrual cycles
- Hemorrhaging
- Ulcerated conditions
- Diarrhea
- Digestive disorders, such as high stomach agni, indigestion, excess thirst or hunger
- Jaundice disorders
- Chest injuries
- Severe asthmatic conditions
- Gout and leprosy
- Heart disease
- Eye diseases or weakened vision
- Diseases of the scrotum
- State of intoxication
- Before or after sexual activity

Seasonal Svedana Guidelines for Each Body Type

Temperate and Tropical Schedule

Pitta disorders:	early and late spring: (March 15 to May 15)	early evening
	summer:	early evening
	autumn:	mid-morning
Vata disorders:	rainy season, early part: (July 15 to August 15)	early evening
	late spring: (April 15 to May 15)	mid-morning or early evening
	summer:	early evening
	autumn:	mid-morning
Kapha disorders:	late spring: (April 15 to May 15)	mid-morning
	summer:	early evening
	early and late winter: (November 15 to March 15)	mid-day

Svedana Therapy: Proper Times and Seasons
- During the cold season, the soft type of svedana therapies are generally used.
- During the warm and cool seasons, the sharp type of svedana therapies are generally used.

Svedana Therapy: Improper Times and Seasons
- As a general rule, svedana should not be performed during excessively hot or cold days when all three doshas are generally easily aggravated.

Observing the Subject During Therapy
During the svedana therapies, it is vital to remain alert to the signs and symptoms of the sudated subject. The attendant must remain nearby throughout the entire period of sudation. If certain adverse symptoms are experienced by the subject during therapy, the treatment must stop immediately. These symptoms include: no sign of perspiration; the subject experiences coldness; increase of bodily pain; and any sign of discomfort or intolerance. Warm, unctuous foods should be served with warming teas such as cardamom, cinnamon, ginseng and ginger. If high Pitta symptoms are present, such as fainting, burning sensation, uncontrollable thirst, weakness of voice or limbs, bluish tinge to the skin or fever, serve sweet, cooling and unctuous foods, e.g., barley or wheat porridge, fruits, water and cooling teas such as saffron, coriander, and fennel.

For severe adverse Pitta symptoms, resulting from svedana therapy, the astringent therapy, sthambana, may be administered.

When the svedana therapies are performed successfully, ample perspiration is produced, all bodily coldness disappears, bodily pains are alleviated or significantly reduced, softness of body is observed; and there is a desire for cold fluids.

Characteristics of Svedana Substances
Like the snehana therapies, svedana is accompanied by a vast Ayurvedic pharmacopoeia of herbs, oils and substances used to stimulate and invigorate the body through perspiration. The qualities of substances used for svedana are hot, sharp, mobile, unctuous, dry, liquid, stable, heavy and subtle, the ingredients have a strong fire and water element component to them.

The unctuous property of the ingredients used in this therapy provides wetness and softness to the body, allowing it to relax and open its vital pores. The heavy character of the ingredients adds strength to the body and breaks down waste matter through external heat, both dry and wet in nature. The hot quality penetrates the skin and stimulates kledaka water to release her waste through the fat tissue. Heat is essential to all tissues and is life supporting to the Vata and Kapha doshas as well.

188

The sharp quality of svedana substances permeates deeply into the concentric layers of bodily tissue and changes the organism into a state of motility necessary for the expulsion of bodily waters and toxins. Sharpness also creates a burning sensation in the body, which facilitates the elimination of excess Kapha. The liquid quality allows excess doshas to join forces with the waste matter exiting the body. Liquification of bodily matter is essential to the organism under the stress of sudation. It helps the body and mind to remain flexible and alert.

The dryness of svedana substances, when applied directly, counteracts the wetness remaining from the preceding snehana therapy, thus reducing the moisture in the organism before svedana actually begins. If the body is excessively laden with water, the heat created from svedana therapy may be detrimental to the tissues, since water is a massive conductor of both heat and cold. The firm quality allows the body to maintain its stability during the heightened state of unrest caused by svedana therapy. Stability is very important to the organism during this period of cleansing. Because the pancha karma therapies are fundamentally eliminatory, the body needs the ample reassurance of warmth, wellness, and so on during treatment. The ingredients' firm factor helps to establish these feelings in the subject.

The subtle, atomic, fine and penetrating property of svedana substances, referred to as *suksma*, maintains the intrinsic balance within the body's most minute particles. Innate to all life, suksma is a principle of the subtle bodily fire, called *tejas*. This most subtle quality in the ingredients used in the therapy under discussion operates through the subtlest channels of the body, called *nadis*. Tejas helps the body maintain its metabolism while producing combustion. It carries the vital essences of radiance, color and luminosity to every cell in the body. The essence of tejas becomes most active at the point when the subtle property, carried in the ingredient, reaches the body's atomic particles, igniting self-cognition through our cellular memory.

Precautionary Measures

Due to the intense heat generated by most svedana therapies, precautions are taken to protect those areas of the body that cannot sustain excessive heat, namely the area surrounding the heart, the eyes, groin and vaginal areas of the male and female respectively.

Traditionally, a pearl necklace inserted into a cotton pouch or a fresh wet lotus flower was placed directly over the subject's heart during fomentation procedures. These items, which are the best protection for the heart, should still be used if at all possible. If, however, neither is available, a cold wet 4-inch cotton pouch filled with sandalwood paste should be placed directly over the heart and remain there for the entire duration of the treatment.

To protect the eyes, two small pouches the size of ping-pong balls, filled with soft whole wheat dough, are placed on the closed eyelids during treatment. This precaution is absolutely essential, especially during sauna or steaming svedanas, to protect the eyes from the intense heat.

An ancient apparel still used today is the loin cloth, which is looser and more flexible than underwear. The loin cloth is recommended for both male and female subjects to protect the delicate groin and vaginal areas during sudation therapy.

Note: Since these items are used in most of the svedana therapies, instructions and illustrations are included in Appendix D.

Having provided a general introduction to fomentation therapy, each method of treatment will now be discussed in detail. The formulas referred to below are set out at the end of this chapter.

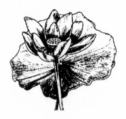

PART TWO

Application of Svedana Therapies
Upanaha: Poultice Therapy

PINDA SVEDA - ENTIRE BODY POULTICE

Upanaha sveda is the generic term for these svedana therapies that use poultices and plasters. As mentioned earlier, pinda sveda is a more recent adaptation of the sankara form of sveda therapy, in which a bolus, pinda, the size of a large orange and made from grains, herbs, and milk, is used to firmly massage the entire body. Like most svedana therapies, pinda sveda helps to awaken cellular memory through the intense stimulation caused by sweating. It is also an excellent relief for many illnesses and is considered especially superb for diseases such as paraplegia and poliomyelitis, which result in the wasting away of muscular tissues.

Prior to the actual pinda treatment, the subject's head and body are thoroughly massaged with the appropriate medicated oil. A preparation of herbal buttermilk is then applied to the head, following the same procedure as outlined in the masthiskya treatment (see pg. 142). The subject's head is shaved before pinda sveda is applied, preferably on the evening of the full moon, with the treatment beginning the next morning. Totally invigorating to the system, this therapy, like most of the rejuvenative treatments in Ayurveda, is beneficial to both the giver and receiver, since its methodical application induces a sense of great harmony.

Tree bark and leaves were used by the ancients as massage ingredients to maintain healthy gums, skin, and hair. So, too, in pinda sveda, the leaves of the coconut palm or castor plant are used to shave the poultice from the skin. Some leaves are used for their volatile qualities, others for their astringency; the antiseptic quality of all medicinal leaves, when used externally, encourage the pores of the skin to close. The fresh leaves used in Ayurvedic therapy are much more than physically healing—lying on a bed of *kusha* grass, for instance, is nothing less than a celestial experience!

Pinda sveda is excellent for Vata and Kapha disorders since both doshas are innately cold in nature and the excessive heat stimulates the fat tissues and releases sweat through the skin, generating a total euphoria of warmth throughout the organism. Due to the heat producing nature of pinda sveda, Vata disorders may also be treated. Pinda sveda should be performed in the early morning for Kapha and Pitta disorders, and in the early evening for Vata disorders.

191

Pinda Sveda

Season: use seasonal guidelines

Body Type: all types

Duration of Treatment: 7 to 14 days; 1 1/4 hours each day

Time: early morning or early evening; begin on first day of the full moon

Conditions

Vata disorders:* arthritis; emaciation; weakness of muscular functions; facial paralysis; dryness of skin; loss of memory; insomnia; mental stress; stiffness of joints; paraplegia; poliomyelitis

Kapha disorders: phlegmatic disorders (colds, coughs, congestion); bronchial asthma; headaches; rheumatoid arthritis; anemia; obesity;* water retention; anorexia; heaviness of body, lethargy

Pitta disorders:* bilious disorders; blood disorders

Use soft-to-moderate pressure for these conditions.

Benefits

In addition to relieving the conditions listed above, this therapy has the added benefit of revitalizing the entire body, giving energy and mobility. It also relieves stress, restoring the appetite and sleep patterns.

Necessary Aids

- Two attendants
- 4 clean cotton napkins, 18 inches square, to wrap the poultice in
- Medium-size clay pot, tightly covered, containing the hot bala decoction and 4 boluses*
- Small stainless steel bowl, covered with a hot damp towel, containing the warm amalaki buttermilk paste for the head treatment
- Small stainless steel bowl, covered with a hot damp towel, containing the heating herbal paste for the head treatment
- Small covered pottery bowl containing the appropriate massage oil
- Eye pads*
- 4 leaves from the castor plant or coconut palm
- 2 pieces of cotton gauze, 48 inches long and 4 inches wide, to bandage the head
- 5 clean, damp cotton hand towels
- 3 clean cotton sheets, 2 to spread on the treatment table and 1 to use for covering the subject
- 3 dry hand towels for attendants' use
- Loin cloth*
- Clean bath towel

- Large stainless steel bowl in which to empty the boluses
- Large bucket of water for attendants to wash their hands
- Large empty bucket to discard used treatment items
- One-burner portable gas stove to keep the bala decoction warm (optional)
- Bathtub

See Appendix D

Note: Arrange all the necessary preparations for the head treatments, body massage as well as pinda sveda before beginning therapy.

Preliminaries to Pinda Sveda

Full-body Massage

For best results, pinda sveda should be preceded by a full body massage with the appropriate oil. The subject should then be allowed to rest for 15 minutes before proceeding.

Head Treatment

- Spread a clean cotton sheet on the treatment table. Have the subject undress and lie down on his/her back.
- Spread a clean cotton sheet over the subject.
- Using the appropriate oil, massage firmly into the head.
- Using his/her hands, one attendant spreads the amalaki buttermilk evenly over the subject's head. The paste should be approximately 1/4 inch thick.
- To apply to the back of the head, gently lift the head.
- Place a piece of cloth under the subject's head and rest it back down on the table.
- The second attendant evenly spreads the warm herbal paste, about 1/8 inch thick, on the strip of gauze.
- The first attendant, after washing the buttermilk off his/her hands, wraps the gauze around the subject's head, keeping the buttermilk paste in place (Fig. 26, Chapter Five).
- Bandage the head loosely with another piece of gauze to prevent the paste from seeping through.
- Let the subject rest for a few minutes. During this time, the attendants may clean the paste containers and so on.

Pinda Treatment

The subject assumes seven postures through the duration of the treatment.

1. Sitting Position

- Have the subject assume a sitting position with the legs extended.

- Cover the groin or vaginal area with the loin cloth.
- Coordinating their movement on either side of the subject, both attendants take a freshly heated bolus. Beginning with the subject's hands, rub the bolus against the skin, using long upward strokes, up the arms to the shoulders.
- Encourage the subject to let his/her arms hang loosely during the rubbing procedure.
- Then, using shorter upward and downward strokes, "scrub" along both arms until they are massaged completely.
- The rubbing time spent on the arms should be 5 minutes.
- As soon as the boluses begin to cool, return them to the hot decoction and take out the heated ones. Before applying to the subject's arms, test the temperature of the bolus on your hands to make sure it is bearable.

2. **Lying on the back**
- Have the subject lie on his/her back.
- With fluid co-ordination and freshly heated boluses, both attendants begin to rub the chest from the waist up, using long upward strokes.
- For female subjects, massage gently around the breasts without applying any pressure.
- Then using short upward and downward strokes, as you would to brush the skin, rub the entire area of the chest, again taking the same precaution on the breast area of female subjects.
- Then move to the legs and hips. Replace the boluses with freshly heated ones, test the temperature, and, beginning from the top of the toes, and using long upward strokes, rub up the front of the legs to the knees.
- Then use short upward and downward strokes, as you would to brush the skin, to rub the front of the lower legs thoroughly.
- Repeat the same procedure from the knees to the groin or vaginal area, without rubbing the groin or vaginal area.

3. **Lying on the left side**
- Gently guide the subject to his/her left side. Move the right arm slightly forward to expose the right side of the body. Have the subject bend the knees slightly so that the position is more comfortable.
- With freshly heated boluses, one attendant begins at the side of the right foot and rubs up the calf to the right knee, while the second attendant begins at the knee and rubs along the right thigh, over the hip, and up to the waist.
- Begin with the long upward slide and then follow up with short upward and downward brushing movements.
- Using a fresh bolus, one attendant then rubs up the right side of the

body from the waist to the armpit. Use gentle circular movements in the armpit and rub for no more than a few seconds.

- At the same time, the second attendant, using a fresh bolus, rubs the area around the right shoulder and up the side of the neck. Use small circular movements for this area of the body, and while rubbing the neck, maintain a gentle stroking motion.

4. Lying on the right side

- Gently guide the subject to his/her right side, bending the knees slightly for a more comfortable position.
- Using fresh boluses, repeat as for the left side.

5. Lying on the stomach

- Have the subject turn onto his/her stomach.
- Standing on either side of the subject, and coordinating their movements, both attendants rub the entire back as follows:
- Using long upward strokes and beginning from the back of the heels, rub up the calves to the backs of the knees; then rub the same area with short upward and downward strokes.
- Continue the same stroking procedure from the back of the knees to the buttocks.
- Lift the loin cloth and rub the buttock area firmly in a circular clockwise motion. Rub the sides of the hips as well, using the same circular clockwise motion. Remember to use freshly heated boluses as necessary.
- One attendant then rubs the kidney area between the buttocks and waist, using short upward and downward movements, for approximately 3 minutes. At the same time, the other attendant rubs the back of the neck for a few minutes, using gentle short strokes along the back of the neck to the center of the shoulder blade.
- With freshly heated boluses in hand, both attendants continue the symphony of rubbing strokes along the back. Beginning at the waist and going up to the shoulders, use long upward strokes, then follow with short upward and downward brushing movements.

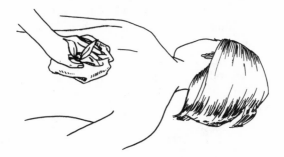

Figure 41: Bolus Application on Back

195

- Rub the shoulders for a few minutes, using small back and forth strokes along the shoulders, starting from the center of the scapulae and continuing to rub outward towards the arms.
- Put the boluses back in the pot of hot decoction. Cover the subject with a sheet and allow him/her to rest for a few minutes.

6. **Lying on the back**
- Gently guide the subject onto his/her back. Remove the covering sheet.
- Repeat the procedures in (2) above.

7. **Sitting position**
- Help the subject sit up and have him/her extend the legs.
- Repeat the procedures in item (1) above, rubbing the arms for one minute.
- Then rub the chest, back, and legs, for no longer than one or two minutes each. Use the same procedures as in (2) and (5) above, except that the subject remains sitting.
- Finally, with freshly heated boluses, rub the palms of the hands gently in small circular motions, and the soles of the feet firmly with both circular and short upward and downward strokes.

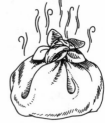

- Place all four boluses into the hot decoction and allow them to re-heat for a few minutes.
- Remove the boluses form the pot and unwrap them. Put the poultice contents in a large stainless steel bowl and place it within your reach.

Figure 42: Bolus

- With your hands, apply a thin layer of poultice to the subject's body while he/she is still sitting.
- Then, using the coconut or castor plant leaf, gently scrape the poultice off the skin in a shaving gesture, using long downward strokes. Begin from the nape of the neck and shave down the back; then shave from the throat down the chest, from above the thighs down to the toes, from the buttocks down to the heels and, finally, from the shoulders down to the finger tips.
- Using the damp towel, wipe the body clean of all remaining poultice, maintaining a general downward stroke.
- While one attendant begins to clean up the remains of the treatment, the other removes the double layer of bandage from the subject's head in one brisk swoop.
- Use a clean damp towel to wipe off the rest of the buttermilk and paste from the subject's head. Then pat the head dry with a towel.
- Run a warm bath and pour the remaining bala decoction, which

kept the boluses warm, into the bath water. Allow the subject to relax in the bath for 10 minutes, while he/she washes the poultice, paste, and oil off his/her body. Do not use soap.

- Provide the subject with a clean bath towel to dry off.
- Have the subject put on warm clothing.
- Cover the treatment table with a clean sheet.
- Have the subject rest on his/her back for 15 minutes.
- Place the cooling eye pads over each eye.
- Remove all of the treatment apparatus, while maintaining a general air of quietude.
- Wrap the subject's head (see procedure in Appendix D) and discuss the need to keep the head wrapped while outdoors to guard against exposure to coldness or dampness. This procedure is to be maintained throughout the period of treatment and for the same length of time after the completion of treatment.
- Advise the subject to refrain from taking cold foods or drinks and cold baths or showers, again for the same period of time as the treatment time.

Pinda Sveda Massage Oils, Pastes and Poultice

In each of the following recipes, it is important to remember to prepare sufficient oil or poultice for that day's use only. This will avoid waste, as old oils or poultices should not be used for treatment, nor should poultices ever be re-used.

Season: use seasonal guidelines

Narayana Oil

Body Type: Vata disorders

For head massage:

> 2 tbs Narayana oil (or the same amount of pinda, dhanvantari or dashamula oil)

In a small stainless steel saucepan, warm oil. Pour into a small pottery container and cover securely to keep warm.

197

Sandalwood Oil

Body Type: Pitta disorders

For head massage:

> 2 tbs sandalwood oil (or the same amount of
> ksheerabala oil)

Pour oil into a small pottery container and cover to keep at room temperature.

Amavathahara Oil

Body Type: Kapha disorders

For head massage:

> 2 tbs amavathahara oil (or the same amount of kottumcukadi oil)

In a small stainless steel saucepan, warm oil. Pour into a small pottery container and cover securely to keep warm.

Sesame Oil

Body Type: Vata disorders

For body massage:

> 1 cup sesame oil

In a small stainless steel saucepan, warm oil for approximately 2 minutes over low heat. Pour into a pottery container and cover securely to keep warm.

Ghee-Oil

Body Type: Pitta disorders

For body massage:

> 1/2 c pure ghee
> 1/2 c sesame oil

In a small stainless steel saucepan, melt ghee over low heat. Remove from heat and pour in sesame oil. Let mixture cool and then pour into a pottery container. Cover securely to maintain the cool temperature.

Sesame Oil-Ghee

Body Type: Kapha disorders

For body massage:

> 3/4 c sesame oil
> 1/4 c pure ghee

In a small stainless steel saucepan, melt ghee over low heat. Add sesame oil and let warm for 5 minutes. Remove from heat and pour mixture into a pottery container. Cover securely to maintain the heat.

Pinda Sveda Amalaki Buttermilk Paste

Body Type: all types

For use as a first course of treatment for the head. Use freshly-made warm paste for all body types.

> For recipe, see Milk Products Recipe, Appendix F.

Buttermilk paste used for treatment should be no more than 3 days old. Never re-use the same batch of buttermilk paste for more than one treatment.

Pinda Sveda Warm Herbal Paste

Body Type: all types

For head wrap

> 1 1/4 c sesame seeds
> 2 tsp cinnamon powder
> 1/2 c bala powder
> 1 tbs shatavari powder
> 2 tsp purnarnava powder
> 1 tbs mustard seeds
> 1 tbs cardamom seeds
> 1/4 c hot water

In a medium cast-iron skillet, roast sesame seeds over medium low heat for 5 minutes. Shift the seeds occasionally with a flat wooden spoon to prevent burning. Grind to a coarse powder in a suribachi, then place in a medium-size stainless steel bowl. Retrieve all the powder from the crevices of the suribachi with a small brush or a clean napkin. In the same skillet, roast cardamom and mustard seeds over low heat for a few minutes. Remove from heat and grind to a coarse powder in the suribachi; then combine with the sesame powder and add bala, shatavari, cinnamon, and purnarnava powders. Add the hot water and mix with a spatula to

199

form a soft paste, thick enough to spread on the gauze. Cover with a hot, damp towel to keep the paste warm. Make fresh paste for every treatment.

Pinda Sveda Poultice

Body Type: all types

2 c dried bala root

8 pt water

2 c certified raw milk

3/4 c short grain brown rice (substitute hulled barley for Kapha disorders and wheat berries for Pitta disorders)

4 clean cotton napkins (18 inches square)

Note: Sixty-day-old brown rice is recommended, i.e., 60 days from the time the rice was harvested.

In a large stainless steel pot, bring the water to a boil and add bala roots. Cover and simmer on medium heat for approximately 4 hours, or until 3/4 of the liquid has evaporated. Carefully strain the hot liquid through a colander into a medium-size stainless steel pot. Return the used roots to the earth. The liquid yield should measure about 4 cups. Pour 2 cups into a heavy pot. Cover and let sit on a warming stove while the poultice porridge is being prepared.

Add the milk to the remaining decoction. Bring to a boil, then add brown rice. Cover and simmer on medium low heat for 1 1/2 hours, or until it becomes the consistency of a thick porridge.

Spread the four napkins on a counter; when the porridge is still piping hot, place a ladle full (approximately 2/3 cup) in the center of each napkin. Carefully pick up two opposite edges of each napkin and tie into as tight a single knot as possible, while keeping the porridge inside. Tie the remaining two ends of each napkin in the same way; then take the two ends of the first knot and tie them securely into a finishing second knot. Repeat with the remaining two ends. The end result should be four firmly tied balls or boluses of porridge with knotted ends on the top to serve as handles while massaging the subject (Fig. 43). Each bolus should be approximately 3 1/4 inches in diameter, the size of a large orange.

Add any remaining porridge to the hot bala decoction and pour into a heavy pottery container. Put the four boluses into the container and cover securely to retain maximum heat for the pinda sveda treatment. Take a large ladle along with the pottery container into the treatment room to lift the boluses out of the pot when needed. Since they are to be kept

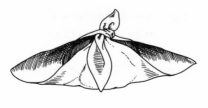
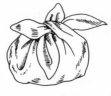

Figure 43: Bolus Wrapping

very hot, the boluses are likely to be too hot to handle with bare hands. Let them sit for a few minutes and then test them before applying. Pick the bolus up by its knotted end and use the ball portion to rub on the subject's body.

BANDHANA SVEDA - LOCALIZED POULTICE APPLICATION

Bandhana sveda is a brief form of svedana therapy where a poultice made from herbs is tied onto the affected area of the body. Traditionally, a wrapping of leather or silk is used as a bandage. Neither material breathes well and thus facilitates proper sudation of the affected area. This therapy is used to alleviate pain, heaviness, and stiffness in various areas of the body, as well to relieve localized pain, swelling, cysts, ulcerations, and fat accumulation. Poultices are never applied to areas surrounding the scrotum, vagina, eyes, or heart. This therapy may also be performed at home, with the aid of a family member or friend, if necessary.

Season: use seasonal guidelines

Body Type: all types

Time: early morning or early evening

Duration of Treatment: 7 or 14 days; 1 1/2 hours daily

Conditions

Vata disorders: pain or stiffness in joints; arthritic conditions in various joints; dry, hard cysts

201

Pitta disorders: ulceration/inflammation of skin; skin rashes (eczema, psoriasis, and so on); acne; inflamed cysts and swellings; stiffness in jaws or limbs

Kapha disorders: rheumatoid arthritis; swellings; heaviness in limbs; water retention; acne; fatty deposits

Benefits
In addition to relieving the conditions listed above, this treatment has the general effect of alleviating stiffness and inflammation in the body, as well as removing putrid flesh and fatty deposits.

Necessary Aids
- Small sterilized stainless steel bowl containing the herbal plaster
- Sterilized stainless steel spatula
- Medium sterilized stainless steel bowl containing witch hazel solution
- 4 pieces of cotton gauze, 4 inches square, on a stainless steel tray
- Pair of sharp sterilized scissors
- Surgical tape, if treatment is to be applied to the face or buttocks
- Pair of sterilized rubber gloves
- 6-inch-wide sterilized wrapping of soft leather (preferably deer hide) or silk fabric; cut length according to the size of the area to be bandaged

Bandhana Treatment
- If the affected area is on the upper body, have the subject sit on an upright chair.
- If the affected area is on the face or lower body, have the subject lie on the treatment table.
- Take the clean piece of cotton gauze, soaked in witch hazel solution, and scrub the affected area of the body. If the condition is very inflamed or painful, use a gentle touch to cleanse it.
- Apply the herbal paste on the affected area, using a sterilized stainless steel spatula, using short upward strokes. Spread the paste evenly, approximately 1/2-inch thick.
- Wrap the pre-cut piece of silk or leather wrapping over the area in a clockwise direction, making sure that the bandage is at least four layers thick.
- With sharp scissors, split the end 12 inches of the bandage up the center to tie the bandage in place.
- If the affected area is around the jaws, tie the bandage under the

chin, far enough back to cover the affected area, and wrap it around the top of the head to secure it.

- Let the subject rest in a quiet, warm place for 1 1/2 hours and check on him/her occasionally.
- Help the subject to assume the most appropriate posture for unwrapping the bandage.
- Using a clean damp face towel, scoop the plaster off and discard into the bucket.
- With gauze soaked in the witch hazel solution, wipe the area clean; adjust the amount of pressure to the degree of pain or inflammation.
- Wrap the area with a clean piece of gauze before the subject leaves.

Before preparing the following formulas, follow sterilization procedures found in Appendix E. These measures are to be used in all snehana and svedana therapies involving the application of pastes, poultices, or plasters directly to inflamed, ulcerated, open sores, and for other physical conditions which could easily become contaminated. Before making the paste or poultice, sterilize all utensils used in its preparation and application, as well as all containers that will hold the ingredients.

Witch Hazel Solution

2 fl oz witch hazel

4 c water

In a small sterilized pot, bring the water to boil. Cover and simmer on medium heat until half the water has evaporated. Remove from heat and let sit for 10 minutes. Add witch hazel while water is still warm. Use to wash your hands before treatment and to clean the affected areas of the subject's body before applying the paste.

Bandhana Sveda Formulas

Season: use seasonal guidelines

Bandhana Sveda - Vata and Kapha Paste

Body Type: Vata and Kapha disorders

> 1/4 c amalaki buttermilk (see recipe for Takra Dhara, pg. 143)
> 1/4 c dashamula powder
> 1/4 c castor root powder
> 1/4 c sesame seeds
> 1/4 c sesame oil
> 4 tbs ground rock salt
> 10 drops essential oil of eucalyptus or ginger

In a small sterilized bowl, pour in freshly made amalaki buttermilk. Grind the sesame seeds to a fine powder in a sterilized suribachi and add to the amalaki buttermilk, using a sterilized rubber spatula. Add the herbal powders, salt, and essential oil.

In a small, sterilized saucepan, warm sesame oil and pour into the buttermilk mixture. Thoroughly mix buttermilk, powders, salt, and oil together, using the sterilized spatula, until it becomes a smooth, thick paste. Cover the bowl with a sterilized plate and take directly to the treatment room.

Bandhana Sveda - Pitta Paste

Body Type: Pitta disorders

> 1/4 c amalaki buttermilk (see recipe pg. 143)
> 1/4 c pure ghee
> 2 tbs calamus root powder
> 2 tbs coriander powder
> 2 tsp castor root powder
> 2 tbs jatamansi powder (Indian spikenard)
> 2 tbs ground rock salt
> 10 drops of essential oil of coriander or sandalwood

In a small sterilized bowl, pour in freshly made amalaki buttermilk. In a small sterilized pot, warm ghee and add to the buttermilk. Add herbal powders and rock salt and stir into a smooth paste, using a sterilized spatula. Mix in the essential oil and cover with a sterilized plate. Take directly to the treatment room.

PRASTHARA SVEDA - POULTICE BED FOMENTATION

A bed of poultice made from corn, mung beans, milk, and herbs is covered with arka leaves and wheat grass. The subject lies on the leaf-covered poultice and is covered with silk sheets and woolen rugs. A vessel containing boiling herbal water, covered with a cotton cloth, is placed next to the reclining subject.

Prior to the prasthara sveda treatment, a full body massage is required. For best results, the appropriate oils for each body type or disorder should be used. After the massage, let the subject rest for 15 minutes while you wash your hands and prepare for the main therapy.

Season: use seasonal guidelines

Body Type: all types

Time: early morning and early evening

Duration of Treatment: 7 days; 1 hour each day

Conditions

Vata disorders: arthritis; emaciation; dryness of skin; weakness of muscular function; nervous disorders; facial paralysis; loss of memory; insomnia; mental stress; joint stiffness

Kapha disorders: phlegmatic disorders (colds, coughs, congestion); bronchial asthma; headaches; rheumatoid arthritis; obesity; water retention; anorexia; heaviness of body; lethargy

Benefits

This treatment not only alleviates the disorders listed above, but also has the effect of revitalizing the entire body, restoring sleep patterns and relieving stress. It also reduces bodily fat and excess water and gives energy and mobility.

Necessary Aids

- Large covered stainless steel pot to hold 6 gallons of poultice
- Large stainless steel pot, 18 inches in diameter and 12 inches high, containing the boiling amla decoction and covered with a piece of cotton cloth, 24 inches square
- Bag the size of a pillowcase filled with fresh or dried wheat grass
- Small covered pottery bowl containing the massage oil
- 2 clean cotton hand towels for the attendants' use
- Clean cotton sheet to spread on the treatment table under the poultice
- Clean silk sheet
- 2 clean woolen rugs, approximately 6 feet square

- Clean bath towel
- Loin cloth*
- Heart pad*
- Eye pads*
- Bathtub
- Portable table top one burner gas stove
- Cleaning area and large utility sink
- 2 large wooden or metal paddles, 4 inches wide and 30 inches long, to scrape the used poultice off the surface of the treatment table
- Large plastic container, approximately 24 inches in diameter and 30 inches tall, to hold the used sheets and towels

* *See Appendix D*

Preparation for Prasthara Treatment
To apply the poultice on the treatment table:
- Spread a clean cotton sheet over the surface of the treatment table.
- Pour the poultice contents from the large pot onto the center of the treatment table.
- Using the wooden paddles, spread the hot poultice evenly over the surface of the table. The poultice bed should be at least 2 inches thick.
- Place the paddles in the empty pot. They will be used again to remove the used poultice after treatment.
- Spread the grass over the poultice bed, making sure that the surface of the poultice is completely covered. Optionally, a silk sheet may then be put over the leaves before the subject lies down. If the grass is not available, spread the silk sheet directly over the poultice.
- By the time the poultice has been spread, it should be cooled sufficiently to provide the subject with a comfortable and bearable sudation.

Prasthara Sveda Treatment
- Have the subject lie down on his/her back on the poultice bed. The subject should be still wearing only the loin cloth put on for the preliminary massage treatment.
- Cover the subject with a silk sheet, allowing only the head to be exposed.
- Place two woolen rugs over the silk sheet, making sure that the subject is securely tucked in.

206

- Place the cooling eye pads over the eyes to protect them from the heat.
- Place the protective heart pad directly over the heart.
- Place the vessel with the steaming amla decoction on a small table at the subject's feet.
- Administer the sudation for one hour, checking periodically to ensure that the subject is relatively comfortable.
- Just before the treatment time is over, run a warm bath and pour the amla decoction into it. Immerse the tied handful of wheat grass in the decoction, in the bath water. Be sure to remove the wheat grass from the bath water before the subject enters the bath. Do not use soap in the bath.
- Provide the subject with a clean bath towel to dry off after the bath.
- Have the subject put on warm clothing.
- Have the subject rest on his/her back for 15 minutes on a clean treatment table.
- Place the cooling eye pads over the eyes again.
- Remove all the treatment utensils and the poultice bed from the treatment room, while maintaining an air of quietude.
- Before the subject departs, advise him/her to wear warm clothing and to cover the head outdoors in order to protect the body from exposure to coldness or dampness. This precaution is to be exercised throughout the period of treatment and for the same length of time following treatment.
- Advise the subject to refrain from taking excessively cold foods or drinks and cold baths or showers for the same period of time.

Cleaning the Treatment Table
- After the treatment has been administered, remove the cotton sheet, keeping the poultice intact.
- Using the paddles, carefully scrape the used poultice off the sheet into the large poultice pot.
- Place the used sheets and towels into the plastic container and remove all the treatment utensils and materials from the therapy room.

Prasthara Formulas

Season: use seasonal guidelines

Prasthara Poultice

Body Type: all types

>   4 gal milk
>   4 gal water
>   7 lbs dried cracked corn kernels
>   4 lbs urad dhal
>   7 lbs millet
>   1/2 c dried ginger powder
>   1/2 c black pepper powder
>   1/2 c pippali powder
>   2 c brown sugar

In a ten-gallon stainless steel pot, combine milk and water and bring to a boil over medium-high heat. Add cracked corn, urad dhal, millet, powdered spices and brown sugar. Cover and simmer over medium low heat for 3 hours, or until 1/4 of the liquid has evaporated. The consistency will be that of a thick porridge. Do not use a thin or runny porridge for this treatment; if the porridge is somewhat thin after cooking, blend in enough buckwheat flour to give it a thick, doughy consistency.

Let the porridge sit on very low heat until you are ready to use it. The porridge should be piping hot when you begin to spread it out on the treatment table. Make fresh porridge daily for this treatment.

Amla Decoction

Body Type: all types

>   5 gal water
>   5 oz dried wheat grass
>   1 c amla powder

In a large stainless steel pot, bring water to a boil over medium heat. Gather wheat grass and tie securely into a small bundle. Place wheat grass and amla powder into the boiling water. Cover and simmer over low heat for 1 1/2 hours, or until 1/4 of the water has evaporated. Remove from the stove and cover with a piece of cotton cloth, approximately 24 inches square, to allow the steam to filter through. Take directly to the treatment room and place it on the portable stove over low heat. Make fresh decoction for each day's application.

Prasthara Massage Oil for Vata

Body Type: Vata disorders

For body massage:

    1 c sesame oil

    20 drops essential oil of almond

In a small stainless steel saucepan, warm oil for approximately 5 minutes over low heat. Pour into a pottery container and add essential oil. Cover the container securely to keep the oil warm. Massage the whole body with the warm oil immediately before the prasthara treatment

Prasthara Massage Oil for Kapha

Body Type: Kapha disorders

For body massage:

    3/4 c sesame oil

    1/4 c ghee

    10 drops essential oil of geranium

In a small stainless steel saucepan, melt the ghee over low heat. Add the sesame oil and let warm for 5 minutes. Remove from heat and pour into a pottery container. Add essential oil and cover container securely to keep the oil warm. Use to massage the whole body.

Wheat Grass to Cover the Poultice

    1/4 bale of dried or fresh wheat grass (enough to fill one pillow case)

Gather grass in a large bag the size of a pillow case and take directly to the treatment room. Arka and urbaka leaves may also be used to cover the poultice bed. If these ingredients are not available, you may use a pure silk sheet to cover the poultice instead.

STHAMBANA SVEDA - COOLING POULTICE THERAPY

Sthambana therapy is used mainly as an antidote for over sudation and for excess Pitta conditions such as fevers, ulcerations, inflammation of the skin or tissues, weakness of the limbs, excess thirst and so on. This therapy cools and constricts the body while dissipating the flow of heat, gradually restoring normal body temperature and relieving the various disorders. The characteristics inherent in ingredients used in sthambana therapy poultices are sweet, astringent, and bitter, with cold, soft, rough, smooth, sluggish, liquid, stable, light, and subtle qualities.

Sthambana Therapy

Season: use seasonal guidelines

Body Type: Pitta disorders

Time: early morning or directly after excess sudation occurs

Duration of Treatment: 3 days, 1 1/4 hours daily

Conditions

Excess sudation; burning sensation; excess thirst; bluish eruptions on skin; inflammation of the skin; tissue ulceration; weakness of voice; weakness of limbs and joints; fevers; stiffness of the body; stiffness in the jaws

Benefits

This treatment alleviates the conditions listed above, relieving thirst and fever by restoring normal body temperature. It also has the effect of alleviating excess Pitta.

Necessary Aids

- Large stainless steel bowl containing sthambana astringent plaster
- Small bowl containing sandalwood powder
- 12 cold wet hand towels
- 2 clean light cotton sheets
- Bath towel
- Upright chair
- Shower

Sthambana Treatment: Cooling Poultice Therapy
Antidote for Excess Sudation

- Quickly remove the subject from exposure to heat. Remove all clothing and/or coverings.
- Have the subject sit on an upright chair, then apply wet, cold towels to the subject's body.
- Have the subject lie down on the treatment table.

- Have the subject assume postures described below while you plaster the body completely with cooling herbal paste.
- Have the person put on a light cotton treatment gown and instruct him/her to sit in a cool shaded spot by a stream, river, or any natural running water. If you cannot provide such a location, advise the subject to spend a few hours daily sitting by a body of water (good for all excess Pitta conditions.)

Sitting with the Legs Extended
- Beginning at the lower back, apply the plaster with your hands, using short upward brushing strokes. Plaster the entire back.
- Moving to the right arm, beginning at the fingers, use the same upward strokes to plaster the entire arm, excluding the armpits and the palms of the hands. Gently lift the arm as necessary to apply the paste evenly.
- Moving quickly to the left, repeat the same plastering procedure on the left arm.

Lying on the Back
- Have the subject lie down carefully on his/her plastered back.
- You may use a light sheet to cover the subject to the waist while applying the remaining plaster.
- Beginning from the navel, apply the plaster to the chest, using the same even upward strokes.
- For females, gently apply a light application on the breasts without covering the nipples.
- Continue applying the plaster until the entire chest and neck are covered.

Lying on the Left Side
- Remove the covering sheet and have the subject turn onto his/her left side, with the knees slightly bent and forward for comfort.
- Starting from the toes, plaster the exposed leg, using long upward strokes, lifting the leg up slightly to spread the plaster evenly.
- Continue up the thighs and over the right hip.
- Lifting the subject's right arm gently, spread the plaster evenly on the right side of the rib cage, making sure the entire area is covered.

Lying on the Right Side
- Have the subject turn onto his/her right side with the knees slightly bent and forward for comfort.
- Apply plaster to the subject's left side as for the right.

Lying on the Stomach

- Have the subject turn onto his/her stomach.
- Touch up the areas on the back that need plaster.
- Starting from the upper thighs, apply the plaster with short upward strokes over the buttocks to meet the plastered areas of the lower back.
- Have the subject turn over onto his/her back once more.

Lying on the Back

- Spread the sheet over the person and let him/her rest for 15 minutes.
- Open the windows to let in the fresh air.
- Leave the room for a brief spell to wash yourself.

Sitting with the Legs Extended

- After the rest period, have the person sit up on the treatment table with legs extended.
- Using a cold, wet hand towel, firm pressure, and a downward stroking motion, wipe the dried paste from the body, beginning with the back.
- Taking a fresh cold, wet towel, remove the plaster from the right arm and then the left arm, using a consistent downward motion.
- Change towels as needed.
- Have the subject assume the same positions as during the application process, and wipe the plaster off his/her body completely, remembering to maintain downward strokes while removing the plaster.
- After all the plaster has been removed, allow the subject to take a cold shower, without soap.
- Provide a bath towel for the person to dry the body after showering.
- Have the subject sit in a chair, and, using your hands, sprinkle a profuse amount of sandalwood powder over the subject's entire body.
- Have the person get dressed.
- Before the subject leaves, advise him/her to avoid excess heat and to use cooling, sweet, unctuous, and bitter foods and beverages.

Sthambana Formula (for excess sudation)

    Season: use seasonal guidelines

    Body Type: Pitta disorders

Sthambana Astringent Plaster

    2 lb whole mung beans

    4 c water

    1/4 c dried wild cherry bark

    1 tbs brahmi powder

    1 tbs bala powder

    1 tbs bamboo powder

    2 fl oz witch hazel

Grind the beans to a fine powder, using a hand operated food grinder. In a medium-size stainless steel pot, bring water to a boil and add wild cherry bark. Cover and simmer for 40 minutes on low heat, or until half the water has evaporated. Strain through a small colander into a medium-size stainless steel bowl. To the bark water, add ground mung beans, herbal powders and witch hazel. Using a rubber spatula, mix into a soft, smooth paste.

ANNA LEPA SVEDA - DIRECT POULTICE APPLICATION

Applying warm poultices directly onto the body without using boluses is called anna lepa, a therapy as timeless in its use as pinda sveda. Anointing the body with the appropriate oil before the poultice is applied is recommended. This therapy may also be performed at home, with the aid of a family member or friend, if necessary.

    Season: use seasonal guidelines

    Body Type: all types

    Time: early morning or early evening

    Duration of Treatment: 7 or 14 days

Conditions

Bodily pains; arthritis; rheumatoid arthritis; consumption; severe congestion; colds; weakness of muscular functions; gout (use soft to moderate pressure when applying poultice)

Benefits

In addition to alleviating the conditions listed above, anna lepa has the effect of giving strength to the muscles and limbs, nourishing the skin and invigorating the whole body.

Necessary Aids

- 2 attendants
- 2 medium-size pottery containers containing the poultice, securely covered to maintain the heat (in this treatment, each attendant uses his/her own container of poultice to facilitate prompt and harmonious application)
- Medium pottery container holding the hot herbal decoction for the bath, tightly covered to maintain the heat
- 2 medium pottery bowls containing the warm massage oils, covered to keep the oil warm (each attendant uses his/her individual container of oil to facilitate prompt and harmonious application)
- 2 clean cotton sheets
- 2 heavy woolen blankets
- Bath towel
- 2 dry hand towels for attendants' use
- Large bucket of water for attendants to wash their hands
- Eye pads*
- Heart pad*
- Loin cloth*

See Appendix D

Anna Lepa Treatment

- With one attendant on either side of the subject, apply a handful of poultice to the feet.
- Coordinating the hand movements of each attendant, firmly, but swiftly, rub the poultice on the feet and legs, using short upward strokes, until the upper surfaces of both legs are plastered.
- Continue to apply the poultice from the thighs up to and over the chest, using consistent daubing strokes.
- For female subjects, apply the poultice lightly around the breasts and do not rub or otherwise apply any pressure in this area.
- When the chest and neck are completely covered with poultice,

214

begin to daub the arms, starting from the hands and going upward, both attendants plastering and moving simultaneously.

- When the arms are completely covered with poultice, have the subject turn over on his/her stomach.
- Repeat the plastering process, using short upward strokes, beginning at the heels and moving up to the calves, the thighs, over the buttocks, and up the nape of the neck.
- While one attendant finishes by rubbing the back of the subject's neck with the poultice, the other washes up and prepares to cover the subject.
- Have the subject turn over and lie on his/her back. Place the cooling pad over the heart and the cooling eye pads over the eyes.
- Spread a fresh cotton sheet over the subject and then 3 heavy woolen blankets over the sheet.
- One attendant then quickly removes the treatment utensils from the room, while the other attendant remains in the room to observe the subject during sudation.
- Turn the lights off, or lower the shades, while the subject becomes sudated.
- Allow the subject to sudate for 1 hour.
- Prepare a hot bath and pour in the herbal decoction.
- Turn on the lights or raise the shades.
- Remove the blankets, sheets, eye pads and heart pad.
- Quickly guide the subject to the hot bath. Test the bath water to make sure that the temperature is bearable.
- All doors and windows should be tightly closed in the bathroom.
- Allow the person to sit in the bath for 15 - 20 minutes, or until the water turns lukewarm. Do not use soap.
- Advise the subject to wash off the poultice before coming out of the bath.
- Provide a clean bath towel for the subject.
- Have the subject put on warm clothing.
- Have the subject rest on his/her back for 15 minutes. Again, apply the cooling eyes pads over the eyes.
- Advise the subject to keep the body and head covered to avoid exposure to coldness or dampness throughout the period of treatment and for the same length of time after the treatment is completed.
- Advise the subject to refrain from taking cold foods or drinks and cold baths or showers.

Anna Lepa Formulas

Season: use seasonal guidelines

Body Type: all types

Anna Lepa Massage Oil
Sesame-Bala Oil

1 c sesame oil

1/4 c dried bala roots

4 c water

In a medium stainless steel pot, bring the water to a boil. Add the bala roots and sesame oil. Cover and simmer on medium low heat for approximately 1 hour, or until all the water has evaporated. Strain the oil through a small colander into a large cup. Return the used roots to the earth. Divide the hot oil between two small pottery bowls, one for each attendant. Cover securely to maintain the heat. Apply the oil while still warm.

Anna Lepa Poultice

8 pt water

2 c certified raw milk

1/2 c hulled barley

1/4 c whole urad legume

1/4 c whole horsegram legume

1 c ground sandstone

1/4 c iron powder

In a large stainless steel pot, bring the water to a boil and add the sandstone and iron powder. Cover and simmer on medium heat for approximately 3 hours, or until 3/4 of the liquid has evaporated. Line a large colander with a clean cotton cloth and set it over a medium-size pot, allowing the rim of the colander to rest on the rim of the pot. Carefully pour the hot decoction into the colander, allowing the liquid to strain while keeping the powder residue in the cloth. The liquid collected should measure 4 cups. The residues may be returned to the earth.

Rinse the pot and pour 2 cups of the hot decoction back into it. Add milk and bring to a boil. Combine barley and legumes and add to the milk decoction. Cover and simmer on medium low heat for 1 1/2 hours, or until the barley and legumes are cooked into a thick porridge. Cover the pot containing the remaining decoction and place on a warming stove until the poultice porridge is ready.

Directly before the therapy begins, pour the hot decoction into a pottery container. Cover it securely to maintain the heat and take it to the treatment room for the bath at the end of treatment.

Remove porridge from the heat and with a ladle carefully scoop it into two medium size pottery containers with large enough openings to allow easy access during therapy. Cover the containers and take them directly to the treatment room. Allow the poultice to cool slightly in order to make the temperature bearable for application.

PACA KIZHI SVEDA - GREEN LEAF POULTICE APPLICATION

Paca kizhi, a light variety of pinda sveda, is the application of a warm bolus made from green leaves. Like most sveda treatments, oiling the body is necessary prior to applying paca kizhi. Paca kizhi is especially excellent for Kapha disorders such as asthma, bronchitis and phlegmatic conditions.

Season: use seasonal guidelines

Body Type: Kapha disorders

Time: early morning

Duration of Treatment: 7 days; 1/2 hour daily

Conditions

Bronchitis; asthma; rheumatoid arthritis; mucus expectoration; colds, coughs, flu; indigestion; suppression of digestive fire; obesity; heaviness of body

Benefits

In addition to relieving the conditions listed above, this treatment has the effect of invigorating and warming the body, giving lightness to body and mind.

Necessary Aids

- Heavy cast-iron pot, amply oiled with neem or castor oil.
- Medium-size pottery container, covered, containing warm massage oil.
- 4 clean cotton napkins, 18 inches square
- Eye pads*
- Heart pad*
- Loin cloth*
- 2 clean cotton sheets
- 5 clean damp cotton hand towels
- 3 dry hand towels for attendants' use
- Large stainless steel bowl to empty the boluses into

217

- Large bucket of water for washing the attendants' hands quickly
- Clean bath towel
- Large empty bucket for used treatment items
- Portable one-burner gas stove
- Bathtub

* *See Appendix D*

Paca Kizhi Treatment
Follow the same procedure mentioned in pinda sveda treatment, omitting the head treatment.

Paca Kizhi Formulas

Season: use seasonal guidelines
Body Type: Kapha disorders

Paca Kizhi Massage Oil
3/4 c sesame oil
1/4 c pure ghee
4 tbs eladi (cardamom) oil

In a small stainless steel saucepan, melt ghee over low heat. Add sesame oil and let warm for 5 minutes. Remove from heat and add eladi oil. Pour into a medium-size pottery container with a tight lid to maintain the heat. Apply to the body while still warm.

Paca Kizhi Poultice
4 tbs sesame oil
1/2 lb fresh castor plant leaves
1/2 lb fresh grated coconut
2 oz tamarind pulp (or paste)
2 oz dill seeds
2 oz fenugreek seeds
1/2 c castor oil or neem oil

In a cast-iron skillet, heat the oil. Finely shred the castor leaves and add to the warm oil, along with the grated coconut. Mix in tamarind paste. Cover and simmer on low heat. Grind the dill and fenugreek seeds to a fine powder in a suribachi. Mix into the heated paste. Let warm for an additional 5 minutes.

218

In a separate cast-iron pot that has a cover, pour the castor or neem oil. Using a clean cloth, spread the oil around the pot. Warm over medium heat. Turn the heat off, cover the pot, and let sit on the stove. Remove the poultice mixture from the stove. Spread the four napkins on a clean counter and, using a large spoon, divide the poultice into four equal portions and place each portion in the center of a napkin. Wrap as in pinda sveda (see pgs. 200-201). Place the four boluses in the hot oiled cast-iron pot. Cover and take directly to the treatment room. Place on a small, portable stove to keep the boluses warm during treatment.

PART THREE
Ayurvedic Steam Therapies

PARISHEKA SVEDA - WARM DECOCTION SHOWER

A unique system of showering the body with mostly warming and sometimes cooling fluids, parisheka sveda has been practiced for over 5000 years in India. The vessel traditionally used for parisheka therapy is a large metal pitcher, equipped with holes on the bottom, which are fitted with spouts made from bamboo. Like the shirodhara treatment, this treatment requires two thoroughly trained svedana attendants who exemplify patience and who have steady hands and strong bodies. The attendants allow the fluid to flow from the many spouts on the bottom of the pitcher onto the subject's body, ensuring an even and consistent flow of decoction throughout the therapy from a regulated distance of 10-12 inches above the subject's body. For Vata disorders, this treatment may last for as long as two hours.

The traditional design for the treatment table, known as a *droni*, has various slopes to provide optimum patient comfort while draining excess decoction from the table into a container. The droni is made from the wood of an appropriate tree, i.e., sandalwood, neem, bilva, khadira, arjuna, pippali, ashoka, and so on, since the energy of certain metals and trees are vital to restoring optimal health.

Parisheka therapy is effective in the cure of diseases such as paraplegia, nervous disorders, tumors, enlarged spleen and prostate, as well as abdominal pains, ulcers, constipation, and lethargy. Like all svedana treatments, parisheka enhances the lightness of body and induces calmness of mind.

The following conditions must be observed while administering this therapy. A consistent flow of decoction over the subject's body from a distance of 10 to 12 inches is essential. The fluids used should be neither too hot nor too cold. If this therapy is improperly administered, conditions such as internal bleeding, hemorrhaging, burning sensation, nausea, hoarseness, excessive physical weakness and fevers may result. Should any adverse conditions arise during therapy, desist treatment immediately. For mild forms of fevers, burning sensation, nausea, hoarseness and weakness of body, administer the Cooling Poultice Therapy, pg. 210.

Traditionally, adverse conditions resulting from svedana therapy were treated with a mild form of pancha karma, beginning with gargling, kavalagraha and gandusa; followed by nasal insufflation, nasya; enema therapy, vasti; and, finally, parisheka therapy.

Note: Traditionally, parisheka therapy is administered by six svedana attendants: one to refill the pitchers during treatment, one to perform parisheka on the head, and four to administer parisheka simultaneously over the entire body, two attendants on either side. All five attendants shower the whole body from head to toe at the same time. Here, a milder form of parisheka treatment is introduced, one more suitable to modern use and requiring only three attendants.

Parisheka Sveda

Season: use seasonal guidelines

Body Type: all types

Time: Pitta and Kapha disorders: early morning
                   Vata disorders: early evening

Duration of Treatment: 7 days

Vata disorders:	2 hours daily
Pitta disorders:	4 hours daily
Kapha disorders:	36 minutes daily

Conditions

Vata disorders: nervous disorders; constipation; cysts and tumors; weakness of muscular function; bodily pain; paraplegia; arthritis; insomnia; injuries caused by accidents

Pitta disorders: cysts and tumors; ulcers; abdominal pain; enlarged prostate; enlarged spleen; abscess; prickling pain in the body; injuries caused by accidents

Kapha disorders: cysts and tumors; anorexia; lethargy; phlegmatic disorders; obesity; injuries caused by accidents

Benefits

In addition to relieving the various conditions listed above, this therapy has the effect of giving a healthy appetite, promoting strength, enhancing virility, and reversing aging. It also calms the mind and body, increases the ojas, and gives lightness to the body. Due to the precise nature of parisheka sveda, a treatment time chart is provided for each body type.

Parisheka Treatment Time

	VATA	PITTA	KAPHA
Total time: (in minutes)	120	45	36
front of head	15	5	5
solar plexus	2	1	1
shoulders, arms, chest	15	7	10
front of lower body	15	7	5
knees	5	2	1
back of head	15	2	3
center (lower) back	15	3	1
upper back	15	10	7
back of lower body	20	7	3

Necessary Aids

- Three attendants
- Large stainless steel pot, covered, containing the parisheka decoction
- Small pottery bowl containing the appropriate massage oil
- Two large parisheka pitchers* with two large stainless steel bowls
- Small parisheka pitcher* with a small stainless steel bowl
- 5 clean damp cotton hand towels
- Clean cotton bath towel
- 4 clean dry hand towels (3 for attendants' use)
- Fresh, cool, damp cotton face towel
- Eye pads*
- Heart pad*
- Loin cloth*
- Bathtub
- Portable one-burner gas stove
- Cleaning area with a large utility sink
- A traditional droni,* if possible

See Appendix D

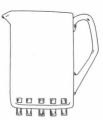

Parisheka
Pitcher

Cleaning the Treatment Table

Use a clean, warm, damp rag to thoroughly wipe the oils and decoction off the droni. Expose the droni to two hours of direct sunlight after cleaning.

Cleaning the Parisheka Pitchers and Bowls

Drain the remaining decoction and oils from the pitchers by sitting them upside down in the utility sink for 15 minutes. Wash the pitchers and bowls thoroughly in warm water to which a tablespoon of witch hazel and a teaspoon of lemon juice have been added. Dry the pitchers thoroughly with a clean cloth and store in a cupboard for future use.

Parisheka Sveda Treatment

- Have the subject lie on his/her back on the treatment table.
- The subject should be wearing only the loin cloth.
- Place the protective heart pad directly over the subject's heart.
- Place the cooling eye pads on the eyes.
- One attendant refills the pitchers while the other two attendants work on either side of the subject, administering the treatment simultaneously.
- The refilling attendant must remain alert to the needs of the operating attendants. The refilled pitchers are handed to the operating attendants one at a time, the bowl remaining under the spouts until the pitcher exchanges hands. The bowl is quickly slipped from under the pitcher and kept ready, while the operating attendants direct the even and continuous flow of decoction over the subject's body.

Shoulders, Arms and Chest

- The two operating attendants begin at the subject's shoulders and work towards the feet. Both attendants maintain a 10 inches distance between the surface of the subject's body and the bottom of the pitcher at all times.
- Allow the fluids to shower the shoulders, arms, and chest. Move simultaneously, making sure that the body is thoroughly showered as you gradually proceed downward. Refer to the parisheka time chart for length of treatment time.
- After saturating the upper body, move to the lower body.

The Hara (solar plexus)

- For Pitta disorders, the attendant on the left side prepares to shower the area surrounding the navel, *hara*, while the attendant responsible for filling the pitchers takes the small pitcher filled with decoction and stands directly behind the subject's head.
- Keeping as closely synchronized as possible, both attendants begin to shower the head and hara at the same time. Because the head treatment lasts longer than the hara treatment, the hara attendant

223

waits until the head attendant has finished, after which both attendants move to the lower body.

- To shower the hara, keep the pitcher 12 inches above the hara and use small, slow, circular, counter clockwise motions around the navel. Refer to parisheka time chart for length of treatment.
- For Vata and Kapha disorders, the attendant on the right side of the subject receives a filled pitcher and begins to shower the hara. The pitcher is kept 12 inches above the hara, but the small, slow, circular motions are to be in a clockwise direction.

The Head

- Place a clean dry towel over the cooling eye pads to absorb any excess decoction flowing from the head during treatment.
- Shower the head by using small, circular, counter clockwise motions for Pitta disorders and clockwise motions for Vata and Kapha disorders.
- The spot 2 inches behind the center of the forehead should be the epicenter of the circular motion employed in this treatment. Refer to the parisheka time chart for length of treatment.
- Remove the soaked towel covering the eyes. Replace the eye pads with fresh ones.

The Lower Body (front)

- Both attendants assume their positions on either side of the subject, receive the refilled large pitchers and proceed to shower the lower body, maintaining an even 10-inch distance above the body.
- Carefully tuck the loin cloth between the subject's legs to protect the groin and vaginal areas during the shower.
- The pitchers are moved simultaneously in a slow, clockwise motion over the hips and thighs, circling directly over the knees, then moving down over calves and feet, thoroughly showering the front of the lower body in the process.

The Shoulders, Arms and Back

- Remove the eye and heart pads and have the subject turn gently onto his/her stomach, resting the neck over the wooden roll of the droni, the face resting comfortably downwards.
- Cover the eyes with a cool damp towel, tucking it in place between the face and the treatment table.
- Shower the shoulders, arms and upper and middle back, using a consistent and simultaneous slow downward motion. Remember to hold the pitcher 10 inches above the surface of the body and to co-ordinate the showering activity with receiving the refilled pitchers.

The Center of the Lower Back and Back of the Head

- Maintaining the pitcher 10 inches above the center of the lower back and using a circular counter clockwise motion for Pitta disorders and a clockwise motion for Vata and Kapha disorders, slowly shower the center of the lower back (refer to parisheka time chart for length of treatment).
- After the back has been thoroughly showered, prepare for the parisheka procedures on the lower back and head.
- Before the lower back is showered, the spare attendant receives a filled small head pitcher and stands directly behind the subject's head.
- For Pitta disorders, the attendant on the left side receives a refilled pitcher and showers the center of the lower back. For Vata and Kapha disorders, the attendant on the right side does this.
- Both attendants begin to shower the back of the head and the center of the lower back at the same time and in synchrony with one another.

The Back of the Head

- Maintaining the small head pitcher at a distance of 12 inches from the back of the head, shower the head, using small circular motions, moving in a counter clockwise direction for Pitta disorders and in a clockwise direction for Vata and Kapha disorders. Use the soft center spot at the back of the head as the epicenter of the circular motion.
- Shower the head slowly and calmly (see the parisheka time chart for length of treatment). When the head shower is complete, replace the soaked towel under the subject's face with a fresh, dry one.

The Lower Body (back)

- Again, two attendants assume their positions on either side of the subject, receive the large pitchers and continue to shower the lower body from an even 10 inches distance above the body.
- Carefully tuck the loin cloth between the subject's legs to protect the groin and vaginal areas from the shower.
- Move the pitchers simultaneously in a slow, downward motion, lightly showering the buttocks, thighs, legs, and heels, to complete the treatment.
- While the excess decoction is draining from the droni, remove the towel from under the subject's face and have him/her turn over on the back. Using clean damp towels, briskly mop up any excess fluid and oil from the body. Use cool towels for cool temperature decoctions and warm towels for warm temperature decoctions.

225

- The refilling attendant prepares the bath (cool or warm, depending on the nature of the treatment) and pours the remaining decoction into it.
- Have the subject bathe for 10 minutes without soap.
- While the subject is in the bath, the refilling attendant cleans the treatment room and utensils, while the operating attendants take a brief rest.
- Provide the subject with a clean bath towel.
- Have the subject get dressed and rest briefly before departing.
- Before the subject leaves, advise him/her to wear appropriate clothing (warm or cool, depending on the nature of the treatment) and, if the treatment is of a warming nature, to cover the head to guard against exposure to dampness and cold. This precaution is to be taken throughout the period of treatment and for the same length of time after the treatment has been completed.

Parisheka Formulas

Season: use seasonal guidelines

Parisheka Sesame Oil-Ghee Decoction

Body Type: Vata disorders

>2 pt sesame oil
>1 oz gold piece
>2 pt pure ghee

Pour oil into a large stainless steel saucepan. Add a 1 ounce piece of gold (to be removed after the treatment), and bring to a boil over medium heat. Remove from heat and add ghee. When ghee is melted, cover the pot and take directly to the treatment room. Let sit for 15 minutes, or until mixture is lukewarm. For Vata disorders, four pints of Narayana oil may also be used instead of the oil/ghee decoction. Generally, a warm decoction is used for Vata conditions.

Parisheka Sandalwood Oil Decoction

Body Type: Pitta disorders

>   1 pt certified raw milk
>   1 pt water
>   1/2 pt sunflower oil
>   1/4 c sandalwood powder

Bring the water and milk to a boil in a large stainless steel pot. Add oil and stir in powder. Cover and simmer over low heat for 1 1/2 hours, or until 1/3 of the liquid has evaporated. Let cool to lukewarm, then pour into a large stainless steel container, keeping sediment in the pot. The sediment may be used in the bath following treatment. Cover the container securely to maintain the temperature and take directly to the treatment room. Parisheka sveda fluids used for most Pitta disorders should be administered lukewarm.

Parisheka Herbal Decoction (Vata)

Body Type: Vata disorders

>   1 gal water
>   1 pt sesame oil
>   1/2 c dashamula powder

Bring water to a boil in a large stainless steel pot. Add oil and herbal powder, stirring briefly. Reduce heat and cover the pot. Simmer for 2 hours, or until half the water has evaporated. Let cool to lukewarm. Carefully pour the fluid into a large stainless steel container, retaining the powdered sediment in the pot. The sediment may be used in the bath following treatment. Cover the container securely to maintain heat and take directly to the treatment room.

Parisheka Ghee Decoction

Body Type: Pitta disorders

>   2 pt pure ghee

Pour the ghee into a large silver or silver plated saucepan. Bring to a boil and remove from heat. Let cool to lukewarm. Cover the saucepan securely to maintain the temperature and take directly to the treatment room. The oil or ghee used in parisheka sveda for most Pitta disorders should be administered lukewarm. Equal amounts of ksheerabala or chandana (sandalwood) oil may also be used instead of ghee for Pitta disorders.

Note: If a silver or silver-plated saucepan is not available, place 10 silver coins into a saucepan while ghee is heating. These coins are removed after the treatment.

Parisheka Sesame Oil Decoction

Body Type: Kapha disorders

    1 1/2 pt sesame oil (eladi oil may be used instead)

Pour oil into a large copper saucepan and bring it to a boil. Reduce heat to low, cover and simmer for 5 minutes. Remove saucepan from heat and let cool to lukewarm. Take directly to the treatment room. Oils used for Kapha disorders should also be administered lukewarm.

Note: If a copper vessel is not available, place 20 copper pennies in the saucepan while oil is heating. These coins are removed after the treatment.

Parisheka Herbal Decoction (Kapha)

Body Type: Kapha disorders

    3 pt water
    3/4 pt sesame oil
    1/8 c cardamom powder
    1/8 c cinnamon powder
    4 tbs jatamansi powder (Indian spikenard)
    4 tbs valerian powder

Bring water to a boil in a large stainless steel pot. Add oil and powders, stirring until powders are dissolved. Reduce heat to low, cover and simmer for 1 1/2 hours, or until 1/3 of the liquid has evaporated. Cool to lukewarm and take directly to the treatment room. When filling the parisheka pitcher, let the powdered sediment remain undisturbed at the bottom of the pot.

Note: The temperature of the decoctions used in parisheka sveda for Kapha disorders is usually warm.

Decoction Antidote for Parisheka

Body Type: all types

Duration of Treatment: 45 minutes

Conditions

Fever, hemorrhaging, internal bleeding, burning sensation, hoarseness, and nausea (either as an existing condition or as a result of improper or excess svedana treatment)

> 2 pt certified raw milk
> 2 pt water
> 1 pt sunflower oil
> 1/4 c sandalwood powder
> 1/8 c licorice powder
> 1/8 c purnarnava powder
> 1/8 c shatavari powder

Bring the milk and water to a boil in a large stainless steel pot. Add oil and stir in the powders. Reduce heat, cover and simmer for 1 hour, or until 1/4 of the liquid has evaporated. Let cool completely. Cover the pot and take directly to the treatment room. When filling the parisheka pitchers, leave the powdered sediment undisturbed at the bottom of the pot.

Note: The fluids used as an antidote for the above conditions should be between 65° and 70° F when administered.

SAMVAHANA SVEDA -
SHOWERING THE BACK WITH WARM DECOCTION

The samvahana treatment is a modification of the parisheka treatment, where only the back of the subject is showered. Samvahana is used primarily to alleviate Vata conditions, nervous disorders, insomnia, tension in the groin area, stiffness and pain in the lower back, and to soothe the mind. Use all of the same procedures, body type specifications and appropriate decoctions as for parisheka. The treatment time for samvahana is 20 minutes.

Only one attendant is required for this treatment (the therapy may also be performed at home with the aid of a family member or friend). Place the pot containing the decoction within easy reach in order to facilitate refilling your pitcher when necessary. Have the subject lie on his/her stomach and shower the back thoroughly, following the instructions for shoulders, arms, and back described in parisheka sveda.

NADI SVEDA - LOCALIZED STEAM APPLICATION

Nadi sveda, practiced since Vedic times, is the topical application of steam on a specific part of the body to alleviate pain. Traditionally, a tube approximately 36 inches in length and 2 inches in diameter, was made from the leaves or wood of the bamboo, arka, or karanja tree and was attached to one side of a pitcher, like a spout, and filled with hot water. The tube is slightly curved in order to regulate the vapors. These tubes are still being used in India.

This therapy may also be performed at home, with, if necessary, the aid of a family member or friend. A simple homemade apparatus for nadi sveda may be constructed by attaching a rubber or plastic hose to the spout of a kettle. The kettle is then filled with a hot decoction made from leaves such as bamboo, arka, and karanja. The steam collected through the hose is then diffused to the injured or painful area of the body.

In ancient times, a procedure called *baspa sveda* was used to steam the entire body. A huge wooden tub with a slotted head board kept the subject's head out of the steam area. A giant hose, seven foot long and three feet in diameter, was used to sudate the subject's body. If available, the distillery apparatus used to make essential oils may also be used in nadi sveda.

This therapy should not be administered directly on the face, over the heart, or in the vaginal and groin areas. Nadi sveda is mostly used locally to alleviate painful swelling of the joints, back pain, stiffness or heaviness of the neck and limbs, arthritic pain, muscular cramps, atrophy of limbs, spraining of the joints and other such conditions.

Season: all year

Body Type: all types

Time: early morning and early evening

Duration of Treatment: 7 days for mild conditions

14 days for serious conditions

Note: For conditions of the head and face, nadi sveda is applied to the sides of the feet for 7 1/2 minutes each side.

Mild Conditions

Moderate bodily aches and pains; stiffness or heaviness of joints and limbs; muscular cramps; backache; mild headaches; tensions of head, face, eyes

Serious Conditions

Chronic bodily aches and pains; chronic backache; extreme pain in joints and limbs; swollen joints, limbs and tissues of body; extreme muscular cramps; arthritic pain; atrophy of limbs; sprains

Benefits

In addition to relieving the conditions listed above, nadi sveda has the added benefit of inducing lightness of body and mind.

Necessary Aids

- Nadi vessel* containing the hot karanja and arka decoction
- Massage oil for the preliminary full body massage
- 2 clean cotton sheets
- 2 clean cotton hand towels for the attendant's use
- Portable gas stove

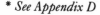

Nadi Vessel

* See Appendix D

Nadi Sveda Treatment

- Place the nadi vessel on the portable stove approximately 2 feet away from the area of the body to be treated.
- Have the subject lie on the treatment table, either on the stomach or back, so that the afflicted area is exposed for treatment.
- Cover the subject with a clean covering sheet, exposing only the area to be treated.
- Allow the nadi hose to curve while steaming the afflicted body part with it. The more curved the hose, the less potent the steam.
- Before proceeding, remove the cork from the treatment end of the hose and test the temperature of the steam on the affected area to ensure the heat is bearable.
- Keeping the outpouring steam 6 inches away from the affected area, steam the area, using a clockwise circular motion.
- Apply the steam to a circumferential area approximately 8 inches from the epicenter of the affected area.
- Continue steaming the affected area for 30 minutes.
- Remove the nadi vessel and have the subject rest on his/her back for 15 minutes.

Nadi Sveda Formulas

Season: all year

Body Type: all types

Strong Decoction

Serious Conditions

> 4 gal water
> 4 c sesame oil
> 1 c dashamula powder
> 4 c milk
> 1 oz dried bamboo leaves
> 1 oz dried arka leaves
> 1 oz dried leaves of karanja (Indian beech)

In a large stainless steel pot, combine the water and oil and bring it to a boil over medium heat. Add the dashamula powder and milk. Cover and simmer over low heat for 2 hours, or until 1/4 of the liquid has evaporated. Add dried leaves, cover, and continue to simmer over low heat for an additional 1 1/2 hours.

Before filling it with the hot decoction, prepare the nadi vessel by attaching the rubber hose to the spout and plug the open end with a cork. Pour the hot decoction, leaves and all, into the nadi vessel. Cover and carefully transport it to the treatment room. Place it on the portable stove over very low heat. Position the extended rubber hose so as to avoid direct contact with the heat.

Mild Decoction

Mild Conditions

> 3 gal water
> 1 oz dried leaves of bamboo
> 1 oz dried leaves of arka
> 1 oz dried leaves of karanja (Indian beech)

In a large stainless steel pot, bring the water to a boil over medium heat. Add dried leaves, cover the pot and simmer over medium low heat for 1 hour, or until 1/3 of the liquid has evaporated.

Ayurvedic Earth Sauna Therapies

JENTAKA SVEDA - SWEAT LODGE SUDATION

There are several forms of svedana therapy involving the use of dry heat, much like the sauna method of sudation. These therapies are generally used for Kapha body types and mostly for Kapha disorders such as phlegmatic conditions and obesity. However, Vata and Pitta types may occasionally use the earth svedas to promote invigoration, providing they are physically healthy.

Many of these therapies have become extinct due to non-use. Vedic therapies are known for their precise and technically detailed instructions, harmonically rooted to the energy matrix of nature. When the earth became modern and humans began to travel on conveyances other than their feet, they left nature behind, forsaking the memory of many numinous ancient practices. Reclaiming the sacred through these arts is an essential means for restoring cognitive memory. Through the practice of the fundamental healing sadhanas discussed in this book, we may begin to garner the necessary globules of earthly memory that are so essential if we are to reclaim the sacred largess bequeathed to us by the seers who have gone before.

The ancients lived in harmony with nature and regarded the gods and children as nature's true heroes. They roamed freely on the plains and plateaus surrounding their villages where the buffalo too roamed along the horizon without obstruction. They bathed in the clean, pure streams and lived where the whole village existed as one family, and the entire village raised each child. In the autumn, the villagers gathered in small groups in the sweat lodge to dispel their bodily wastes together; on the harvest moon, they gathered and celebrated in exhilaration.

In a universe where nothing is constant, change is inevitable. However, change does not have to be detrimental to the pure, simple, idyllic joys we humans are capable of experiencing. If we can gather as a community and build a community sweat lodge to the specifications of a jentaka structure, we may once more ignite the luminous spirit of invigoration originally shared among the human family. A family who sweats together *is* together.

The jentaka and kuti methods of svedana are two examples of what we have relinquished and may still reclaim. Both the jentaka and kuti svedas were practiced even before the time of Buddha.

The classic invitation to enter a sweat lodge, delivered by an Ayurvedic physician, according to Charaka Samhita (Sutra 14/46), is as follows:

O noble and kind one
Enter the room for the sake of your well being
Cure your disease.
Come in and lie down on the bench comfortably
Turn from side to side as necessary
Even if you feel faint, do not leave the bench
You may not be able to reach the door and
you may die inside the room.
When you are without obstructions, and sweat is
drained from your body, all the channels
become light and free.
When you are free of stiffness, numbness, pain,
heaviness
Then you may leave the bench and walk through
the door.
Do not apply cold water to your body or face when
you leave the lodge.
If you do, it may adversely affect your eyes.

Jentaka Sweat Lodge: Traditional Structure

The jentaka sweat lodge, circular in structure, 118 feet in diameter and 12 feet high, was originally constructed on a sacred site, facing east or north where the earth was black as the crow, or golden red like a fallow deer. Because water is the source of cooling energy, the lodge was situated on the leveled bank of a pond or water reservoir, either south or east of the sweat lodge. The walls were 2.6 feet from the water's edge and had circular apertures, 18 inches in diameter, spaced evenly around the lodge, in place of windows. There was only one doorway, curved at the top, 5 feet high and 3 feet wide. The walls were one foot thick and covered with mud inside and out. A bench, 1 1/2 feet wide and 1 1/2 feet high, made from such woods as mahanimba or khadira, was along the inside wall of the lodge, its ends on either side of the doorway. A clay oven, columnar shaped, 5 feet in diameter and 4 feet high, stood in the center of the lodge. It had four round apertures, 6 inches in diameter, spaced evenly around its circumference and slightly below

234

its center line. This oven had one main opening, 18 inches above the surface of the stone floor and 18 inches wide. A wood kindling fire was kept burning in it during the jentaka sveda. A 1-inch deep oil container hung suspended from the top aperture into the oven. The container had a wide rim that rested on the top circular ledge of the oven.

In preparation for treatment, one pint of khadira oil, mixed with asvakarna oil, was placed in the oil container and ignited. After the oils burned completely and the smoke subsided, a fire made from khadira wood kindling remained burning in the clay oven.

Once the fire was burned in the clay oven, the subject was invited to enter the sweat lodge.

Jentaka Sweat Lodge: The Contemporary Alternative

Although the proper location is required to achieve a jentaka sudation, a contemporary alternative may be achieved as follows:

Locate a carpenter who is experienced in constructing the wooden sweat lodges used by the Native American people. The windows can be slotted spacings between the logs or boards. A heavy canvas may be used to drape the lodge's entrance during sudation. A conventional door should not be used. The procedure of daubing mud on the inside and outside walls may be eliminated. Instead, large vessels of water may be placed inside the lodge during sudation.

A contemporary fireplace may be erected in the center of the lodge and properly vented by means of a chimney extending through the apex of the lodge. The container of oil may be placed on the fireplace while the fire is burning.

Jentaka Sveda

Season: use seasonal guidelines

Body Type: Kapha

Vata types use only for the specific disorders listed below. Pitta types use only as an occasional invigorating therapy, when mild conditions exist (see list below). Do not use if serious Pitta conditions exist.

Duration of Treatment: 7 days

Time:		
Kapha types:	early morning, 25 minutes daily	
Vata types:	early morning or early evening, 15 minutes daily	
Pitta types:	early morning, 10 minutes daily	

Conditions

Kapha disorders: phlegmatic disorders (colds, coughs, mucus and so on); bronchial asthma; headaches; rheumatoid arthritis; obesity; water retention; anorexia; heaviness of body; lethargy; indigestion; suppression of digestive fire; and as a seasonal cleansing therapy when in good health

Vata disorders: arthritis; stiffness of joints; bodily aches and pain; indigestion; suppression of digestive fire; nervous tension; and as a seasonal cleansing therapy when in good health

Pitta disorders (mild conditions only): headaches; bodily aches and pains; excess bodily oils; indigestion; suppression of digestive fire; nervous tension; and as a seasonal cleansing therapy when in good health

Benefits
In addition to relieving the conditions listed above, this therapy has the additional benefit of calming the mind and body, while reviving the mind and spirit.

Necessary Aids
- Fully equipped jentaka sweat lodge (see pg. 234)
- Khadira oil and asvakarna oil
- Small covered pottery bowl containing appropriate massage oil for each body type
- Sufficient khadira wood kindling or substitute (see pg. 447, Appendix A) to last for the length of treatment time; two bundles of kindling will last for approximately 45 minutes
- Box of fireplace matches, 8 - 10 inches long
- 2 clean cotton bath towels
- Loin cloth*
- Eye pads*
- Heart pad*
- String bandages*

See Appendix D

Jentaka Treatment
- Let the subject rest for 20 minutes after the massage, before inviting him/her into the sweat lodge.
- While the subject is resting, prepare the lodge by burning the oils in the clay oven and allowing the smoke to subside.
- Place half a bundle of wood kindling in the oven and light with a long match.
- Spread a clean towel on the sweat bench and invite the subject into the sweat lodge to receive sudation.
- Have the subject lie down on the prepared bench. The subject should be wearing only the loin cloth worn during the preliminary

massage. Ask the subject to tuck the loin cloth between his/her legs to protect the vaginal or groin area from heat.

- Place the cooling eye pads over the subject's eyes and the protective heart pad over the heart area, using the string bandage to secure both the eye pads and the heart pad comfortably around the head and the chest. This will keep them in place when the subject turns from side to side during fomentation.
- Leave the lodge while the subject receives sudation, returning at 15-minute intervals to restock the kindling and ensure that the fire is burning.
- While in the lodge, check on the subject for any abnormal condition or sign of excessive fomentation.
- After the appropriate time period for sudation has elapsed, enter the lodge, gently remove the eye pads and heart pad, and assist the subject to rise and leave the lodge.
- Guide the subject to the shower or bath for a brief wash with lukewarm water.
- Provide the subject with a clean towel.
- The subject may then get dressed.

Cleaning Aids
- A large metal fireplace shovel and a broom are needed to remove the completely cooled ashes from the oven. Ashes should be thrown directly on the earth outside the sweat lodge.
- A preparation area with a utility sink, built outside the sweat lodge, is a necessary adjunct to jentaka sveda. A shower or bath, located outside the sweat lodge, is also essential.
- Clean rags are needed to wipe the soot and oil off the oil container which is placed in the clay oven. The oil container may be rinsed in warm water afterwards.

ASHMAGHNA SVEDA - ASH SUDATION ON A STONE SLAB

This treatment is one of the most ancient of the svedana therapies. A stone slab, 6 feet long by 4 feet wide, is heated by building a fire right on it. A few piles of wood kindling and sveda herbs are strategically placed over the surface of the slab. The piles are then lit, and the fire is allowed to burn until reduced to ashes. The hot ashes are then carefully removed from the slab, and the remaining ash dust is brushed off. Cool water or herbal decoction, i.e., amla decoction, is sprinkled on the stone's surface to moderate the heat of the stone. Woolen blankets are then laid out on the stone and the subject lies on the stone, covered with silk or woolen sheets. The hides of such animals as deer and antelope, acquired after they had succumbed to a natural death, were traditionally used to cover both the slab and the subject during ashmaghna sveda.

The therapy is generally conducted in a simple wooden sweat lodge or mud hut. It may also be administered in a secluded spot outdoors during the warm weather.

Like all svedana therapies involving the use of dry heat, i.e., the sauna effect, ashmaghna sveda is most suitable for Kapha types and conditions. Brief treatments may be taken by Pitta and Vata types if they are in a healthy condition or exhibit mild disorders, such as bodily aches and pains, nervous tension and low digestive fire.

Season: use seasonal guidelines

Body Type: Kapha

> Vata types use only for the specific disorders listed below. Pitta types use only as an occasional invigorating therapy, when mild conditions exist (see list below). Do not use if serious Pitta conditions prevail.

Duration of Treatment: 7 days

Time:

Kapha types:	early morning, 25 minutes daily
Vata types:	early morning or early evening, 15 minutes daily
Pitta types:	early morning, 10 minutes daily

Conditions

Kapha disorders: phlegmatic disorders (congestion, cough, mucus accumulation); bronchial asthma; headaches; indigestion; rheumatoid arthritis; obesity; water retention; anorexia; heaviness of body; lethargy; suppression of digestive fire; and as a seasonal cleansing therapy when in good health

Vata disorders: arthritis; stiffness of joints; bodily aches and pains; indigestion; suppression of digestive fire; nervous tension; and as a seasonal cleansing therapy when in good health

Pitta disorders (mild conditions only): headaches; bodily aches and pains; indigestion; suppression of digestive fire; nervous tension; excess bodily oils; and as a seasonal cleansing therapy when in good health

Benefits

In addition to relieving the conditions listed above, this therapy makes the body supple, giving energy and mobility. It has the added benefit of reviving the mind and spirit while calming the mind and body.

Necessary Aids

- Small simple wooden structure, or sweat lodge, approximately 12 feet square
- Stone slab 6 feet long, 4 feet wide and at least 2 inches thick (Slate is an ideal stone for this treatment, although any large stone with a fairly smooth surface will suffice. The stone slab should be placed on a stone, concrete or brick floor in the center of the room with one end towards the east; if the flooring is made of wood, it should be protected by a covering of stone or brick, 8 feet long and 5 feet wide, centered under the stone slab.)
- 3 bundles of khadira wood kindling or substitute (see pg. 447)
- Fresh or dried herbs: 1 oz mistletoe, 1 oz rue, 1 oz lemon balm and 1 oz sage
- Small covered pottery bowl containing the appropriate massage oils
- Box of fireplace matches, 8 - 10 inches long
- 4 woolen blankets
- Silk sheet
- Clean cotton bath towel
- Clean wet towel to moisten attendant's face while tending the fire
- Loin cloth*
- Eye pads*
- Heart pad*
- String bandages*

See Appendix D

Ashmaghna Treatment

- Let the subject rest for 20 minutes after the massage before inviting him/her onto the heated stone.
- While the subject is resting, prepare the heated stone.
- Mix the fresh or dried herbs together and spread them on the surface of the stone, making sure the area where the subject will lie is covered with herbs.
- Arrange the kindling in three piles, stacking the brambles and wood pieces in the shape of a pyramid (Fig. 44). Do not place the kindling too close to the edge of the stone. Allow approximately 8 inches on all sides.
- Set fire to each pile and tend the blaze so that no hot kindling pops off the slab of stone.

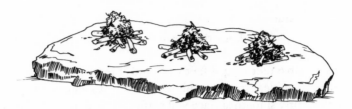

Figure 44: Kindling Piled on Stone

- Use the wet cool towel to wipe your face, arms, and so on while you tend the fire. Stand as close to the entrance way as possible while tending the fire to avoid dehydration.
- When the kindling has been reduced to ashes, carefully remove the ashes with the long-handled fireplace shovel and the long-handled brush or broom.
- Place the ashes into the large bucket or aluminum washtub and set aside to allow it to cool.
- Brush the remaining ash dust off the stone, collecting it in the dust pan.
- Sprinkle cool water on the surface of the stone, approximately 5 cups.
- Let the stone cool down for approximately 5 minutes before spreading the blankets on it.
- Spread two woolen blankets on the heated stone.
- Invite the subject into the sweat lodge and have him/her lie on the covered slab with the head towards the east. If the temperature of the stone is too hot for the subject, have him/her get up, remove the blankets and sprinkle the stone with more cold water.
- When the stone is a bearable temperature, continue with the sudation.
- The subject should be wearing only the loin cloth worn during the preliminary massage. Ask the subject to tuck it between his/her legs to cover the vaginal or groin area.
- Secure the cooling eye pads over the subject's eyes using the strip bandage.
- Secure the protective heart pad over the heart area, using the strip bandage.
- Cover the subject, first with the silk sheet and then with the two additional blankets, making sure that the head and face are left uncovered.
- Tuck the edges of the blankets securely under the subject, allowing ample room for turning to each side.
- Advise the subject to turn from side to side as necessary, to receive comfortable sudation of the whole body.

- Leave the lodge and let the subject receive a peaceful sudation.
- Return at 15-minute intervals to check on the subject. Make sure that there are no abnormal conditions or signs of excessive fomentation.
- After the appropriate time has elapsed, enter the lodge, remove the covers and pads, and gently assist the subject in getting up.
- Guide the subject to the shower or bath for a brief wash with lukewarm water.
- Provide the subject with a clean towel.
- The subject may then get dressed and rest a while if desired.

Cleaning Aids
- Use a long-handled fireplace shovel and a long-handled broom to carefully remove the hot ashes from the stone slab. Put the hot ashes in large buckets or aluminum washtubs and let them cool before throwing them directly on the earth outside the sweat lodge.
- Use a soft broom and fireplace shovel to brush off the remaining ash dust from the surface of the stone.
- A utility sink, located outside the sweat lodge, is a necessary adjunct to an ashmaghna sweat lodge. A shower or bath, located outside the sweat lodge, is also required, as is a treatment table, located in a separate area or room.

KUMBHIKA SVEDA - SUDATION FROM A PITCHER OF HERBAL DECOCTION

Among the ancient svedana practices, kumbhika svedana is a simple procedure whereby a large pitcher of steaming hot herbal decoction is half buried in the earth, and a small cot made from ropes or canvas is placed over it. The subject then rests on the cot and receives sudation. In a nearby fireplace, iron balls or stones are heated until they are red hot, then placed in the pitcher to maintain the heat of the decoction throughout the course of the treatment.

As a convenient practice at home, this therapy may be performed in a clean, uncluttered treatment room, with the pitcher half submerged in a box of sand under a cot. Instead of using hot stones or iron balls, the decoction may be kept on a stove and the pitcher refilled as needed.

Season: all year

Body Type: all types

Duration of Treatment: 7 days

Time:	Kapha types:	early morning, 25 minutes daily
	Pitta types:	early morning, 10 minutes daily
	Vata types:	early morning or early evening, 15 minutes daily

Conditions

Nervous disorders; nervous tension; headaches; anxieties or fears; phlegmatic disorders; colds; coughs; flu; congestion; mucus accumulation; bronchial asthma; lethargy

Benefits

In addition to relieving the conditions listed above, kumbhika sveda has the added benefit of restoring calmness of mind.

Necessary Aids

- A 12-foot-square area of cleared flat space on the earth
- Canvas or rope-string cot,* 7 feet long, 4 feet wide, 4 feet high
- Small covered pottery bowl containing the appropriate massage oils
- 2 gallon stainless steel pitcher, 12 inches tall, containing the hot herbal decoction
- Clean cotton sheet
- Clean damp cotton bath towel
- Dry cotton bath towel
- Clean silk sheet
- 2 bundles of cut wood
- Massage table
- Box of fireplace matches, 8 - 10 inches long
- 10 iron balls, 1 inch in diameter, or 10 stones, approximately 1 inch in diameter
- Small shovel
- Large long-handled pair of tongs
- Loin cloth*
- Eye pads*
- Heart pad*
- String bandages*

* See Appendix D

Kumbhika Treatment

- Let the subject rest for 20 minutes while you prepare for the svedana treatment.
- In a cleared spot on the earth, near the kumbhika treatment area,

build a strong fire with the wood. Place the iron balls or stones directly into the fire and let them become red hot.

- On the cleared earth area designated for the kumbhika sveda, using the shovel, dig a hole 12 inches in diameter and 6 inches deep.
- Place the pitcher of herbal decoction into the hole.
- With your hands, pile the dirt snugly around the half-exposed pitcher.
- Wash your hands and place the cot directly over the pitcher so that the pitcher is located underneath the center of the cot.
- Fold the cotton sheet and spread over the cot so that the sides of the sheet do not obstruct easy access to and from the pitcher.
- Invite the subject, wearing only the loin cloth, to lie down on the cot.
- Secure the cooling eye pads and heart pad with the string bandages.
- Cover the subject with the silk sheet.
- Tuck the ends of the sheet securely, allowing enough room for the subject to move from side to side.
- Leave the head and face uncovered.
- Retrieve the iron balls or stones one at a time from the fire, using the long-handled tongs. Carry them in the tongs with your arm extended away from your body.
- Place five hot balls or stones, one at a time, into the pitcher, leaving the remaining five balls or stones in the fire.
- Once the steam from the decoction begins to dissipate, remove the balls or stones from the pitcher with the tongs and return them to the fire.
- Retrieve the other five balls or stones from the fire and place them, one at a time, in the decoction.
- Continue this process throughout the treatment.
- Once the required treatment time has elapsed, gently help the subject get up.
- Remove the eye and heart pads, and guide the subject to the portable massage table or to a blanket on a comfortable, shaded spot on the grass or ground.
- Give the subject the damp and dry towels to wipe the sweat off his/ her body; you may assist the subject with this procedure.
- The subject may rest for a short while before getting dressed. If the treatment is conducted far away from an indoor space, locate a secluded spot, behind a tree perhaps, where the subject may get dressed.

The Kumbhika Decoction

Season: all year
Body Type: all types

> 3 gal water
> 1/2 oz dried bala root
> 1/4 oz dried peppermint leaves
> 1/4 oz dried lotus root
> 1/2 oz dried sage leaves
> 1/2 oz dried eucalyptus leaves

In a large stainless steel pot, bring the water to a boil. Add the dried roots and leaves; cover and simmer on low heat for 1 1/2 hours, or until 1/3 of the water has evaporated. Remove from heat and, while the decoction is still hot, carefully strain it through a large colander held over a large pot. Cover the pot and take the decoction directly to the treatment area.

If the treatment is conducted outdoors on the earth, prepare this kumbhika decoction over the wood burning fire, on a 3-foot-high grated iron table placed directly over the fire. Reduce the simmering time to 3/4 hour.

BHU SVEDA - AN EARTH SVEDA

True to the meaning of the word "bhu," belonging to the earth, this sveda is performed directly on the earth. Like kumbhika, holaka, kupa and karshu, bhu sveda is another ancient Ayurvedic practice.

There are no substitutes for the therapies that use mud or that are administered on the earth. The earth's magnetic and healing properties lend themselves completely to rejuvenation for the person receiving svedana. Therapies performed directly on the earth invoke feelings of connectedness to Mother Nature and are a vital stimulant for awakening cognitive memory.

Although the basic necessities for the earth svedanas are not readily available in the Western hemisphere as yet, there are thousands of excellent locations, and scores of herbs and kindling available to perform these svedas among small groups of Ayurvedic enthusiasts. A sequestered area of private property or the sites used for camping and hiking can suffice for the practice of earth svedas. Of course, adherence to the proper observances concerning private property and forestry fire regulations goes without saying.

Similar to ashmaghna therapy, bhu sveda is performed on the heated surface of the earth. A cloistered 12-foot square area is chosen, free from dust and wind. In Ayurvedic practice, an auspicious area is chosen for all earth svedas, meaning that it must be free from high winds and dust, it may be close to a stream or a holy river, or it may be on the consecrated grounds of a temple. In the Western

Hemisphere, divination can be employed to ascertain sacred and powerful grounds, i.e., where the matrix of energies are gathered. The grounds used in the past by the indigenous people for their ceremonies are ideal for these practices. A simple, cleared and private ground, which is not polluted and has rich, fertile soil, may also be used for these earth svedas.

Certain cleaning practices, applied to the surface of the earth, are essential before therapy may be performed. The designated area must be flat, compact and dry, and cleared of all bushes and brush. A layer of clay may then be daubed on the surface and allowed to dry in the sun in preparation for the treatment.

Wood kindling and sveda herbs are placed in small piles across a 6-foot square area of the earth's surface. The piles are lit and burned to ashes. The hot ashes are then carefully removed from the heated ground and the surface is sprinkled with an herbal decoction to cool it slightly. Woolen blankets and/or the hides of animals such as the deer, acquired after it has succumbed to a natural death, are used to layer the heated surface before the subject lies down. The subject is also covered with layers of blankets before receiving sudation.

Like ashmaghna sveda, the drying effect of bhu sveda is most suitable for Kapha disorders. Brief treatments may be taken by Pitta and Vata types if they are in general good health, or exhibit only mild disorders, such as bodily aches and pains, nervous tension and low digestive fire.

Season: use seasonal guidelines

Body type: Kapha

> Vata types use only for the specific disorders listed below. Pitta types use only as an occasional invigorating therapy, when mild conditions exist (see list below). Do not use if serious Pitta conditions are present.

Duration of Treatment: 7 days

Time:

Kapha types:	early morning, 25 minutes daily
Pitta types:	early morning, 10 minutes daily
Vata types:	early morning or early evening, 15 minutes daily

Conditions

Kapha disorders: phlegmatic disorders (congestion, colds, coughs, mucus accumulation, etc.); bronchial asthma; headaches; indigestion; rheumatoid arthritis; obesity; water retention; anorexia; heaviness of body; lethargy; suppression of digestive fire; and as a seasonal cleansing therapy when in good health

Pitta disorders (mild conditions only): headaches; bodily aches and pains; indigestion; suppression of digestive fire; nervous tension; excess bodily oils; and as a seasonal cleansing therapy when in good health

Vata disorders: arthritis; stiffness of joints; bodily aches and pains; indigestion; suppression of digestive fire; nervous tension; and as a seasonal cleansing therapy when in good health

Benefits

In addition to relieving the disorders listed above, this therapy has the benefit of giving energy and mobility, while reviving the mind and spirit. It also has the effect of calming the mind and body of the subject.

Necessary Aids

- A suitable 12-foot-square cleared ground, daubed with three buckets of clean, smooth mud, if possible
- 4 bundles of khadira wood kindling or substitute (see pg. 447)
- Dried herbs: 1 oz sage; 1 oz rosemary; 1 oz basil; 1 oz oregano; 1 oz mugwort
- Large stainless steel bucket filled with the cool Amla Decoction (see Amla Decoction formula, pg. 208)
- Small covered pottery bowl containing appropriate massage oil
- Box of fireplace matches, 8 - 10 inches long
- 4 clean woolen blankets
- Clean silk sheet
- Portable massage table
- Loin cloth*
- Eye pads*
- Heart pad*
- String bandages*
- Clean damp cotton bath towel
- Clean dry cotton bath towel

* *See Appendix D*

Bhu Treatment

- Have the subject rest for 20 minutes after the preliminary massage, while you prepare the heated sveda ground.
- The designated ground must be cleared (and optionally daubed with mud and sun dried) before the subject arrives for treatment.
- Mix the dried herbs together on the cleared ground and scatter them to cover an area about 6 feet long and 4 feet wide.
- Arrange kindling in four small pyramidical piles on the scattered herbs, stacking the wood pieces and brambles strategically, and covering the 6-foot length of ground.
- Light the piles and tend the fire, until the kindling is reduced to ashes.
- While the ashes are still hot, carefully remove them from the ground,

using the long-handled fireplace shovel and long-handled broom.

- Place the hot ashes in the large aluminum washtub.
- Set the tub out of the way and let the ashes cool before discarding them directly on the earth.
- Sprinkle the amla decoction directly onto the heated surface of the ground.
- Allow the steaming vapors from the heated surface to subside and then spread two of the blankets on the heated ground.
- Test the heat of the ground to ensure that the temperature is bearable before inviting the subject to lie down.
- The subject should be wearing only the loin cloth worn during the preliminary massage.
- Ask the subject to tuck the loin cloth between his/her legs to protect the vaginal or groin area from excess heat.
- Secure the cooling eye pads and heart pad with the string bandages.
- Cover the subject first with the silk sheet and then with the two blankets.
- Tuck the edges of the blankets securely under the subject, allowing room for him/her to turn on each side.
- Leave the subject's head and face uncovered, except for the cooling eye pads.
- Leave the person undisturbed to receive a comfortable and peaceful sudation.
- Remain close by to check for any abnormal conditions or signs of excess fomentation.
- After the appropriate treatment time has elapsed, remove the blankets and sheet.
- Guide the subject to a sitting position and quickly remove the eye and heart pads.
- Assist the subject to the portable massage table or to a blanket spread out nearby on flat ground and invite the subject to lie down.
- Wipe the sweat off the subject's body, using the damp cotton towel.
- Pat the subject's body using the dry towel. If the subject is able, he/she may be given the towels to wipe down and dry off.
- The subject may rest for a brief while before getting dressed. If the treatment is conducted far away from an indoor space, find a secluded spot, behind a tree perhaps, where the subject may get dressed.
- Before the subject leaves, caution him/her to wear warm clothing and to cover the head when outdoors, in order to protect the body from the cold and damp. This precaution applies throughout the course of the treatment.

Cleaning Aids
- Large aluminum washtub
- Long-handled soft broom
- Fireplace shovel

The hot ashes must be carefully removed from the heated ground with a long-handled fireplace shovel and long-handled broom; store the ashes in the aluminum washtub until cool.

KARSHU SVEDA - ANOTHER EARTH SVEDA

The karshu form of treatment is very powerful in that it takes us back into the womb of the earth where we may replenish our vital energies and restore synchronicity with our Earth Mother. The ancients held the earth to be dear and precious, the fertile womb that gave birth to all species of animals, humans, plants, birds, fishes and so on. They practiced being buried alive in the earth overnight to rid the physical mind and body of all fears and to keep the memory of human immortality alive.

Lying on the sweating surface of the earth stimulates our cognitive memory of our journeys throughout time. To lie in the earth is to be put back into the primordial soil where both embryonic stillness and dynamic fluency prevail; it is to gather all the senses and limbs into a mute entity. It is to become a seed again, sheltered by the massive earth until it implodes into fresh life; it is to relearn the true human spirit of full cognition. Essentially, to lie in the earth is a powerful means of rebirth, rejuvenation and revival.

For karshu sveda, a pit is dug in an auspicious area free from high winds and dust. The standard pit is 6 1/2 feet long, 2 1/2 feet wide and 1 1/2 feet deep. In it, a fire is built from wood kindling which is burned to ashes. The ashes are then removed, and the earth is sprinkled with an herbal decoction made with milk or water. Fresh or dried herbal leaves are then spread on the heated earth. A blanket is spread over the herbs, and the subject lies down in the heated pit.

This therapy may also be performed in a smaller but deeper pit in which the kindling burns into a smokeless fire. A cot is then straddled over the pit, and the subject receives fomentation lying on the cot.

Season: use seasonal guidelines

Body Type: Kapha

Vata types use only for the specific disorders listed below. Pitta types use only as an occasional invigorating therapy, when mild conditions exist (see list below). Do not use if serious Pitta conditions exist.

Duration of Treatment: 7 days

Time:	Kapha types:	early morning, 25 minutes daily
	Pitta types:	early morning, 10 minutes daily
	Vata types:	early morning or early evening, 15 minutes daily

Conditions

Kapha disorders: phlegmatic disorders (congestion, colds, coughs, mucus accumulation); bronchial asthma; headaches; indigestion; rheumatoid arthritis; obesity; water retention; anorexia; heaviness of body; lethargy; suppression of digestive fire; and as a seasonal cleansing therapy when in good health

Pitta disorders (mild conditions only): headaches; bodily aches and pains; indigestion; suppression of digestive fire; nervous tension; excess bodily oils; and as a seasonal cleansing therapy when in good health

Vata disorders: arthritis; stiffness of joints; bodily aches and pains; indigestion; suppression of digestive fire; nervous tension; and as a seasonal cleansing therapy when in good health

Benefits

In addition to relieving the conditions listed above, this therapy has the added effect of giving energy and mobility, while reviving the mind and spirit. It also has the effect of calming the mind and body of the subject.

Necessary Aids

- Suitable 12-foot-square cleared ground—refer to the location specifications in the introduction to bhu sveda
- A pre-dug pit: 6 1/2 feet long, 2 1/2 feet wide, 1 1/2 feet deep
- 3 bundles of khadira wood kindling or substitute (see pg. 447)
- Stainless steel bucket containing the cool amla decoction (see formula, pg. 208)
- Dried or fresh herbs: 3 oz bilva leaves; 3 oz bala leaves; 3 oz peppermint leaves; 3 oz sage leaves (see pgs. 448-449, Appendix A, for other suitable herbs)
- Small covered pottery bowl containing the appropriate massage oil
- 4 woolen blankets
- Clean silk sheet
- Portable massage table
- Loin cloth*
- Eye pads*
- Heart pad*
- String bandages*
- Clean damp cotton bath towel
- Clean dry cotton bath towel

* See Appendix D

Preparation of the Karshu Sveda Pit

Necessary Aids
- 2 strong men
- 2 shovels
- Stone or iron roller
- Measuring tape
- Level ground, 12 feet square

Directions
- Dig the pit 6 1/2 feet long, 2 1/2 feet wide, and 1 1/2 feet deep.
- Clear away the dug out earth.
- Even out the surface of the pit, using a heavy iron or stone roller.

Additional Aids
- Box of fireplace matches, 8 - 10 inches long
- Large aluminum washtub to collect the hot ashes

Lighting the Pit
- Pile the wood kindling in three pyramidical piles and light each pile.
- Burn the kindling to ashes.
- Carefully remove all the ashes from the pit, using the shovels.
- Ashes may be placed in a large washtub and cooled before discarding on the earth.
- Sprinkle the amla decoction in the hot pit and let the steam vapors settle.
- Sprinkle the herbal leaves on the ground of the hot pit, sparsely covering the entire surface.
- Spread a blanket on the layer of herbal leaves.

The pit is now ready to receive the subject for fomentation.

Karshu Directions
- Have the subject rest for 20 minutes after the preliminary massage, while the sveda pit is prepared (refer to preparation of the karshu sveda pit, above).
- Test the pit to ensure it is of a bearable temperature before inviting the subject to lie down.
- The subject should be wearing only the loin cloth worn during the preliminary massage.
- Secure the cooling eye pads and cooling heart pad with the string bandages.

- Have the subject climb into the pit, without getting in yourself, and cover him/her with the silk sheet and then the two blankets.
- Leave the subject's head and face uncovered.
- Leave the subject undisturbed to receive comfortable and peaceful sudation.
- Remain close by to check for any abnormal conditions or signs of excess sudation.
- After the appropriate treatment time has elapsed, remove the covers and guide the subject out of the pit.
- Remove the eye and the heart pads and assist the subject to the portable massage table or to a blanket spread out nearby and invite the subject to lie down.
- Wipe the sweat off the subject's body, using the damp towel.
- Pat the subject's body using the dry towel. If the subject is able, he/she may be given the towels to wipe down and dry off.
- The subject may rest for a brief while before getting dressed. If the treatment is conducted far from an indoor facility, find a secluded spot, behind a tree perhaps, where the subject may get dressed.
- Before the subject leaves, caution him/her to wear warm clothing and cover the head when outdoors to protect the body from exposure to cold and damp. This precaution is to be taken throughout the course of treatment.

Maintaining The Karshu Pit

Like the bhu sveda grounds, the karshu sveda pit may be cleared after the treatment is finished. The herbal leaves may be thrown back on the earth. For continuous use of the karshu sveda pit, it should be covered with a tarpaulin during rainy weather; otherwise, it should be left exposed to the natural elements to maintain its full earth potency. A net may be placed over the pit to prevent leaves and debris from accumulating in it.

KUTI SVEDA - ANOTHER SWEAT LODGE SUDATION

Like jentaka sveda, the kuti sveda is a dry, sauna-type form of sudation therapy. The kuti sweat lodge is similar to the jentaka structure, except that it is not necessarily close to water. Dome shaped, this lodge faces east and is 78 3/4 feet in diameter and 12 feet high. It has a small doorway, 5 feet high and 3 feet wide, the top corners of which are curved instead of square. The walls of the lodge are 1 inch thick. The inside wall is daubed with mud mixed with dried kushta root pieces or powder. If mud is not available, the dried herb may be burnt in each furnace with the wood kindling during sudation.

Four small wood-burning furnaces are situated in a circle and approximately 6 feet apart. Each furnace is 2 feet tall and approximately 2 feet wide. The openings of the furnace boxes are kept closed while the wood burns into a smoldering fire. Like all furnaces, these need to be properly vented according to local municipal or rural codes. Contemporary wood-burning furnaces may also be used.

A bench made from such wood as mahanimba or khadira is placed in the center of the room. One end of the bench points toward the east. The bench is 1 1/2 feet wide, 1 1/2 feet high, and 7 feet long, and covered with three layers of cotton or silk sheets. It is approximately 6 feet away from the surrounding furnaces.

Season: use seasonal guidelines

Body Type: Kapha

> Vata types use only for the specific disorders listed below. Pitta types use only as an occasional invigorating therapy, when mild conditions exist (see list below). Do not use if serious Pitta conditions exist.

Duration of Treatment: 7 days

Time:

Kapha types:	early morning, 25 minutes daily
Pitta types:	early morning, 10 minutes daily
Vata types:	early morning or early evening, 15 minutes daily

Conditions

Kapha disorders: phlegmatic disorders (congestion, colds, coughs, mucus accumulation); bronchial asthma; headaches; indigestion; rheumatoid arthritis; obesity; water retention; anorexia; heaviness of body; lethargy; suppression of digestive fire; and as a seasonal cleansing therapy when in good health

Pitta disorders (mild conditions only): headaches; bodily aches and pains; indigestion; suppression of digestive fire; nervous tension; excess bodily oils; and as a seasonal cleansing therapy when in good health

Vata disorders: arthritis; stiffness of joints; bodily aches and pains; indigestion; suppression of digestive fire; nervous tension; and as a seasonal cleansing therapy when in good health

Benefits

In addition to relieving the conditions listed above, this therapy has the effect of giving energy and mobility and reviving the mind and spirit. It also calms the mind and body of the subject.

Necessary Aids

- Fully equipped sveda sweat lodge (for details, refer to kuti introduction)
- 12 ounces of dried kushta herbs
- Small covered pottery bowl containing the appropriate massage oil
- Sufficient khadira wood kindling for each treatment (two bundles of kindling last for approximately 45 minutes in each fireplace—see pg. 447 for other suitable kindling)
- Box of fireplace matches, 8-10 inches long
- 3 clean cotton or silk sheets
- 1 clean cotton bath towel
- Loin cloth*
- Eye pads*
- Heart pad*
- String bandages*

See Appendix D

Kuti Directions

- Have the subject rest for 20 minutes after the preliminary massage before inviting him/her into the sweat lodge.
- While the subject is resting, prepare the lodge by burning 3 ounces of the kushta herbs in each fireplace.
- After the herbs have burned to ashes, place half of a bundle of kindling in each fireplace.
- Spread three sheets on the treatment bench.
- Light the fires in each fireplace and invite the subject into the lodge.
- Have the subject lie down on his/her back on treatment table.
- Secure the cooling eye pads and heart pad with the string bandages.
- The subject should be wearing only the loin cloth worn during the massage.
- Ask the subject to tuck the loin cloth between his/her legs to protect the vaginal or groin area from excess heat.
- Have the subject turn from side to side to receive a comfortable sudation.
- Leave the person undisturbed to receive a comfortable and peaceful sudation.
- Return at 15-minute intervals to replace the kindling and ensure that the fires are burning.
- While in the lodge, check for any abnormal conditions or signs of excessive fomentation in the subject.

- After the appropriate time has elapsed, enter the lodge and gently help the subject rise. Remove the eye pads and heart pad.
- Guide the subject to a shower or bath, where he/she may wash with lukewarm water.
- Give the subject a clean towel to dry off.
- The subject may then get dressed and rest for a few minutes if necessary.
- Before leaving, discuss the necessity of wearing warm clothing and covering the head when outdoors to protect the body from exposure to cold and damp. This precaution is to be taken throughout the period of treatment.

Cleaning Aids
- Utility sink outside of the sweat lodge
- Shower or bath outside of the sweat lodge
- Fireplace shovel
- Broom

After the ashes have completely cooled, they must be removed from the fireplaces, using the large metal fireplace shovel and broom. These ashes should be thrown directly on the earth outside the sweat lodge.

KUPA AND HOLAKA SVEDAS -
DUNG AND MUD SWEAT LODGE SUDATION

Since ancient times, the dung of animals, such as the cow and elephant, has been used to sustain the habitats and lifestyles of the native people. Even today in India, Africa, and South America, people in rural areas build their huts from grass and mud and daub mineral rich, unpolluted dung on the walls of their serene abodes to a simple matted finish.

Known for its antiseptic qualities, the dried dung provides a cooling atmosphere amid the summer's heat and is also used as fuel to keep the cooking fires burning and the home warm. Covering the porous structure of the grass and mud habitats, the dung increases the inner oxygen level and also wards off bacteria and germs. The flooring of these structures is the natural earth, covered and wiped with the life enriching dung.

As part of the daily cleaning ritual, the inside walls of the hut, as well as the mud stove, are also daubed with fresh dung. These simple people, skilled in nature's ways, extend Mother Earth above the surface and live within her warm and nurturing womb.

The Ayurvedic practice of both kupa and holaka svedanas has sustained the native wisdom of using healthy animal dung to restore balance within the human body. Ayurveda considers the bodily waste, malas, of all species to contain sustaining minerals. As the so-called wastes make their way out of the body, they synthesize essential elements in the tissues. Essentially, healthy tissues produce a healthy body, which, in turn, produces the healthy wastes so vital to replenishing svedas like kupa and holaka. Healthy waste is scarce today. Due to the enormous contamination of our natural resources, which influences the foods of humans and animals alike, our bodily wastes, like our tissues, are becoming increasingly polluted. Today, the dung of animals is being contaminated by the deliberate addition to their feed of toxic chemicals and cancerous growth hormones. Poisoned and polluted dung cannot be used in these therapies.

Hope still flickers strong, however, as a small but significant number of people practicing natural animal husbandry and farming has recently sprouted up in various areas of the Western Hemisphere. With the revitalization of these farms and the wholesome treatment of the animals, especially the cows, we may once again be able to avail ourselves of the therapies that depend on the dung of healthy animals.

In kupa sveda, a deep pit, resembling a well, is dug in an auspicious area free from high winds and dust and suitable for the earth svedas. The pit is filled with the dried dung of such animals as the elephant, cow, camel, horse, and donkey and set to burn. Ingredients, i.e., the husks of grains, paddy, fine sand, and the leaves, roots and seeds of herbs, i.e., hibiscus, cassia and coriander, are then thrown into the burning pile of dung.

After half the dung is burnt and the smoke of the fire subsides, a cot is straddled over the fire pit, and the subject lies on it to receive fomentation.

In holaka sveda, the dried dung is placed directly on a cleared, leveled ground, identical to the site used in bhu sveda. The same ingredients and herbs mentioned above are added to the dung pile, which is then ignited. After the dung has been burnt to ashes, a herbal decoction is sprinkled on the ashes and the steam vapors allowed to settle. Layers of blankets or animal hides are placed on the warm ashes and the subject lies on them to receive sudation.

Kupa Sveda

Season: use seasonal guidelines

Body Type: Kapha

> Vata types use only for the specific disorders listed below. Pitta types use only as an occasional invigorating therapy, when mild conditions exist (see list below). Do not use if serious Pitta conditions exist.

255

Duration of Treatment: 7 days

Time: Kapha types: early morning, 25 minutes daily
           Pitta types: early morning, 10 minutes daily
           Vata types: early morning or early evening,
           15 minutes daily

Conditions

Kapha disorders: phlegmatic disorders (congestion, colds, coughs, mucus accumulation); bronchial asthma; headaches; indigestion; rheumatoid arthritis; obesity; water retention; anorexia; heaviness of body; lethargy; suppression of digestive fire; and as a seasonal cleansing therapy when in good health

Pitta disorders (mild conditions only): headaches; bodily aches and pains; indigestion; suppression of digestive fire; nervous tension; excess bodily oils; and as a seasonal cleansing therapy when in good health

Vata disorders: arthritis; stiffness of joints; bodily aches and pains; indigestion; suppression of digestive fire; nervous tension; and as a seasonal cleansing therapy when in good health

Benefits

In addition to relieving the disorders listed above, this therapy has the benefit of regulating the digestive fire, giving energy and mobility, and reviving the mind and spirit. It also calms the mind and body of the subject.

Necessary Aids

- Suitable 12-foot-square cleared ground (refer to the location specifications in the introduction to bhu sveda)
- Pit dug to these specifications: 4 feet long, 4 feet wide, 8 feet deep
- Sufficient organic animal dung to fill 2/3 of the pit
- Gallon bucket of paddy husks
- Gallon bucket of fine, clean sand
- Fresh or dried herbs: 3 oz cilantro leaves, 3 oz cassia leaves and 3 oz echinacea flowers or leaves (see pgs. 448-449, Appendix A, for other suitable herbs)
- Small covered pottery bowl containing the appropriate massage oil
- 3 clean woolen blankets
- Clean silk sheet
- Portable massage table
- Loin cloth*
- Eye pads*

- Heart pad*
- String bandages*
- Clean damp cotton bath towel
- Clean dry cotton bath towel

See Appendix D

Preparation of the Kupa Sveda Pit

Necessary Aids
- 4 strong men
- 4 shovels
- Measuring tape

Digging the Pit
- An appropriate leveled ground, 12 feet square, is necessary.
- Dig a pit, 4 feet deep, 4 feet wide and 4 feet long, with the earth cleared away from the pit.

Lighting the Pit
- A box of fireplace matches, 8 - 10 inches long, is needed.
- Pile the dried dung into the pit until it is 2/3 filled.
- Throw the husks, sand and herbal leaves on top of the dung.
- Light the dung pile.
- Allow the dung and other substances to burn. When the fire has become smokeless and burned down halfway, the treatment cot may be placed over the pit.
- After the treatment is finished, the cool ashes may be cleared from the pit and thrown back on the earth.

Kupa Directions
- Have the subject rest for 20 minutes after the preliminary massage.
- Place the cot over the burning pit.
- Cover with a blanket, folded to keep it from hanging over the edges of the cot.
- Assist the subject onto the cot.
- The subject should be wearing only the loin cloth worn during the massage.
- Secure the cooling eye pads and cooling heart pad, using the string bandages, before he/she lies down in the pit.
- Guide the subject to the cot and cover him/her with the silk sheet and the two blankets.
- Leave the subject's head and face uncovered.

257

- Leave the person undisturbed to receive a comfortable and peaceful sudation.
- Check periodically to make sure that there are no abnormal conditions or signs of excessive sudation in the subject.
- After the appropriate treatment time has elapsed, remove the covers and help the subject out of the pit.
- Remove the eye and heart pads and assist the subject to the portable massage table or to a blanket spread out nearby on flat ground and invite the subject to lie down.
- Give the towels to the subject and ask him/her to wipe the sweat off the body with the damp towel and dry off with the dry towel; you may assist the subject with this, if necessary.
- The subject may rest for a brief while before getting dressed. If the treatment is conducted far from an indoor facility, find a secluded spot, behind a tree, perhaps, where the subject may get dressed.
- Before the subject leaves, discuss with him/her the importance of wearing warm clothing and covering the head when outdoors to protect the body from exposure to cold and damp. This precaution is to be taken throughout the course of treatment.

Maintaining the Kupa Pit

For continuous use of the kupa pit, it should be covered with a tarpaulin during rainy weather; otherwise, it should be left exposed to the natural elements to maintain its full earth potency. A net may be placed over the pit to prevent leaves and debris from accumulating in it.

Holaka Sveda

Season: use seasonal guidelines

Body Type: Kapha

> Vata types use only for the specific disorders listed below. Pitta types use only as an occasional invigorating therapy, when mild conditions exist (see list below). Do not use if serious Pitta conditions exist.

Duration of Treatment: 7 days

Time:

Kapha types:	early morning, 25 minutes daily
Pitta types:	early morning, 10 minutes daily
Vata types:	early morning or early evening, 15 minutes daily

Conditions

Kapha disorders: phlegmatic disorders (congestion, colds, coughs, mucus accumulation); bronchial asthma; headaches; indigestion; rheumatoid arthritis; obesity; water retention; anorexia; heaviness of body; lethargy; suppression of digestive fire; and as a cleansing seasonal therapy when in good health

Pitta disorders (mild conditions only): headaches; bodily aches and pains; indigestion; suppression of digestive fire; nervous tension; excess bodily oils; and as a seasonal cleansing therapy when in good health

Vata disorders: arthritis; stiffness of joints; bodily aches and pains; indigestion; suppression of digestive fire; nervous tension; and as a seasonal cleansing therapy when in good health

Benefits

In addition to relieving the conditions listed above, this treatment has the added effect of calming the mind and body of the subject. It also gives energy and mobility and revives the mind and spirit.

Necessary Aids

- Suitable cleared ground, 12 foot square (refer to the location specifications in the introduction to bhu sveda)
- Pit dug to these specifications: 4 feet long , 4 feet wide, 8 feet deep
- 40 pounds of dried organic animal dung
- Gallon bucket of paddy husks
- Gallon bucket of fine, clean sand
- Fresh or dried herbs: 3 oz cilantro leaves, 3 oz cassia leaves and 3 oz echinacea flowers or leaves (see pgs. 448-449, Appendix A, for other suitable herbs)
- Small covered pottery bowl, containing the appropriate massage oil
- 3 woolen blankets
- Clean silk sheet
- Portable massage table nearby
- Loin cloth*
- Eye pads*
- Heart pad*
- String bandages*
- Clean damp cotton bath towel
- Clean dry cotton bath towel

* See Appendix D

Preparation of the Holaka Sveda Ground

Necessary Aids
- Box of fireplace matches, 8 - 10 inches long
- Broom
- Heap of dung along a piece of ground 6 feet long and 3 feet wide

Directions
- Scatter the husks, sand and herbal leaves over the dung.
- Light the pile and let it burn to ashes.

Holaka Treatment
- Have the subject rest for 20 minutes after the preliminary massage.
- Spread the blanket over the ashes while they are still warm.
- Ensure that the temperature of the ashes is not too hot for the subject.
- Have the subject lie on the covered ashes.
- The subject should be wearing only the loin cloth worn during the preliminary massage.
- Ask the subject to tuck the loin cloth securely between his/her legs to protect the vaginal or groin area from excess heat.
- Tuck the blankets securely under the subject, allowing enough room for him/her to turn on each side.
- Leave the subject's head and face uncovered.
- Remain close by to check for any abnormal conditions or signs of excess fomentation.
- Remove the blankets and sheet from the subject after the appropriate treatment time.
- Guide the subject to a sitting position and quickly remove the eye and heart pads.
- Assist the subject to the portable massage table, or to a blanket spread on the ground.
- Give the subject towels and instruct him/her to wipe the sweat from the body and dry the body afterwards; you may assist the subject with this procedure if necessary.
- The subject may rest for a short while before getting dressed. If the treatment is conducted far away from an indoor facility, find a secluded spot, behind a tree perhaps, where the subject may get dressed.
- Before the subject leaves advise him/her to wear warm clothing, and to cover the head when outdoors to avoid exposure to cold and damp. This precaution is to be taken throughout the course of treatment.

AVAGAHANA SVEDA - HOT TUB SUDATION

A variety of hot tub baths have been formulated in Ayurveda to relieve bodily aches and pains and to regenerate bodily tissues. The avagahana method of svedana, an Ayurvedic hip bath, has been practiced for over 4000 years and is prescribed for conditions such as hemorrhoids, urinary tract infections, disorders of the bladder and kidneys, and for nervous disorders and insomnia.

The body is thoroughly rubbed with Ayurvedic oils, such as ksheerabala or sesame oil, before it is immersed in a warm decoction generally made from dashamula, a formula consisting of ten herbal roots especially soothing to nervous disorders. Various oils may also be added to the decoction. The bath solution may be tempered with ghee and/or milk for Pitta types.

Although this therapy is mild, it is essential to be free from your regular schedule of activities for the duration of the treatment, in order to allow the body, mind and spirit to be restored.

Season: all year

Body Type: all types

Duration of Treatment: twice daily for 7 days

Time: early morning and early evening, 20 minutes each

Conditions

Hemorrhoids; cramps in the legs; tension of the groin; pain in the scrotum; constipation; pain in the hips or thighs; stiffness of the back; bladder disorders (urinary tract infections); vaginal infection; kidney infection; nervous disorders; insomnia

Benefits

In addition to relieving the conditions listed above, this therapy has the effect of soothing the nerves, inducing sleep, and calming the mind and body.

Necessary Aids

- Small covered pottery bowl containing warm oil
- Small covered pottery bowl containing oil to be applied topically on hemorrhoids
- Large stainless steel pot containing warm decoction for the bath

- Clean cotton bath towel
- Clean cotton robe
- Clean floor mat
- Bathtub

Preliminary Body Rub

For best results a self-rubdown of the entire body should be performed with ksheerabala oil before immersing yourself in the avagahana hip bath. For hemorrhoids, apply two tablespoons of warm kaseesadi oil to the hemorrhoids with a clean hand before getting into the bath.

Avagahana Sveda Treatment

In a clean, uncluttered bathroom, half fill the bath tub with hot water. Close the bathroom door to keep the heat in the room. Spread a clean floor mat or large, clean bath towel on the floor. Undress completely and sit on the mat in a comfortable position. Spread the oil liberally over the surface of your entire body. Add the hot decoction to the bath water, just before getting into the bath. Test the bath with your hand to ensure that the temperature is bearable before getting in. Sit back in the tub and allow your mind to empty itself of its thoughts. Close the eyes and rest in the tub, while your pains and tension slip away.

After fifteen or twenty minutes, when the bath water has cooled, step out of the tub and wipe yourself dry with a bath towel. Slip into a comfortable robe and observe a period of quiet and rest until your evening bath. Repeat the same procedure as above, including the preliminary body rub and the observance of quiet afterwards.

Avagahana Sveda Formulas

Season: all year

Avagahana Vata and Kapha Bath Decoction

1 gal water
1 c dashamula (dried roots) or 1/4 c dashamula powder

In a large stainless steel pot, bring the water a to boil over medium heat. Add the dried roots or powder; cover and simmer over low heat for 1 hour, or until 1/4 of the liquid has evaporated. Remove from heat.

Straining or settling procedure for the decoction: If dried herbs were used, carefully strain the hot decoction through a large colander placed over a large pot. Cover the pot and carry it carefully to the bath area. If

262

powdered roots were used, carefully transport the covered pot directly to the bath area and allow the powdered sediment to settle. Pour the decoction into the bath water directly before getting in. Allow most of the sediment to remain in the pot.

For the required second bath of the day, you may re-use the dried roots or powder along with an addition of 1/4 cup of unused dried roots or 2 tablespoons of unused powder to freshen up the decoction.

Avagahana Pitta Bath Decoction

2 qt water
2 qt certified raw milk
1 c dashamula (dried roots) or 1/4 c dashamula powder

In a large stainless steel pot, bring the water and milk to a boil. Add the dried roots or powder; cover and simmer on low heat for 1 hour, or until 1/4 of the liquid has evaporated. Remove from heat.

Use the straining or settling procedures mentioned above.

Oil for Hemorrhoids

2 tbs kaseesadi oil

Warm oil in a small stainless steel sauce pan over low heat. Pour into a small pottery bowl and cover to maintain heat. Take directly to the bath area. Wash your hands thoroughly with warm water and apply the oil with your hand directly onto the hemorrhoids after your body rub and directly before getting into the bath.

Avagahana Rubbing Oil

Body Type: all types

1/2 c ksheerabala oil

Warm oil in a small stainless steel sauce pan over low heat. Pour into a small pottery bowl and cover to maintain heat. Take directly to the bath area for your body rub.

Ayurvedic Cleansing Therapies:

PANCHA KARMA

CHAPTER SEVEN

INTRODUCING PANCHA KARMA

SHODHANA: THE MAIN ACTIONS OF PANCHA KARMA

*The function of pancha karma is to preserve
the equilibrium of the doshas, promote lessening
of the doshas, pacify aggravated doshas, and
eliminate advanced doshas.*

—Sushruta

Today, we find there is a major resurgence of this unique genre of healing therapies, not only in India but also throughout the world. Pancha karma is considered the font whose essence can make us fully alive again. An infinite number of healing practices accompany this central science of rejuvenation.

The practice of pancha karma requires a proper knowledge of timing, application techniques, and procedures for eliminating the body's excesses and toxins. The five phases of pancha karma are designed to penetrate vital tissues of the body in order to uproot the source of aggravation and dislodge unwanted accumulations. The primary intention of pancha karma—to restore the body's natural processes through the vital forces whose task it is to rid the body of its wastes—must be kept in mind at all times. The body must first be nourished with preparatory procedures, such as massage and fomentation, so that its flow of natural "valium" may be activated. Essentially, the body is cajoled, by pancha karma therapies, into simultaneously letting go of its excesses and retrieving its essences.

Pancha karma belongs to the shodhana group of therapies comprising five essential parts: *vamana*, emesis; *virechana*, purgation; *niruha vasti*, medicated enema; *anuvasana vasti*, unctuous (oil) enema; and *nasya*, nasal insufflation.

267

In ancient practice, the two enema procedures, medicated and unctuous, were considered as two phases within one action; and *rakta mokshana*, blood letting, was recognized as the fifth part of pancha karma therapy, especially where Ayurvedic surgical procedures were involved. Later, Charaka's followers considered the two enema processes as two separate actions within pancha karma, and rakta mokshana was observed as a completely separate therapy practiced outside of the pancha karma group. This is still the popular view today.

Four Selective Actions in the Medicines of Pancha Karma

Ayurvedic pharmacology is steeped in the three predictable actions of a substance: *rasa, virya* and *vipaka*. Although rasa has many meanings in Ayurvedic medicine, for our purposes, let us simply define it as the initial taste of a substance; for example, the pungency of the ginger root would be its first taste. Virya refers to the energy of the substance in terms of its innate heating or cooling properties; to use the same example, the energy of ginger root is heating in nature. Vipaka is the post-digestive taste of the substance, which can differ from its initial taste; again, the after-taste of ginger root is sweet rather than pungent.

Ayurveda is renowned for exceptions to its rules, and the substances used in the pancha karma therapies are no exception. For example, the general rule governing the six tastes in Ayurveda implies that: sweet substances are generally cooling and remain sweet in their post-digestive form; sour substances are usually heating and remain sour after digestion; pungent substances are heating and remain pungent after digestion; salty substances are heating but turn sweet after digestion; bitter substances are cooling and turn pungent after digestion; and astringent substances are cooling and also turn pungent after digestion. Exceptions to such general rules are called *prabhava*.

In Ayurvedic pharmacology, the prabhava, or variance of action within a substance, also plays an imperative role. Rasa, virya, vipaka and prabhava, referred to as the selective actions of the medicinal substance, provide the physician with the necessary means for implementing a specific treatment. Prabhava is present when there is variance from the predictable sequences of rasa, virya and vipaka of the six tastes, or when drugs similar in rasa, virya and vipaka differ in action. An example of the first type of prabhava is found in sesame seeds. Used extensively in pancha karma, sesame seeds have a sweet rasa and vipaka, but their virya is heating instead of cooling and thus is at variance with the energy usually carried by the sweet taste. Peppermint, also used extensively in Ayurvedic remedies, is pungent in taste but is cooling instead of heating. Both substances, therefore, demonstrate prabhava qualities.

Although many emetic and purgative drugs have the same rasa, virya and vipaka, their prabhava actions differ, and thus one group of substances will produce nausea when digested and the other will produce purgation. An example of the second type of prabhava may be found in the use of chitraka and danti; these

268

two medicines having the same rasa, virya and vipaka, but chitraka stimulates impulses of nausea, while danti produces purgation.

In addition to their intrinsic qualities, medicinal substances are also influenced by the condition of the physical organism into which they are introduced, as well as by the timing and mode of application. A drug's virya or energy potency can be radically changed if the drug is not suited to the condition and/or if the timing or mode of application is inappropriate.

Proper Timing

The timing of pancha karma treatment must be finely tuned to both the condition of the person receiving treatment and to the seasons. Aggravated doshas experience a period of accumulation before they extend themselves beyond their sites of origin. The only appropriate time to apply the elimination aspects of therapy is when the vitiated doshas become fluent in the body, which usually occurs towards the end of the season in which a particular dosha tends to become disturbed. According to Charaka, " Only when the doshas become liquified can they be reduced to the impotent state of bodily waste, which can then be eliminated from the body." The dosha's disturbance must be in an advanced state before it can be removed.

Likewise, the bodily tissues must also be approached when they are most relaxed and willing to let go of the excesses and toxins lodged within them, usually at the junctions between seasons. Essentially, once the disturbed dosha or doshas have advanced to their most fluent state, and just prior to their rooting themselves in the tissues as disease, they are ready to be plucked and eliminated. The tissues ripen simultaneously, i.e. at the junction between seasons, when one of the vitiated doshas is ready to be removed.

Bodily wastes, malas, are removed from the body during pancha karma. When out of order, the doshas are also considered bodily waste. Ayurveda does not consider malas to be useless. In fact, the word "mala" is derived from the Sanskrit verbal root *dharane*, "to sustain." While existing in a timely manner within the organism, the bodily wastes are considered helpful to the body's nourishment. The quantum of malas is balanced within the body by its fire, *agni*, and its air, *vayu*. When agni and vayu are functioning properly, the dhatus are amply fed with the essences of food, leaving just enough malas to synthesize essential tissue elements as they make their way out of the body. When agni and vayu are not functioning properly, the production of malas increases in the body and begins to consume live tissues, causing degeneration. According to the principle of natural cessation, the deranged tissues affected by excessive bodily waste, unable to revert back to life, are excreted from the body as malas. Pancha karma is designed to assist the body in its elimination of both tissue waste and dosha waste in order to allow the natural regeneration of vital tissues within an environment of healthy doshas.

Classic Pancha Karma Treatment Schedule

The order in which pancha karma is performed is also of vital importance. When the mandala of therapies are all performed together, the process would take approximately one month. The classic schedule which follows is recommended when all five actions of pancha karma are required; depending on the nature of the condition being treated, fewer therapies may be administered. However, whatever treatment is prescribed is administered only after the initial preparatory procedures of snehana and svedana, all of which is accompanied by the use of a healing diet throughout the course of treatment and for a short period thereafter. The classic schedule of treatments must be maintained whether one pancha karma treatment is being administered or the entire course of pancha karma treatments is given. For instance, if only vamana and virechana are prescribed, then the sequence of procedures to be followed is: snehana, svedana, vamana, virechana, along with the observance of healing diet appropriate to the season and the doshas' condition.

Classic Pancha Karma Treatment Schedule

30 Days	Treatment
1st - 3rd day	Abhyanga and Snehana
3rd - 6th day	Svedana
7th day	Vamana
8th - 10th day	Observance of rest and healing diet
10th - 14th day	Snehapana (internal oelation)
15th day	Virechana
16th - 23rd day	Vasti (niruha and anuvasana)
24th - 26th day	Observance of rest and healing diet
27th - 30th day	Nasya

A brief description of the five pancha karma therapies follows.

Emesis Therapy: Vamana

Excess Kapha is brought to the stomach for elimination by means of two preparation procedures, Ayurvedic oil massage and fomentation therapy. Vomiting is then induced to cleanse the body's upper pathways, Kapha's main location. In addition to its generic use in pancha karma, vamana is employed specifically to cleanse Kapha disorders from the body. This therapy should only be used as part of the pancha karma therapies and under proper supervision. A full description of the vamana therapies is presented in the pancha karma section of this chapter.

270

Purgation Therapy: Virechana

The elimination of excess Pitta is promoted through the use of Ayurvedic purgatives. In this way, Pitta excesses, such as blood and bile disorders, are extracted from the stomach (Pitta's main location in the body), moved into the large intestines, and then removed in the form of feces. Virechana therapy is used in pancha karma specifically for Pitta disorders, and only when the necessary preparation procedures, i.e., Ayurvedic oil massage and sweat inducing therapy, have been performed. Virechana in its milder forms may also be used independently of the pancha karma group of therapies. A full description of the virechana therapies is given in the pancha karma section of this chapter.

Enema Therapy: Vasti (Niruha and Anuvasana)

The two main types of enema used in Ayurveda employ either oils or herbal decoction. They are most often used successively during vasti therapy; however, in some instances, the herbal decoction enema is used alone. The oil enema called anuvasana generally consists of an unctuous substance such as sesame oil, occasionally medicated with Ayurvedic herbs, whereas the herbal decoction known as niruha is a tea brewed with specific Ayurvedic herbs. The decoction or unctuous substance is introduced into the colon, Vata's main seat in the body, to extract excess Vata. Vasti is the primary cleansing therapy for Vata disorders and may occasionally be used without the complete course of pancha karma therapies. A full description of the vasti therapies is presented in the pancha karma section of this chapter.

Nasal Insufflation: Nasya

Insufflation is the procedure in which a medicated liquid or powder is introduced into the body through the nasal passage. When snuff, the powdered form of the substance prescribed, is used, the therapy is called *sirovirechana*. The use of unctuous substances—ghee with salt, for example—is called nutritional nasya. This form of nasya is administered for Vata disorders. Medicated oil nasya may be used by Vata, Pitta, and Kapha types, the substance used as medication depending on the specific dosha to be treated and the nature of its disorder. Medicinal roots such as ginger and calamus are generally used. Nasya may also be performed apart from pancha karma itself.

Nasya therapy belongs to both the snehana, or oelation group of preparatory therapies, as well as being the final treatment of the pancha karma therapies.

A word of caution: the pancha karma therapies contained herein should be administered *only* under the supervision of a qualified Ayurvedic practitioner, except for those that have been adapted for home use and are so indicated.

271

Application techniques and procedures for four of the five pancha karma therapies are presented in detail in the remainder of this chapter. The fifth pancha karma, nasya, is not included here because it is discussed at length in Chapter Five.

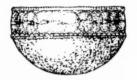

PART ONE
Emesis Therapy: Vamana

Emesis therapy, or vamana, to give it its proper name, is the first of the five prin-ciple therapies in the mandala that is pancha karma. Considered to be an excellent therapy for both Pitta and Kapha excesses, vamana may also be used occasionally to treat Vata disorders. Vamana is the process of eliminating waste from the body through the upper pathways. Prior to determining the efficacy of emesis treat-ment, the practitioner must ascertain the degree of strength or weakness of both the physical and mental disposition of the patient, the nature and condition of disease, the patient's constitution, the doshas involved, the climate, the patient's age, cultural background, and so on. To treat a weakened patient with a serious disor-der with pancha karma is not advised because the extractive nature of vamana, for instance, weakens the body for a period of time. Thus, pancha karma, mostly a series of depleting therapies, is designed to be used under specific conditions; when this stipulation is violated, both the disease and the physical disability of the patient could be intensified.

The Vata dosha, due to its temperamental nature, is generally at risk during these therapies; therefore, a gingerly and knowledgeable approach is necessary when administering these cleansing procedures. Emesis therapy is rarely admin-istered to alleviate excess Vata. There are many rejuvenative procedures, non-depleting in nature and not belonging to the pancha karma therapies, recom-mended in Ayurveda for the pacification of delicate conditions such as aggravated doshas, physical weakness, pregnancy, traumatic diseases such as extreme obesity or emaciation, malignant tumors, serious heart conditions, AIDS, inflammation or swelling of the prostate glands and spleen, bleeding from the upper pathways of the body and for patients who are very old or very young. All of these conditions are contra-indicated for emesis therapy.

Fasting, considered to be a very important medicine in Ayurveda, is one of the alternative procedures used instead of emesis therapy. Fasting allows the body to digest accumulated toxins, rekindles digestive fire, and clears bodily channels while drying excess moisture from the tissues. The timing of the fast is usually determined by the particular disorder and/or body type. Other palliative methods used to restore strength while clearing the body's excesses are herbal and mineral therapy; abhyanga, snehana and svedana therapies; acupressure and/

or acupuncture; aroma therapy; flower and gem essences; potentiated remedies such as those used in homeopathy; and exercise therapy, such as yoga and tai chi, used concurrently with spiritual practices, such as charity and praying. These measures serve to regulate the digestive fire and dissolve toxins. They may also be used to treat disorders which occur in seasons unsuited for pancha karma cleansing.

Emesis, considered a cleansing therapy due to its depleting nature, is the purification of bodily waste through a process of therapeutic vomiting. When conditions such as lung congestion, bronchitis, cough, cold and asthma exist, emesis is administered to relieve excess Kapha from the stomach and upper pathways of the body. This therapy may also be used to relieve many Pitta disorders. Like all pancha karma therapies, it is vital to administer emesis within the proper season and time of day for specific disorders, and with due consideration to body type.

PREPARATION FOR VAMANA THERAPY

Before emesis therapy is begun, oil massage, followed by fomentation therapy, is absolutely essential. Traditionally, the patient is massaged, oiled, and sudated for three days until he/she becomes totally tranquil. Only then is emesis therapy administered. These necessary precautions safeguard the patient from traumatic reactions during therapeutic vomiting and also make the internal and external body flexible. Of the pancha karma therapies, emesis is the one to which the human system is the least habituated. Therefore, it requires the practitioner to be extremely patient and to have the necessary knowledge as well as the willingness to provide the patient with the preliminary nurturing and comforting that will induce calm vibrations in the bodily tissues and the mind of the patient.

Before the commencement of any aspect of pancha karma, the traditional observances of cleansing ablutions—a bath, mantra recital, donning clean clothing and prayers to the Lord—are performed by both practitioner and patient (see Chapter Nine). Many of these observances have been discarded by contemporary Ayurvedic practitioners in both India and the west, partly because of the pressure of time and space in modern society and largely because of the decline in human cognitive memory functioning, which has resulted in a lack of faith in the creator and the natural harmony of nature. It is important to re-cognize that these observances are precious and necessary to the healing forces of these therapies and that, essentially, they are the numinous and luminous core of all healing.

Appropriate Conditions for Vamana Therapy
- The subject must be in a tranquil state.
- This treatment must be supervised by a trained pancha karma practitioner.
- The proper seasonal and time schedules for administering emesis therapy must be observed.

274

- The subject must be cautioned to observe celibacy during the entire period of treatment and for one month before and after treatment.
- The subject's body must be fairly strong, i.e., not excessively weakened, emaciated or wasted by disease.
- The subject must be cautioned to observe the healing diet and activities during therapy, and for the same length of time following therapy (see Chapters Eight and Nine).
- The preliminary treatments of oil massage and fomentation must be performed prior to commencing emesis therapy (for details and appropriate massaging oils for each body type, see Chapter Four).
- Observe the Vamana Therapy Schedule, pg. 277.
- While the subject is resting, his/her head should be pointing towards the east.
- Cleansing ablutions are to be observed by both the practitioner and the subject prior to beginning therapy (see Chapter Nine).

Note: The subject must be fully informed about the nature and intention of emesis and be comfortable with the idea of it before such procedures are administered.

Inappropriate Conditions for Vamana Therapy
- Childhood, old age, hunger, and physical or mental debility
- During menstruation or pregnancy
- Periods of studying
- Grieving
- An empty stomach
- Thirst and hunger
- Before or after sexual activity
- Obesity
- Emaciation or exhaustion
- Severe anorexia
- Inappropriate diet
- Excessive eating
- Suppression of natural urges
- Speaking loudly or excessively
- Physical injury
- Constipation (reverse peristalsis)
- Heart disease
- Chest pains
- Worms in the intestines
- Abdominal disease

- Malignant tumors
- Swelling of prostate glands or spleen
- Hemorrhoids
- Urinary disorders causing the retention of urine
- Headaches
- Pains in eyes
- Prickling pain
- AIDS
- Any bleeding in the upper channels
- Sleeping during day
- Remaining awake during night
- Giddiness or fainting
- Hoarseness
- After vasti treatment
- Excess body dryness
- Low digestive fire

Signs of Inadequate Emesis

- Only the decoction is expelled, the food contents and excess doshas remain in the stomach
- The urge to vomit is infrequent and weak
- Obstruction in the flow of the vomitis—the channels are blocked
- Heavy feeling in the heart and body
- Fever occurs during or after emesis

Signs of Excessive Emesis

- Frothing during vomiting
- Blood in the vomit
- Excess thirst
- Excessive pains in the stomach or intestine
- Loss of strength
- Insomnia
- Dark circles around the eyes
- Pain in the throat
- Pain in the heart
- Giddiness
- Burning sensation
- Hemorrhaging as a result of treatment

VAMANA THERAPY SCHEDULE

To be observed *only* when emesis therapy is recommended.

Seasonal Guidelines for Vamana Therapy

Temperate and Tropical Climates

Pitta and Kapha disorders:

Late autumn:	October 20 to November 20
Late winter into spring:	March 21 to April 21

Time: early morning

Classic Schedule

1) Oil massage: 1st - 3rd days
2) Fomentation: 3rd - 6th days
3) Vamana therapy: 7th day
4) Observance of post-therapy regimens, i.e., healing diet, herbal smoking and calming activity: 3-7 days following emesis therapy.

Observing the Subject During Vamana Therapy

Note: The formulas referred to below are set out at the end of this chapter.

During emesis treatment, it is vital to remain attentive and alert to the subject's progress. He/she must become comfortable and be ready to commit to the process of vomiting. Certain natural reactions tend to persist during this procedure. First, the subject may begin to perspire and shudder. The abdomen will then distend and feelings of nausea will follow. If the subject experiences complications during therapy, it must be stopped immediately.

Symptoms of Complications

- Irregular or untimely urges to vomit
- The matter to be expelled is obstructed while the urge to vomit persists
- Bodily weakness or heaviness
- Frothing during vomiting
- Excess pain or cramps occur in the stomach or intestines
- Fainting or heaviness in the head
- Symptoms of Vata vitiation such as fears, insomnia and erratic behavior
- Burning sensation
- Blood in vomitis

Should any of the above conditions appear, wipe the subject's hands and face with a clean cotton towel and have him/her lie down. Serve the subject warm rice porridge and digestive tea to kindle the digestive fires and settle the stomach's disrupted impulses. An atomizer containing warm water, fragranced with a few drops of essential oil of coriander or peppermint, may be placed next to the reclining subject to calm the mind. Rub the subject's feet with a warm, damp towel, then lightly massage the feet while the subject is resting. Observe carefully until he/she has returned to a state of normalcy.

Dosage for Adequate Emesis

A maximum, moderate or minimal therapy requires a specific dosage of decoction: one quart for maximum therapy, one and one half pints for moderate therapy and one pint for minimal therapy. Eight vomitings in maximum therapy, six vomitings in moderate therapy and four vomitings in minimal therapy are considered to be excellent results. Once the decoction is taken, the oral expulsions are expected to occur at a steady and successive pace.

Characteristics of Vamana Substances and Their Actions

All pancha karma therapies are accompanied by a vast Ayurvedic pharmacopoeia of herbs, oils and substances used to stimulate the organism to produce the desired results. Emesis therapy is facilitated by substances that are hot, sharp, diffusing, anti-spasmodic and subtle in nature. The intent of these specific properties is to penetrate the bodily tissues through heat, to circulate through the small and large blood vessels reaching the heart, and to break up accumulated doshas before liquefying them.

The main tastes used in the emesis therapy decoction are pungent and bitter with the secondary tastes of sweet and astringent. The potency of substances used in the decoction is generally heating. The subtle character of emesis substances allows their passage through the minute openings of the channels and pores of the stomach, while sustaining the necessary balance within the body's most minute particles.

An ideal therapy for both Pitta and Kapha disorders, the main action of emesis therapy is centered in the stomach. The preparatory actions of oiling, massaging and fomenting the body help move the excess doshas into the stomach. As soon as the emetic decoction is administered, the bodily air, vyana, which regulates the functions of the entire body, is drawn to the stomach. This air becomes vitiated, thus allowing the decoction to penetrate and irritate the mucous membrane of the stomach. The impulses of discomfort are then transmitted through the air of the throat, udana, which also becomes aggrieved and, in turn, signals the fourth ventricle of the brain, the medulla oblongata, which is the organism's vomiting center. The sympathetic and parasympathetic nerves are then stimulated; and the udana's vitiation is further reinforced, thus expelling the contents of the stomach. In this way, emesis uproots the cause of stomach excesses of a Pitta and especially Kapha nature, thus restoring the doshas to conditions of normalcy.

278

VAMANA THERAPY: APPLICATION

Season: use seasonal guidelines

Body Type: Pitta and Kapha disorders

Duration of Treatment: one treatment

Time: 2 1/2 hours; late morning
               (after massage and fomentation treatments)

Use vamana therapy schedule

Conditions

Kapha disorders: phlegmatic disorders (cold, cough, mucus); asthma; chronic sinusitis; recurring tonsillitis; spasm of throat; muscles; tuberculosis; nausea; loss of appetite; indigestion; anemia; anorexia (early stages); poisoning; toxicity; diabetes (Kapha related); oedema; fever (Kapha related); lymphatic obstruction; vitiation of breast milk; epilepsy; lethargy; mental disorders

Pitta disorders: diseases of the eyes, except cataracts; fevers (Pitta related); skin diseases, including leprosy; gastro-enteritis; diarrhea; chronic indigestion; hemorrhaging; diabetes (Pitta related); epilepsy; mental disorders (Pitta related)

Benefits

In addition to clearing the problems of the head, eyes, ears, nose, and throat, this therapy regulates the blood sugar and stimulates proper digestion. It relieves bleeding through the lower pathways, relieves tension in the blood and re-awakens the heart. It also clears out poisons and toxicity from the system, extracting stubborn substances from the body and mind. By removing the cause of Pitta and Kapha vitiation, and regulating the bodily airs of samana, udana, and vyana, it has the effect of giving lightness and energy to the body and mind, and restoring reality and clarity to the mind and senses.

Necessary Aids

- Two qualified attendants
- Large stainless steel jug containing the emesis decoction
- Large stainless steel jug containing warm water
- Smaller stainless steel jug containing the cool milk
- Three stainless steel tumblers, one for each of the above liquids
- Small stainless steel bowl containing emetic compound preparation
- Medicated herbs for smoking after emesis treatment
- Sterilized smoking pipe
- Matches

- 5 clean damp cotton hand towels
- 3 clean dry cotton hand towels
- Clean cotton emesis bib*
- Clean cotton treatment gown*
- Clean heavy cotton sheet to keep subject warm during therapy

* See Appendix D

Treatment Room
- Treatment table covered with a clean cotton sheet for preliminary oelation and fomentation treatments and for the subject to rest during treatment intervals
- Knee-high chair, well-padded and facing east
- Low table, approximately 12 inches high, placed in front of the chair
- Large spittoon or bucket to collect the vomitis; the bucket's exterior should be pre-marked with measuring lines, denoting 1 pint, 2 pints, 1 quart, 2 quarts and 3 quarts levels to measure vomitis after treatment in order to determine adequacy of therapy results
- Upright chair with a back
- Knee-high service table to be placed within subject's reach; place jugs and other treatment aids on this table
- Half bath with a commode and a sink

Pre-Vamana Procedures
Note: The recipes or diet mentioned below are set out at the end of this chapter.
- Oil massage and fomentation are to be administered consecutively for 3 days prior to the beginning of emesis therapy (see the Classic Pancha Karma Treatment Schedule, pg. 270), the last treatment to be conducted on the morning the therapy is administered.
- Have the subject drink one cup of lukewarm sesame oil twice daily for the first two days of preliminary treatments, one cup in the early morning and one cup in the early afternoon. This procedure moistens the stool, facilitating easy evacuation from the body. It also stimulates the vomiting center of the brain to induce nausea.
- To irritate the Kapha dosha, have the subject eat a Kapha increasing diet for 3 days prior to emesis therapy.
- Two hours before emesis therapy, give the subject an early breakfast of rice and salted yoghurt porridge. Be sure to measure the quantity of porridge the subject takes.

The Seven Phases of Vamana Therapy

1. Give the subject 1 pint of cool milk.
2. Twenty minutes later, give subject the emetic compound preparation with a cup of warm water.
3. Wait for 30 minutes. If the subject does not vomit, then administer the emetic decoction, the quantity depending on whether the therapy is to be maximum, moderate or minimal in nature, as indicated above.
4. After each vomitis, provide the subject with warm water to wash his/her face and to gargle.
5. After 30 minutes, administer the therapeutic smoking of herbs.
6. Ensure that the subject rests comfortably.
7. No food is to be taken for 3 hours after the completion of emesis therapy (see the Vamana Remedial Menu for post-dietary recommendations).

Vamana Therapy in Detail

- After the pre-emesis procedures have been carried out and the subject is feeling comfortably disposed to the expelling process of emesis, treatment may begin.
- Give the subject a comfortable treatment gown to put on.
- Secure the emesis bib around the subject's neck.
- Place the heavy cotton sheet over the subject's shoulders to comfort him/her during the expected shuddering sensation of the therapy.
- Give the subject the pint of milk to drink.
- Have the subject rest for 20 minutes.
- Administer the emetic compound preparation with a cup of warm water.
- Have the subject rest for 30 minutes. If the vomiting sequence does not begin at this point, administer the emetic decoction. The decoction must be measured before it is administered according to the subject's need.
- Encourage the subject to drink glass after glass of the decoction until it is finished.
- Place the chair facing east. Place the spittoon or bucket on the table directly in front of the subject.
- Place the large jug with warm water, the glass and hand towels on the service table close to the subject.
- Before the subject begins to vomit, advise him/her to wash the face with warm water and to gargle after each vomitis.
- After the decoction has been given, have the subject rub the tongue with the index and middle finger of the right hand to more rapidly induce the expulsion of the stomach contents.

- If the subject experiences difficulty vomiting in a sitting position, rub the subject's back firmly while the other attendant holds the subject's forehead and rubs the area around the umbilicus.
- After the urges subside, remove the bib and have the subject wash up and rest for a short while.
- Measure the vomitis in the bucket to evaluate the adequacy of therapy. Contents of the bucket should equal the quantity of the decoction, the milk, and the morning gruel.
- Gently wipe the subject's hands and feet with a warm, damp towel during the post-therapy period. Then rub the feet so that the subject feels comforted and safe.
- After resting for 20 minutes, have the subject sit in an upright chair, with a back.
- Fill the pipe with the herbs, give to the subject, and light it, instructing him/her to begin with shallow inhalations, and deepen them as tolerated. After one pipeful has been smoked, the subject may continue resting for a short while.
- Before the subject leaves, discuss the healing diet and calming activity regimens to be observed for the designated period after treatment.

Vamana Formulas

The following list of uncommon Ayurvedic ingredients used in the formulas set out below are defined here with their English names. Ask suppliers (Appendix G) to provide comparable herbs if these are not available.

Sanskrit	English
agaru wood	eagle wood
dokshi	bottle gourd
jatamansi	Indian spikenard
madana	emetic nut
musta	nut grass

Vamana Decoctions (recipes make one serving)

Season: use seasonal guidelines
Body Type: Pitta and Kapha

Calamus Root Tea (mild)

1 qt water
1 qt milk
1 c dried calamus root
1 pt cold milk

Bring the water and 1 quart of milk to a boil in a large stainless steel pot. Add the calamus root, cover and simmer over medium heat for 30 minutes, or until 1/3 of the liquid has evaporated. Strain through a colander. Let decoction cool, then pour in a large jug. The cold milk should be taken before drinking the decoction.

Licorice and Honey Tea (mild)

1 1/2 qts water
1 c licorice powder
1 tsp honey

Bring the water to a boil in a large stainless steel pot. Add the powder, cover and simmer over medium heat for 30 minutes, or until 1/3 of the water has evaporated. Remove from heat and let cool while the powdered sediment settles to the bottom of the pot. Carefully pour the decoction into a large jug, making sure the sediment remains in the pot. Stir in the honey thoroughly before drinking.

Warm Salt Water Decoction (mild)

One serving:

1 qt water
1/4 c sea salt

In a large stainless steel pot, bring the water to a boil. Add salt and remove from heat. Let cool before drinking.

Note: An equal amount of rock salt may be substituted for the sea salt.

Jatamansi and Valerian Decoction (mild)

1 1/2 qts water
1/4 c valerian root powder
1/4 c jatamansi powder
2 tbs powdered rock salt
2 tbs cardamom powder
2 tbs coriander powder

Bring the water to a boil in a large stainless steel pot. Add the powders, cover and simmer over medium heat for 30 minutes, or until 1/3 of the water has evaporated. Remove from heat and let the powdered sediment settle to the bottom while the decoction is cooling. Keep the decoction in a cool place overnight without refrigerating, then carefully pour into a large jug, keeping the sediment in the pot. Dilute the rock salt in the decoction before drinking.

Note: After preparing the following decoctions and teas, remember to collect the powdered sediment, boiled roots and so on and give them back to the earth or put them into a mulching pile.

Rice Gruel - Licorice Decoction (mild)

One serving:

1 1/2 qts rice gruel (see recipe below)
1 c dried licorice root

Bring the rice gruel to a boil. Use a handstone to pound the roots until they are bruised. Add to the boiling gruel. Cover and simmer over medium heat for 30 minutes or until 1/3 of the mixture has evaporated. Let cool; then remove the cooked roots with a spoon.

Rice Gruel

One serving:

3 qts water
1 c short grain brown rice

In a large stainless steel pot, bring the water to a boil. Add the rice, cover and simmer on medium heat for 1 1/2 hours, or until half the liquid has evaporated. Allow the gruel to cool. Use a hand masher (a flat bottom ladle) and puree the soft cooked rice until the gruel is smooth and fluent.

284

Dokshi Decoction (potent)

One serving:

    1 1/2 qts water
    1/2 c calamus root powder
    2 tbs cardamom powder
    1 tbs neem leaf powder
    1 tbs doshki seed powder

Bring the water to a boil in a large stainless steel pot. Remove from heat and let cool for 15 minutes, then stir in the powders. Cover the pot with a folded piece of clean cotton gauze and let sit in a dry, cool place overnight. Do not refrigerate. In the morning, pour the decoction into a large jar, keeping the sediment in the pot. Drink as directed for emesis therapy.

Vamana Compound

Madana Compound (mild)

Two servings:

    2 tbs madana seeds
    2 tbs sesame seeds
    2 tbs honey
    1 tbs ghee

Place the seeds in a small stainless steel bowl. Cover with a clean piece of cotton gauze and secure it by placing a rubber band around the rim of the bowl. Place in direct sunlight for 3 hours daily for 7 days, until the seeds are completely parched. Place the dried seeds in a suribachi and grind into fine particles using a clockwise motion. Cover the ground seeds and allow to sit for a few hours, then grind again, using the same clockwise motion until the particles are reduced to a fine powder. Allow the powder to sit for an additional hour, and then grind the powder once more. Using a clean piece of cotton cloth, brush the powder out of the suribachi into a stainless steel bowl. Cover once more with a clean piece of cotton gauze and allow the bowl to sit in a cool, dry place overnight. Do not refrigerate.

Directly before administering the therapy, mix the honey, ghee and powder together into a paste or compound. Serve with a glass of warm water.

POST-VAMANA PROCEDURES

Apart from the necessary healing diet and activities which are to be maintained during and after treatment, Ayurveda recommends the additional procedures of inhaling herbal substances, called *snehika dhoomapana*, to soothe the throat, chest and digestive tract. The herbs used for this purpose do not contain any of the harmful properties and side effects of tobacco products. Dhoomapana is Ayurvedically formulated to calm the mucus membranes of the lungs and to stimulate and restore equilibrium to the tissues, while alleviating or eliminating excess Kapha dosha from the body.

Pack the herbs snugly into a pipe as you would tobacco. Sit back, light the pipe and inhale slowly. First-time smokers should take shallow inhalations and gradually increase the depth as you habituate yourself to smoking. These herbs do not contain any of the harmful properties and side effects that tobacco products possess. Dhoomapana is Ayurvedically formulated to calm, alleviate or eliminate excess Kapha dosha.

Dhoomapana: Herbal Smoke

Body Type: Pitta and Kapha disorders
Use after emesis therapy.

Snehika Dhoomapana

Four refills unctuous smoking herbs:
>   1" piece of cinnamon stick
>   1/2 tbs cardamom (green pods)
>   1 tsp licorice root
>   1 tsp lotus
>   1 tsp dried musta leaves
>   1/4 tsp pure ghee
>   1/4 tsp brown sugar

In a small cast-iron skillet, roast all ingredients except ghee and sugar over medium heat for 3-4 minutes. In a hand food grinder, crush the cinnamon stick, cardamom pods and seeds, licorice root, lotus seeds and musta leaves into fine pieces. Store mixture in an airtight jar in a cool, dry place suitable for storing smoking tobacco. Use as needed.

Mix 1/4 teaspoon ghee and 1/4 teaspoon brown sugar together and add this amount to each pipeful of herbs or to the herbs for one cigarette. To prevent spoilage, add directly before the herbs are to be smoked.

Vairechanika Dhoomapana

Four refills eliminative smoking herbs:

     1/2 tsp fennel seeds

     1 tbs cinnamon bark

     1 tsp dried calamus root

     1/2 tsp agaru wood powder

In a small cast-iron skillet, dry roast all ingredients together for 3 minutes over medium heat. Then, in a small hand food grinder, crush everything but the wood powder into fine pieces. Mix in the wood powder and store in an airtight jar in a cool, dry place suitable for storing smoking tobacco. Pack the herbs snugly into a pipe as you would tobacco.

Vamana Remedial Menu

For: Vamana recipients

To induce emesis, breakfast before emesis

Licorice-Rice Gruel

Two servings:

     3 c water

     1/4 c arborio rice

     1/4 c licorice powder

     2 tbs powdered rock salt

     1 c milk

Bring the water to a boil in a heavy, medium size stainless steel pot. Add the rice, licorice powder and salt. Cover and simmer on low heat for 40 minutes, or until the rice is softly cooked. Add milk and cook for an additional 20 minutes. Remove from heat and, using a flat-bottomed ladle, puree the porridge into a thick gruel. Let cool before serving.

Note: Basmati white rice may be substituted for the arborio rice, in equal measure.

Salty Rice and Yoghurt Porridge

To induce emesis, breakfast before emesis.

Two servings:

> 4 c water
> 1 c basmati rice
> 3 tbs powdered rock salt
> 1 c yoghurt

Bring the water to boil in a heavy medium size stainless steel pot. Add rice and salt. Cover and simmer over low heat for 40 minutes, or until the rice is softly cooked. Mix in yoghurt and continue to simmer for an additional 20 minutes. Remove from heat and let cool completely before serving it for breakfast two hours before emesis therapy is to be administered.

Warm Rice Porridge

Use for post-vamana diet.

Two servings:

> 2 c water
> 1/2 c white basmati rice
> 1 tsp cumin seeds
> 1 tbs ghee
> 1/2 tsp cardamom seeds
> 1/2 tsp coriander seeds
> 1/4 tsp powdered rock salt

In a medium-size stainless steel pot, bring the water to a boil. Wash rice and add, along with the salt. Cover and let simmer over low heat for 20 minutes, or until the rice is cooked. Combine the seeds and dry roast in a small cast-iron skillet for a few minutes. Using a suribachi, crush seeds to a coarse powder. Heat ghee in the same skillet and add the powder. Fry for 3 minutes, then pour into the cooked porridge. Mix thoroughly and serve warm.

Digestive Teas

Use for post-vamana diet.

To aid digestion, increase agni, warm the body

All Teas: two servings

Cloves-Ginger-Fennel Tea

Body Type: all types

    2 c water

    1/4 tsp peeled, finely grated fresh ginger

    3 cloves

    1/2 tsp fennel seeds

Add the grated ginger to water in a small stainless steel pot. Bring to a boil over low heat. In a small cast-iron skillet, dry roast cloves and fennel seeds for 3 minutes over low heat. Then, using a mortar and pestle, crush cloves and seeds; add to boiling ginger water. Remove from the heat, cover and steep for 10 minutes. Use a tea strainer to draw the infusion and serve warm.

Black Pepper-Lemon Tea

Body Type: Vata and Pitta

    2 c boiling water

    1/2 tsp black pepper powder

    1/4 pc fresh lemon

    1/2 tsp date sugar

Squeeze the juice from the lemon into the boiling water and add black pepper. Finely grate about 1/8 teaspoon lemon zest into the tea. Add date sugar, stir and serve warm.

Refreshing Spray

Fragrant Atomizer

One treatment:

    1 c warm water

    3 drops of essential oil of peppermint

    3 drops of essential oil of coriander

Pour water and oils into a spray bottle with a fine spray cap. Shake to mix. Use as a refreshing spray for the subject's face, as needed.

PART TWO
Purgation Therapy: Virechana

Purgation therapy, the second of the five main pancha karma therapies, is the process by which bodily wastes are evacuated through the lower pathways of the body. A primary therapy for Pitta disorders involving bile and blood, virechana cleanses Pitta's main site, the stomach and small intestine. This therapy may also be used to clear excess Kapha from the stomach, since one of Kapha's main divisions is also stored in the stomach. Virechana is sometimes also used to restore Vata's vital air, samana, which circulates in the stomach, although the primary treatment for Vata disorders is enema therapy, vasti.

PREPARATION FOR VIRECHANA THERAPY

Prior to purgation therapy, a careful evaluation of the subject needs to be made by an Ayurvedic practitioner. Physical and emotional weaknesses and strengths, whether the condition is mild or serious, the subject's constitution, cultural background and age, timing of the therapy based on the season and time of day, and the appropriate herbs and substances to be used must all be determined before treatment begins. As with emesis therapy, disorders that occur during a season that is contra-indicated for pancha karma may be treated with palliative regimens such as herbal therapy, healing diet, snehana and svedana therapies, potentiated remedies such as those used in homeopathy and so on.

Like emesis therapy, purgation therapy is also considered a cleansing therapy in that it is a purification by elimination process. When certain conditions exist, such as fever, skin diseases, urinary disorders, toxicity, gastro-enteritis, intestinal parasites, anemia, anorexia, jaundice, indigestion, chronic ulcers, external burns, eye disorders, burning sensation in the body and bleeding from the upper pathways, purgation therapy is administered to help restore the body's health.

Like all pancha karma therapies, it is vital to administer purgation therapy only after the required preparatory processes of oil massage and fomentation have been performed. Sushruta stresses that emesis therapy is also necessary before purgation, especially for Kapha disorders. Otherwise, he says, Kapha may become stagnated in the duodenum, causing the patient to suffer from heaviness in the body. The Ayurvedic physician determines the course of treatment and the

290

appropriateness of emesis therapy as a preparatory measure before purgation. Depending on the specific nature of the disorder, *snehapana*, the intake of unctuous substances such as medicated ghee, may be administered after emesis and before purgation (see order of treatment on pg. 270).

Once purgation therapy begins, the subject is examined daily, using such diagnostic procedures as pulse examination to verify the subject's fitness to continue therapy.

Appropriate Conditions for Purgation Therapy

- This treatment must be supervised by an Ayurvedic physician or a trained pancha karma practitioner.
- The proper seasonal and time schedules for administering the therapy must be observed.
- For specific Pitta and Kapha disorders, see Conditions, pg. 296.
- The subject must be fairly strong, i.e., not excessively weakened, emaciated or wasted by disease.
- The subject must not be experiencing any of the contra-indicated or inappropriate conditions listed below.
- While the subject is resting, his/her head should be pointing towards the east.
- The subject must be fully advised of the nature and intentions of purgation therapy before it is begun.
- The subject must observe the healing diet and activity regimen during therapy, and for the same length of time following treatment (see Chapters Eight and Nine).
- The preliminary procedures of oil massage and fomentation therapy must be performed prior to virechana therapy (see Chapter Four.)
- The appropriate massaging oils for each body type are mentioned in Chapter Four.
- The traditional preparatory ablutions should be observed by both the practitioner and the subject prior to the commencement of treatment (see Chapter Nine).

Inappropriate Conditions for Purgation Therapy

- While menstruating or pregnant
- Weak constitution or weakened person
- Ulcers
- Prolapsed rectum
- Bleeding from the lower pathways
- While fasting, thirsty or hungry
- Excessive appetite
- Low digestive fire

- Along with or after vasti, enema therapy
- During disturbed emotional state
- During indigestion
- Directly after feverish condition
- Alcoholism or drug addiction
- Abdominal distention
- Bodily injury
- Excessive fat in body
- Excessive dryness in body or in an emaciated person
- Chronic constipation
- Flatulence
- Children, the aged, physical or mental debility
- Directly before or after sexual intercourse
- Periods of studying
- Busy schedules
- Diarrhea
- Tuberculosis
- Unhappiness
- Heart disease

Signs of Inadequate Purgation

- Constipation
- Obstruction in the lower pathways
- Obstruction of urination
- Indigestion
- Nausea
- Drowsiness or heaviness in the heart and abdomen
- Burning sensations
- Anorexia or loss of appetite after purgation

Signs of Excessive Purgation

- Numbness
- Bodily aches and pains
- Exhaustion
- Tremors
- Blood, bile or watery fluid appearing in stool
- Giddiness or faintness
- Hiccough
- Mental disturbance
- Prolapse of the rectum
- Excessive thirst
- Dark circles around the eyes

- Discoloration of the thighs
- Swelling of the body
- Cramps in the calves

VIRECHANA THERAPY SCHEDULE

Seasonal Guidelines for Virechana Therapy

Temperate and Tropical Climates
Pitta and Kapha disorders:

Late autumn:	October 20 to November 20
Late winter into spring:	March 21 to April 21

Time: early morning

Classic Schedule

The following schedule is observed when only purgation therapy is being administered.

1) Oil massage: 1st - 3rd day
2) Fomentation: 3rd - 6th day
3) Virechana therapy: 7th day
4) Observance of post-therapy regimens, the healing diet and activity for a period of three days to a week after the completion of therapy.

Observing the Subject During Virechana Therapy

While administering purgation, it is important to remain alert to the vital signs of the patient. It is natural for the person to feel repelled by the taste of the purgatives, and a brief sensation of nausea may be experienced. To neutralize this negative reaction, sprinkle cold water on the subject's face and instruct him/her to rinse the mouth with warm water directly after taking the purgative. Provide fresh, fragrant flowers or a small container with aromatic essential oils, such as lime, orange or jasmine, for the subject to inhale during therapy. Provide a warm, clean space for the subject to rest after taking the purgatives. If, after a short while, the person does not experience purgation, he or she should be given hot water to drink. A warm compress should also be applied to the stomach and hands of the subject. After the purgatives have been administered, a successful evacuation will first consist of urine, then stool and flatus, followed by the elimination of Pitta and Kapha in watery form. The bodily channels will then be free of obstructions. Lightness and invigoration will prevail, and the digestive fire will be restored.

Should complications occur during treatment, it must be stopped immediately. Complications may result from improper diagnosis, improper seasonal use of therapy, defective medicine, or inadequate or excessive dosage. Charaka cites ten main complications that can arise during purgation. **Match the symbol preceding each complication with the treatment provided below.**

+bleeding from the lower pathways
+strong abdominal cramps and pain
+exhaustion
>spasms and pain in the chest and heart
>hiccough or uncontrollable coughing
>pain and agitation in the eyes
~spasms in the limbs
~spasms and pains in the gut
~prolapse of the rectum
~stillness of the joints

Sushruta cites five additional complications:
+pain in the anus
+dysentery/excessive discharge of stool and so on
~purgation treatment producing vomiting instead
~constipation during treatment
~retention of the decoction

Treatment for Complications

The formulas referred to below are set out at the end of this chapter, unless otherwise indicated.

~ **To restore normal health:**
1) Thoroughly massage the subject's body with oil and rock salt.
2) For severe complications, apply pinda or prasthara sveda (see Chapter Six).
3) For mild complications, e.g., no purgation ensuing or abdominal cramps and distention, place a hot water bottle on the subject's stomach.
4) Administer niruha vasti with Gotu Kola decoction, pg. 327.
5) Give the subject a Vata healing diet (see Chapter Eight).

+ **To restore normal health:**
1) Have the subject fast for 3 days (see pg. 273).
Administer digestive stimulants, i.e., Cinnamon-Cardamom Tea.
3) Give Kapha healing diet (see Chapter Eight).

> **To restore normal health:**
1) For Vata and Pitta body types, give the sattvic diet; for Kapha body types, give the energizing diet (see Chapter Eight).

294

2) Administer abhyanga with ghee (see Chapter Four).
3) Administer pinda sveda (see Chapter Six).
4) Administer anuvasana vasti with Licorice Medicated Oil, pg. 328.
5) Administer nasya therapy with Sesame-Ginger Oil, pg. 177.
6) Administer mild emesis therapy with Licorice-Rice Gruel decoction (see Vamana Remedial Menu, pg. 287).

Dosage for Adequate Purgation

A specific dosage of a specific purgative substance is required to achieve a maximum, moderate or minimal purgation result. Generally, three purgative elements, e.g., a quarter cup of herbal decoction, two laxative pills and a purgative oil, are given to produce maximum results. Not counting the first two urges, twenty evacuations are considered ideal for maximum therapy. In moderate therapy, a quarter cup only of herbal decoction is given. Fifteen evacuations are considered ideal. For minimal purgation, either the purgative oil or two laxative pills alone are given, and eight evacuations are considered ideal.

During adequate purgation, the bodily wastes, excess doshas and purgative substances evacuate the system in the following order: urination, followed by the bowel movements; then bilious materials, followed by the purgative substances; and, finally, phlegm matter.

Characteristics of Virechana Substances and Their Actions

Like the characteristics of substances used in emesis therapy, purgation also depends on the heating, sharp, diffusing, anti-spasmodic and subtle qualities in the purgatives used. Through their characteristics, the medicines are able to penetrate the tissues, while circulating the heart, opening the channels and infiltrating the most minute cells and organs of the body. The sharp nature of the purgative chases the excess doshas into the stomach. The presence of all five elements, especially the element earth, in the medicines persuades bodily wastes to descend into the large intestines. Moreover, the heating, diffusing and anti-spasmodic properties of purgative substances stimulate the heart.

VIRECHANA THERAPY: APPLICATION

Season: use seasonal guidelines

Body Type: Pitta and Kapha

Time: 3 hours

Use virechana treatment schedule

Conditions

Pitta disorders: fever; skin disease; headache; urinary disorders; bleeding through upper pathways; swelling of spleen; swelling of prostate; cysts/breast tumors; abscess; toxicity; poisoning; parasites/worms in intestines; pains in the chest; painful hemorrhoids; jaundice; epilepsy; mental disorders; faintness; hypo-acidity; abdominal distention; stomatitis; gynecological disorders; insufficient semen; excessive bodily heat; gastro-intestinal disorder; indigestion; intestinal pain; irregular peristalsis; constipation; fleshy moles; nausea; swellings; external burns; chronic ulcers; abscess; inflammation of the eyes; conjunctivitis; burning sensation in anus; burning sensation in penis; burning sensation in nose; burning sensation in ear; burning sensation in eyes; vitiation of breast milk

Kapha disorders: anemia; headache; cysts/breast tumors; parasites/worms in the intestines; painful hemorrhoids; pains in the chest; irregular peristalsis; stomatitis; gastro-intestinal disorder; anorexia; asthma; cough; epilepsy; mental disorders; gynecological disorders; abdominal distention; pain in the intestines; constipation; oedema; bodily swellings; poisoning; toxicity; external burns; burning of the eyes, ears, nose or throat; vitiation of breast milk; vitiation of seminal fluid

Benefits

In addition to alleviating the conditions listed above, this therapy has the added benefit of restoring ojas, clearing the intellect, preventing aging, restoring Pitta and Kapha doshas, and relieving mental disorders.

Necessary Aids

- Service table
- Clean stainless steel jug containing the purgative decoction and a clean glass placed on service table
- Kettle of hot water and a cup
- Purgative oil or tablets, if being administered, also placed on service table with the necessary aids, e.g., a spoon
- Glass of freshly squeezed orange juice combined with a teaspoon of lime juice
- Fresh aromatic flowers or slightly bruised fresh lemons and oranges
- Small pottery bowl containing cold water to sprinkle on the subject's face in the event of nausea
- Essential oils such as lime, orange, or jasmine
- Small bowl containing the pre-roasted pods of cardamom and coriander seeds for post-therapy tea
- Heavy cotton sheet to keep the subject warm during therapy
- Treatment table for the subject to lie on between evacuation urges

- Treatment gown
- Bathroom equipped with a commode, sink and shower stall
- Clean cotton hand towels and an ample quantity of toilet paper
- Clean cotton face cloth
- Fresh bar of sandalwood soap
- Portable one-burner gas stove for making post-therapy tea, and to boil water for the hot compress, if necessary

Pre-purgative Procedures
- The preliminary procedures of oil massage, fomentation and, if necessary, emesis therapy, are to be administered during the appropriate seasons. For emesis therapy, see preceding chapter.

Preparations for Purgation Therapy
- Before administering the purgative, familiarize the subject with the procedures involved, location of the bathroom, towels, and so on.
- Have the subject put on the treatment gown.

Purgation Therapy
- Administer 1/4 cup of purgative decoction, then give the subject a cup of warm water to drink.
- If necessary, laxative tablets, served with a 1/2 cup of warm water, are given right after the warm water is taken.
- If necessary, as a third measure, a tablespoon of purgative oil is also given. Another 1/2 cup of warm water is given to the subject to chase the oil's unpleasant taste.
- Have the subject lie down on the treatment table, located near the bathroom, and cover him/her with the heavy sheet.
- If the subject begins to feel nauseous, give 1/2 glass of fresh orange juice combined with a teaspoon of lime juice. Draw the subject's attention to the fresh aromatic flowers and spray face with water to which an essential oil such as lime, orange or jasmine has been added. Do this throughout the therapy.
- Once the purgatives have been taken, watch for adequate or inadequate therapy results.
- If there is any sign of inadequate or improper therapy results, administer the appropriate treatment for the specific complication. The urge to evacuate should occur within five minutes after the substances have been ingested.
- Advise the subject to go to the commode as soon as the urges begin and to remain there until the urges have completely subsided.

- Examine each evacuation for signs of adequate or improper purgation before flushing the commode.
- Advise the subject to wash the hands with the sandalwood soap after each evacuation.
- After the last evacuation, have the subject rest for thirty minutes, while gently rubbing the feet and hands to soothe the nervous system and restore normalcy to the body.
- After this rest period, serve a cup of warm coriander and cardamom tea to settle the subject's stomach.
- Before the subject departs, discuss the healing dietary and activity regimen to be followed.
- No food is to be taken for two hours after the completion of purgation therapy.

Virechana Formulas

Season: use seasonal guidelines

Body Type: Pitta and Kapha, unless otherwise indicated

Conditions

All listed conditions except where otherwise indicated

The following list of uncommon Ayurvedic ingredients used in the formulas set out below are defined here with their English names. Ask suppliers (Appendix G) to provide comparable herbs if these are not available.

Sanskrit	English
aragvadha	purging cassia
brahma dandi	Mexican poppy
draksha	grape
katuki	gentian
khadira	catechu
kurchi	conessi root
musta	nut grass
nilini	indigo
palasha	flame tree
trivrit	turpeth root
vidanga	embelia

Mild Draksha Decoction

One serving:

     1 c water
     1 tsp draksha powder
     1 tsp aragvadha powder
     1 tsp haritaki powder
     1 tsp katuki powder

In a small stainless steel saucepan, bring the water to a boil. Stir in the powders, cover and simmer on low heat until 1/3 of the water has evaporated. Remove from heat and cool for 10 minutes. Stir before administering.

Aromatic Linctus

Conditions
Urinary disorder, poisoning, toxicity, fever, cough, asthma, hypo-acidity, excessive bodily heat, exhaustion, anemia

One serving:

     1 1/2 c water
     1 tbs brown sugar
•   2 tsp trivrit powder
     1 tsp ginger powder
     1 tsp cardamom powder
     1 tsp pippali powder
     1 tsp black pepper powder
     1/2 tsp cinnamon powder
     1/2 tsp musta powder
     1/2 tsp vidanga powder
     1/2 tsp amalaki powder
     1/2 tsp haritaki powder

Bring the water to a boil in a medium-size stainless steel saucepan. Stir in sugar and boil on medium heat for 5 minutes; then add the ten powders. Stir, cover and simmer on low heat for 20 minutes, or until 3/4 of the water has evaporated and the brew has become a thick syrup. Let cool for 10 minutes before administering.

Trivrit and Triphala Tincture

Conditions

Tumors, spleenic disorders, jaundice

One serving:

       1 1/2 c water

       1/4 c brown sugar

       2 tsp trivrit powder

       1 tsp triphala powder

       1 tsp vidanga powder

       1 tsp pippali powder

       5 drops of milk of arka plant

Bring the water to a boil in a small stainless steel saucepan. Stir in sugar and boil on medium heat for 5 minutes, until syrupy. Mix in the herbal powders and arka. Cover and simmer on low heat for 15 minutes, or until 2/3 of the syrup has evaporated. Remove from heat and allow to cool for 10 minutes. Stir before administering.

Note: If arka is not available, 1/4 tsp of rock salt may be used.

Potent Pungent Pill

Conditions

Hemorrhoids, gastro-intestinal disorder, spleenic disorder, cough, hiccough, abdominal pain, irregular peristalsis

One serving:

       1/4 tsp triphala powder

       1/4 tsp trikatu powder

       1/4 tsp calamus root powder

       1/4 tsp coriander powder

       1/4 tsp pomegranate powder

       1/4 tsp chitraka powder

       1 tsp honey

Mix the powders together in a small pottery bowl. Mix in the honey or ghee, forming a lump. Ask the subject to wash his/her hands thoroughly and, using both palms of the hands, roll the lump into three or four small balls. The perfect size ball for each person will be that which fits comfortably in the hands without crushing. Administer the pill with a glass of warm water.

Note: Pitta types, use 1 teaspoon of ghee instead of honey.

Trivrit Paste

Body Type: Kapha disorders

Conditions
Phlegmatic disorders; delicate bodily conditions

One serving:
> 1/2 tsp ginger powder
> 1/2 tsp pippali powder
> 1/2 tsp trivrit powder
> 1 tsp honey

Mix all ingredients together and divide into two small sticky lumps. Administer with a glass of warm water.

Mild Trivrit-Draksha Paste

One serving:
> 1/2 tsp trivrit powder
> 1/4 tsp draksha powder
> 1/4 tsp dashamula powder
> 1/2 tsp honey

In a small pottery bowl, mix all ingredients into a paste. Administer with a glass of warm water.

Mild Trivrit-Licorice Paste

One serving:
> 1 tsp trivrit powder
> 1/2 tsp licorice powder
> 1/2 tsp brown sugar
> 1/2 tsp water

In a small pottery bowl, mix the powders and sugar together, then add sufficient water to make a soft paste. Administer with a glass of warm water.

Mild Trivrit-Rock Salt Pill

One serving:

> 1 tsp trivrit powder
>
> 1/4 tsp ground rock salt
>
> a few drops of water

In a small pottery bowl, mix the powder and salt together; then add sufficient water to form a pill. Administer with a glass of warm water.

Sweet Purgative Brew

Body Type: Pitta disorders (especially those of a bilious nature)

One serving:

> 1/4 c milk
>
> 1/4 c grape juice
>
> 1/4 c palasha juice or 1 tsp palasha powder
>
> 1 tbs honey
>
> 1 tbs brown sugar

Pour milk into a clean glass jug. Dilute honey and sugar in the milk. Add juices or powders and stir. Administer the full jug.

Mild Castor Oil Purgative

One serving:

> 1 tbs castor oil
>
> 1/2 tsp triphala powder
>
> 1/2 tsp ground rock salt

In a small pottery bowl, combine all ingredients. Serve with a half glass of fresh orange juice, followed by the same amount of warm water.

Sour Fruit Gel

One serving:

> 2 tbs lime juice
>
> 2 tbs amalaki juice or 1 tsp amalaki powder
>
> 2 tbs haritaki juice or 1 tsp haritaki powder
>
> 2 tbs pomegranate juice
>
> 1/4 c water
>
> 1 tsp kudzu starch
>
> 1 tsp trivrit powder

1/2 tsp cinnamon powder

1/4 c pulp of unripened mango

1 tbs honey

Mix juices together in a large cup and dissolve the kudzu in the blend. In a small stainless steel saucepan, heat water and add starch/juice mixture. Stir over low heat until mixture begins to gel. Remove from heat and stir in trivrit and cinnamon powders. In a hand food grinder, puree mango pulp. Add pulp and honey to the juice/gel mixture and stir thoroughly. Administer while still warm.

Note: If fresh fruit is not available, substitute the same quantity of dried fruits. Soak overnight in 1 cup water, then puree with a hand food grinder. The same quantity of soaking water may be used instead of the 1/4 cup of water.

Vidanga-Trivrit Pill

One serving:

1/4 tsp trivrit powder

1/4 tsp nilini powder

1 tsp ginger powder

1/4 tsp vidanga powder

1/4 tsp black pepper powder

1/2 tsp ground rock salt

2 tsp water

In a small pottery bowl, mix powders and the salt together with sufficient water to roll into three or four small pills. Administer with a glass of warm water.

POST-VIRECHANA PROCEDURES

- Observe the pancha karma healing diet for the first three days; the Sattvic Diet for the next two days (see Chapter Eight); thereafter, the diet most suitable to the person's constitution. This dietary observance gradually restores the bodily fire, agni, which is decreased immediately after purgation.
- A mixture called *tarpana*, consisting of 1 tablespoon ghee, 1/2 tablespoon honey and 1/4 teaspoon finely-ground black pepper, may be taken once a day for 3 days directly after purgation.

HOME VIRECHANA THERAPY

Unlike emesis therapy, mild purgation therapy may be self-administered during the appropriate seasons to maintain good health and to relieve Pitta and Kapha excesses. There are also certain instances when Vata disorders, such as emaciation and exhaustion, may be treated with purgation therapy.

The preliminary oil massage and fomentation procedures are to be performed at home for two days prior to administering your purgative treatment (see Chapter Four). Also, the healing dietary and activity regimens are to be observed during therapy and for a period of one week following therapy (see Chapters Eight and Nine).

Virechana: Home Application

Season: use seasonal guidelines

Body Type: all types

Conditions
Mild disorders: headache; hypo-acidity; indigestion; toxicity; poisoning; exhaustion; constipation; pain in the intestines; bodily swelling; burning sensation in the body; heaviness in the body

Home Purgation Formulas

Purgative for Rainy Season

Body Type: Pitta and Kapha
One serving:

> 1/4 tsp trivrit powder
> 1/4 tsp kurchi powder
> 1/4 tsp ginger powder
> 1/4 c grape juice

Pour grape juice in a glass and dilute the powders in it. Stir and drink. Take once in the morning, two hours after an early light breakfast, for two consecutive days.

Early Winter Purgative

Body Type: Pitta and Kapha

One serving:

      1/4 tsp draksha powder

      1/4 tsp musta powder

      1/4 tsp dried ginger powder

      1 tsp honey

In a small pottery bowl, combine powders. Add honey or ghee to form a paste. Take with a glass of warm water once in the morning, two hours after breakfast, for two consecutive days.

Note: Pitta types, use 1 teaspoon of ghee instead of the honey.

Late Winter Purgative

Body Type: Pitta and Kapha

One serving:

      1/4 tsp trivrit powder

      1/4 tsp chitraka powder

      1/4 tsp jasmine powder

      1/4 tsp calamus root powder

      1/8 tsp brahma dandi powder

Mix powders in a half glass of hot water. Let sit for 10 minutes before drinking. Take once in the morning, two hours after an early breakfast, for two consecutive days.

Summer and Autumn

Body Type: all types

Choose one of the following standard Ayurvedic formulas

1. Ayurvedic Trivrit and Barley Wine: Take 1/4 cup in the morning, two hours after an early breakfast, for three consecutive days.
2. Trikatu or Avipattkar Pill, for Vata and Kapha disorders only: Take one 250 mg. pill in the morning with a half glass of warm water, two hours after an early breakfast, for three consecutive days.
3. Icchabhedhi Pill, Drakshadi Pill, Jalodharari Pill, Triphala Pill or Kutajaghana Pill: Take one of the above (250 mg.) in the morning, with a half glass of warm water, two hours after an early breakfast, for three consecutive days.

Note: Refer to Appendix G, Ayurvedic Resources and Suppliers, for all formulas listed above.

Anti-dehydration Purgative

Body Type: all types

One serving:

      1/4 tsp trivrit powder

      1/4 tsp triphala powder

      1/8 tsp pippali powder

      1/8 tsp nilini powder

      1/8 tsp musta powder

      1/8 tsp katuki powder

Mix powders in 1/4 glass of warm water and take in the morning, two hours after an early breakfast, for three consecutive days.

Trivrit-Brown Sugar

One serving:

      1 tsp trivrit powder

      1 tsp brown sugar

Combine powder and sugar in 1/4 glass of warm water. Drink in the morning, two hours after an early breakfast, for three consecutive days.

VIRECHANA REMEDIAL MENU

- For complications after purgation therapy
- To aid digestion, increase agni, warm the body

Trikatu Tea

Body Type: Vata and Kapha

One serving:

      1 c boiling water

      1/2 tsp trikatu powder

      1/2 tsp honey

Add powder to the boiling water. Cover and let sit for 10 minutes. Add honey and serve while still warm.

Cinnamon-Cardamom Tea

Body Type: all types

One serving:

>1 c boiling water
>
>1/2 tsp cinnamon powder
>
>1/2 tsp cardamom powder
>
>5 strands of saffron

Add powders and saffron to the boiling water. Cover and let sit for 10 minutes before serving.

Tarpana Paste

Body Type: all types

To restore digestive fire after virechana therapy.

One serving:

>1 tbs ghee
>
>1/2 tsp honey
>
>1/4 tsp black pepper powder

In a small cast-iron skillet, warm ghee and add black pepper. Remove from heat and add honey. Serve once a day for three days after purgation therapy.

Aromatic Atomizer

Body Type: all types

To alleviate nausea and excess bodily heat during therapy.

One treatment:

>1 c cool water
>
>3 drops essential oil of lemon
>
>3 drops essential oil of jasmine

Pour the water and oils into a small spray bottle with a fine mist spray cover. Shake to mix. Spray on the subject's face during therapy if nausea occurs.

Fresh Orange - Lime Juice

Body Type: all types

To relieve nausea.

One serving:

      1/2 glass fresh-squeezed orange juice

      1 tsp fresh-squeezed lime juice

Mix juices and serve. Instead of the juice, two oranges may be sliced and served.

PART THREE
Enema Therapy: Anuvasana and Niruha Vasti

Enema therapy is used in Ayurveda to cleanse and purify the colon and to nourish the body. The term *vasti* was originally used in Ayurveda for enema therapy since it refers to the bladder of an animal and, traditionally, the enema bag was made from the bladder of certain animals.

Charaka suggests that sixty percent of all diseases are attributed to the Vata dosha, and eighty percent of these disorders may be cured by enema therapy. Operating mainly in the colon, enema therapy is used to maintain or restore equilibrium to the nervous system. It is administered to alleviate stomach disorders such as gastric and peptic ulcers, rheumatoid arthritis, hyper acidity, sexual disorders, chronic fever, heart pain, kidney stones, and so on. Although Vata's primary seat of activity in the body is the colon, the bone and cartilage tissue is another significant site of Vata. Mucus membrane in the colon nourishes the bones, as it is related to the periosteum or outer casing of the bones. Medications used in enema therapy penetrate the intestinal walls and diffuse deeply into the bone tissue, restoring order in bone-related conditions such as arthritis, backache, nervous disorders, and sciatica.

Vasti is considered both an eliminating and a nourishing therapy due to its two-pronged method. Niruha vasti is the use of medicated decoctions in the colon, to remove excess bodily wastes and aggrieved doshas from the colon through the anus. This form of vasti is sometimes called *ashtapana*.

Anuvasana vasti, the second form of enema therapy, uses oils, fats and honey, with nourishing herbs such as bala, bilva, kashmari and patala. This nourishing therapy is used to build up bodily tissues, rather than to deplete them of their excesses. Anuvasana is a term used generically for both unctuous enema and treatment using oil or unctuous substances in combination with herbal decoctions. Usually, one cup of oil is used in the anuvasana enema. Two other forms of enema treatment in the anuvasana group are offered. When only a quarter cup of oil is used, the treatment it called *matra*, and when a half cup of oil or fat is used, the treatment is called *sneha*. Generally, all of the anuvasana enemas may be used without any seasonal restrictions by individuals who are emaciated, exhausted, overexerted or experiencing excess Vata, since they are considered nurturing and replenishing to the body.

Vasti therapy has been used from the beginning of time to cleanse and rejuvenate the systems of both humans and animals. Unlike the superficial and often excessive uses of colonic enema treatment in our modern culture, vasti is used Ayurvedically in four deeply healing ways. Both niruha and anuvasana, administered through the rectum into the large intestine, are considered colonic forms of therapy. The second method functions through the vagina or penis into the bladder. This mode of therapy applies to conditions such as menstrual disorders, sexual disorders (including insufficient seminal fluid and infertility), and inflammation of the urinary tract or bladder. The third method, douching, is used in female disorders relating to the vagina, uterus and cervix to restore a prolapsed uterus and alleviate vaginitis and certain post-partum complications. The fourth method of treatment, aimed at purifying, draining and mending ulcers, is through the opening of the ulcer, rather a painful procedure.

PREPARATION FOR VASTI THERAPY

In the traditional sequence of administering pancha karma therapies, anuvasana is followed by *niruha*. Prior to therapy, the subject must be carefully evaluated, as in all pancha karma therapies. The physical and emotional strength of the subject, the specific condition of the disorder, the subject's constitution, cultural background and age, the appropriate season and time, and the appropriate herbs and substances, all need to be assessed before the mode of treatment can be determined. The preparatory procedures of oil massage and fomentation are absolutely essential prior to enema therapy. Depending on the nature of the disorder and the individual constitution, emesis and purgation may also be administered prior to enema therapy.

Although herbs comprise the bulk of enema recipes, medicinal wines, meat soups, milk and even the raw blood of animals were used in days of yore. Blood transfusions were administered both orally and by enema before the advent of modern intravenous techniques. In ancient practice, the blood of a live sheep was extracted during an auspicious phase of the moon. The fresh blood, churned with "darbha" grass and mixed with rock salt, was used as an enema to enhance the patient's blood tissue. It is not advisable to use the blood or meat of animals today.

Two main qualities are inherent in the panoply of herbs used in both niruha and anuvasana vasti therapies, namely bitter/alkalizing and sweet/desisting. Herbs such as trivrit and vacha are used with ghee, rock salt and/or milk to form the bitter and alkalizing quality. The sweet and desisting characteristics in enema decoction are found in herbs such as udumbara and licorice, combined with oil or ghee. The nature of the disorder, as well as the individual's constitution, are the determining factors when choosing the appropriate substances to be used in the enemas.

Appropriate Conditions for Niruha and Anuvasana Vasti Therapy

- When used as part of pancha karma therapy, must be supervised by a trained pancha karma practitioner.
- After the subject is fully advised of the nature and intentions of vasti procedures.
- At the proper time and season, except for sneha and matra vasti.
- After emesis and/or purgation, if deemed to be applicable.
- While observing celibacy, i.e., during the period of treatment and for the same length of time before and after therapy.
- For most Vata disorders and for certain Pitta and Kapha disorders.
- When the subject is not experiencing any of the contra-indicated or inappropriate conditions (see below).
- While the subject is resting, his/her head should be pointing towards the east.
- While observing the healing diet and activity regimen during and for the same length of time following treatment (see Chapters Eight and Nine).
- After oil massage and fomentation have been administered (see Chapter Four).
- The appropriate massaging oils for each body type are mentioned in Chapter Four.
- After the necessary preparatory ablutions have been observed by both the practitioner and the subject (see Chapter Nine).

Inappropriate Conditions for Niruha Vasti (Decoction Enema Therapy)

- Pregnancy, unless administered on the direction of an Ayurvedic physician
- After sexual intercourse
- Children and the elderly
- After nasya therapy
- Immediately following purgation therapy
- After taking large quantity of foods
- Indigestion
- Fasting
- Exhaustion
- Emaciation
- Excess hunger and thirst
- Immediately after meals
- The use of cold foods or drinks, unless Pitta conditions prevail
- Diarrhea
- Nausea
- Hemorrhoids

- Inflammation of anus
- Abscesses
- Urinary disorders, such as diabetes
- Intoxication
- Anger, fear, mental confusion, anxiety or sorrow
- Insanity
- Hiccough
- Coughing
- Skin disease
- Anorexia
- Dryness of throat
- Chest injury
- Bodily swellings
- Loud noises or activities
- Excess exposure to sunlight

Inappropriate Conditions for Anuvasana Vasti (Unctuous Enema Therapy)

- After sexual intercourse
- After taking large quantity of food
- Urinary disorders, including diabetes
- Obesity
- Acute Fever
- Anorexia
- Colds and flues
- Low agni
- Enlarged spleen or liver
- Insanity
- Unconsciousness
- Diarrhea
- Internal poisoning
- The use of cold foods or drinks
- Fasting
- Loud noises or activities
- Jaundice
- Excess heat in body
- Exposure to direct sunlight
- Heart disease
- Convulsions
- Heaviness in body
- Pain in lower body, especially buttocks
- Toothache or pain in the nails
- Faintness

- Paralysis
- Impairment of breast milk

Signs of Excessive Enema
- Dullness in the body
- Loss of sensation in the sense organs
- Pain in the intestines
- Exhaustion
- Fever
- Bodily tremor
- Temporary paralysis
- Excess sleep
- Weakness
- Blurred vision
- Mental confusion
- Hiccough

Signs of Inadequate Enema
- Bodily pain and stiffness
- Swellings
- Coldness
- Retention of urine
- Anorexia
- Constipation

VASTI THERAPY SCHEDULE

Traditionally, one of the following three primary vasti schedules is observed within pancha karma, depending on the nature of the disease. All three schedules involve the use of both oil and decoction enemas used on alternating days. Each schedule is to be preceded by the preparatory actions of oil massage and fomentation treatment and followed by post-therapy regimens of healing diet and activity.

Seasonal Guidelines for Niruha Vasti Therapy
Temperate and Tropical Climates

Rainy season (early fall):	July 24 to August 7
Late autumn:	October 20 to November 20

Seasonal Guidelines for Anuvasana Vasti Therapy: all year

Yoga Vasti

A series of 8 enemas: for mild conditions

1st - 4th day:	oil enema
5th - 7th day:	decoction enema
8th day:	oil enema

Kala Vasti

A series of 16 enemas: for serious conditions

1st day:	oil enema
2nd - 15th day:	alternate between decoction and oil enemas, beginning with decoction enema
16th day:	oil enema

Karma Vasti

A series of 30 enemas: for serious conditions

1st day:	sneha (i.e. ghee, cocoa butter) enema
2nd - 24th day:	alternate between oil and decoction enemas, beginning with oil enema
25th - 30th day:	five consecutive days of oil enemas

Observing the Subject During Vasti Therapy

Note: Unless otherwise indicated, the formulas mentioned below are set out at the end of this chapter.

- During the administration of enema therapy, it is vital to remain alert to the symptoms of the subject. The maximum length of time the subject should retain the enema substance is forty-eight minutes. If the enema decoction is not expelled during that length of time, the following procedures are to be adopted: apply a hot ginger compress to the subject's lower back and stomach, then administer an enema containing pungent and sour herbs. The Amalaki, Pippali and Black Pepper Decoction may be used. When expulsion of the enema content still does not occur, administer two to three tablespoons of castor oil, followed by a half cup of warm triphala or trivrit decoction.

- Another formula which may be used when repeating the enema therapy is the Potent Dashamula Decoction. Directly afterwards, use the surprise technique of exposing the subject to cold air for a few minutes while firmly rubbing his/her throat. Assist the subject back into the treatment room and give him/her a warm cup of the Khadira Paste Tea to drink. This remedial treatment may also be used in complications resulting from enema therapy, such as pain in the chest or heart.

- In ancient times a scary object, such as a snake, was shown to the subject to induce fear, which would normally result in the release of the bowels. A less dramatic measure, also quite effective in prompting peristalsis movement of the colon, is to give the subject reading material which consists of a riveting subject matter.

- If the decoction is eliminated before the first 15 minutes of retention, it should be administered a second time. No more than three attempts should be made during a single course of treatment.

- Evaluate the contents of the subject's bowel evacuation after each release to determine the effectiveness of treatment. The contents released should equal the quantity of the decoction plus the ingested breakfast.

- If bodily or intestinal pain is experienced by the subject as a result of therapy, administer an oil massage with ksheerabala oil, followed by a ginger compress on the lower back and stomach (see Chapter Four). Finally, serve Warm Milk and Ghee, pg. 330.

- If the subject experiences headaches as a result of therapy, administer the nasya therapy with ginger juice (see Appendix E, pg. 488).

- For hiccoughs or coughing, administer a cup of Pippali and Rock Salt Tea. Ayurvedic herbal smoking may also be observed.

- Should the subject become unconscious during therapy, stop treatment immediately and sprinkle ample quantities of cold water on the subject's face. Apply a gentle massage to the sides and abdomen. As soon as the subject recovers, give him/her a cup of Wide-Awake Brew.

- If complications arise due to excessive therapy, stop treatment immediately and give the subject warm milk and ghee brew to drink. Have the subject rest in a warm place for several hours and then administer the pancha karma healing diet (see Chapter Eight). Advise the subject to rest for one week, while avoiding excess activity, noise, traveling, sexual activity, fasting, coldness, dampness and excessive sunlight. The subject should continue the healing dietary and activity regimen for a period of two weeks following treatment.

- Generally, the subject observes a period of rest after vasti therapy, the normal period being three days.

Signs of Adequate Enema Therapy
- Natural mobility of urine, feces and flatus from the body
- Doshas' equilibrium restored
- Subject feels light and energetic
- Healthy appetite restored
- Quietness prevails in the colon
- Physical strength and mental clarity increase
- Signs of disease disappear
- General feeling of good health prevails

Characteristics of Enema Substances and Their Actions

The characteristics of the herbs and substances used for decoction enema therapy closely resemble those used for emesis therapy. Mostly Vata nurturing in nature, enema decoctions are made from substances that are hot, sharp, diffusing, anti-spasmodic and subtle in nature. These qualities facilitate deep penetration through the mucus membrane of the colon and diffuse their healing vibration into the surrounding tissues. At once, the tissues are persuaded to release any toxins stored within them, which, along with the aggrieved doshas, are eliminated. The subtle properties of enema substances allow their potency to permeate the most minute cells and pores of the cervix.

The tastes used in the decoctions are sweet, sour and salty with a heating potency and unctuous nature, generally nourishing to Vata constitutions. The pungent and bitter tastes, accompanied by their alkalizing effect and heating energy, are generally used in enema decoctions that treat Kapha disorders. Sweet, bitter and astringent tastes, cooling in nature, are generally used to alleviate Pitta disorders.

Because the main action of enema therapy is centered in the region of the colon, it is an ideal therapy for Vata disorders. The preparatory procedures of oil massage and fomentation transfer the dosha wastes into the digestive tract where the downward air, apana, actively draws the dosha wastes into the large intestine so that they can be extracted during enema therapy.

Vasti Equipment

Traditionally enema equipment consisted of two parts, a hose, *vasti netra*, and a bag made from the bladder of an animal, *vasti putaka*. The enema hose was made of silver, copper, tin, bronze, wood or cow's horn. When used by the royal family, the hose was made of gold. The classic length of the hose was 6 inches long for children, 8 inches long for teenagers, and 12 inches long for adults. The enema bag was made by curing the oval shaped bladder of such animals as buffalo and deer. The bladder was then heated with an herbal antiseptic solution and rubbed with oil until it was smooth, pliable and germ free. The narrow end of the bag was then heated and fastened securely to one end of the enema hose. The other end of the hose, used to insert into the rectum, was heated sufficiently to shrink the aperture to the size of a split pea. Today's enema bag is made from rubber and is fifty percent larger, while the hose is three times the length of the original. Modern bags also come with the additional feature of a 6-inch long perforated nozzle for insertion into the rectum. This enema equipment suffices adequately for present day use.

Vasti Dosage

Niruha Vasti

Mild conditions: 1/2 cup - 1 cup decoction
If oil is to be combined with the decoction, use a ratio of 1/2 oil to 1/2 decoction.

Serious conditions: 2 cups decoction
If oil is to be combined with decoction, use 1/2 cup oil to 1 1/2 cups decoction.

Anuvasana Vasti

Mild conditions: 1/2 cup oil or unctuous substance
Serious conditions: 1 cup oil or unctuous substance

NIRUHA VASTI THERAPY: APPLICATION

Season: use seasonal guidelines

Body Type: Vata disorders
Pitta and Kapha disorders (occasional)

Time: 2 1/2 hours; late morning (after massage and fomentation procedures)

Use the Yoga Vasti schedule

Conditions

Vata Disorders: bodily pains; nervous disorders; constipation; heart disease; abdominal distention; bodily tremors; lower backache; sciatica; convulsions; spondylitis; arthritis; urinary disorders; disorders of the uterus; headache; earache; muscular atrophy; pain in the jaw; pains in the joints; pains in the lower body; cramps in the calves; intermittent fevers; intestinal worms or parasites; epilepsy; vitiation of semen; vitiation of breast milk

Pitta Disorders: gastro-intestinal disorders; hyperacidity; abdominal distention; disorders of the uterus; heart disease; fevers; faintness;

317

constipation; intestinal parasites or worms; spleenic disorders; bodily aches and pains; epilepsy

Kapha Disorders: heaviness in the body; gastro-intestinal disorders; abdominal distention; disorders of the uterus; rheumatism; urinary disorders; heart disease; intestinal parasite or worms; bodily aches and pains

Benefits

In addition to alleviating the above disorders, this therapy has the effect of reducing fat and increasing bodily mobility. It restores a healthy appetite and calms the body parts that were previously afflicted. It also gives lightness to the body, restores ojas and soothes the heart.

Necessary Aids

Niruha vasti:

- Small stainless steel pot with a cover containing the enema decoction
- Small pottery bowl containing two tablespoons of warm sesame oil or cocoa butter which is used to smear both the subject's anal area and the nozzle of enema bag
- Mobile post with a knob, or the secure knob of a door, to hook the enema bag onto (Fig 45)
- 4 clean cotton hand towels
- Clean cotton bath towel
- Clean cotton sheet
- Clean cotton blanket
- Clean cotton treatment gown (Appendix D)
- Bathroom equipped with a commode, sink and bath tub
- Ample toilet paper

Note: Niruha Vasti directions are presented below.

ANUVASANA VASTI THERAPY: APPLICATION

Season: all year

Body Type: all types

Time: early morning: summer, rainy season (early fall), autumn

          morning: early winter, late winter, spring

Conditions

Vata disorders: emaciation; excessive bodily dryness; nervous disease; muscular atrophy; exhaustion; obstruction of urine, feces or semen; arthritis; hemorrhoids; stricture in the urethra; gout; lock jaw; earache; pain in the breast; stiffness in body

Benefits

In addition to alleviating the above conditions, this therapy has the effect of giving strength and energy to the body, soothing the nervous system and quieting the heart.

Necessary Aids

Anuvasana vasti:
- Small covered stainless steel pot containing oil
- All aids, other than decoction, listed above for niruha vasti

Pre-enema Procedures

The preliminary procedures of oil massage, fomentation and, if necessary, emesis and purgation therapies are to be administered during the appropriate season.

Ask the subject to evacuate bowels and bladder before treatment begins. If emesis and/or purgation therapies are to be administered prior to enema therapy, have the subject follow the pancha karma diet during treatment (see Chapter Eight).

Directions for Niruha and Anuvasana Vasti Therapy

- After the subject is fully informed of the nature of his/her disorders, based on the examination and diagnosis of a qualified practitioner, and the procedures about to be administered—oil massage, fomentation, and, if necessary, emesis and purgation treatments—are performed. Only then is enema therapy to be administered.
- Before commencing enema therapy, tell the subject where the bathroom is and ask him/her to put on the treatment gown.
- Spread the clean sheet on the treatment table or on a clean wooden floor and invite the subject to lie down on the left side with the head pointing east (west if therapy is being performed in the late afternoon).
- Prop the subject's right leg forward and bend the knee so that it is close to the abdomen.
- Making sure that the clip on the hose is shut off, pour the decoction and/or oil into the enema bag.
- Fasten the nozzle securely onto the hose and then smear it with the sesame oil or cocoa butter. Always fasten the nozzle first before oiling it to keep the oil from the screw end of the nozzle.
- Use the hook provided with the enema kit to hang the filled bag on the mobile post or on the secure knob of a door. The post should be placed on the subject's left side, approximately three feet from

319

the buttocks. The hose should have a two-foot fall from top to bottom (Fig. 45).

- Place the warm towel on the subject's lower back, over the kidney area.
- Smear the area around the subject's anus with the warm sesame oil or cocoa butter.
- Insert the lubricated nozzle into the subject's rectum.
- Release the clip on the hose and allow the decoction or oil to flow.
- Remove the towel from the subject's back and allow him/her to rest in privacy while the decoction is being received into the colon.
- As soon as the enema bag is almost empty, shut off the clip on the hose.
- Using a small hand towel, slowly and gently release the nozzle from the anus. Use a fresh warm hand towel to quickly wipe the oil or cocoa butter from the anal area and lower the right leg.
- While the subject remains on the left side with knees slightly bent, place the small pillow under the left hip.
- Massage the buttocks and thighs to facilitate the upward movement of the decoction into the large intestines.
- Advise the subject to remain very still while retaining the decoction or oil.
- Cover the subject with the blanket and remain in the treatment room to observe.
- After a successful result, draw a warm bath and have the subject sit in it for 15 minutes.
- Give the subject a bath towel and ask him/her to get dressed.
- Serve a cup or two of Cloves-Ginger-Fennel Tea.
- Before the subject leaves, discuss the healing diet and activity regimen to be followed and for how long.

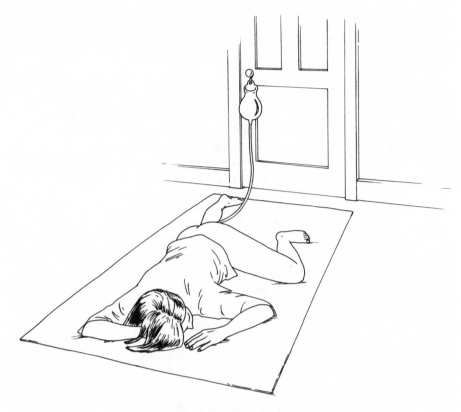

Figure 45: Vasti Procedure

Niruha Vasti Formulas

Niruha Vasti Decoction Preparation

Traditionally, a double boiler is used to prepare enema decoctions. A make-shift double boiler may be devised by immersing a smaller covered pot containing the decoction in a larger pot 1/3 filled with water. In enema therapy, the decoction is always administered while it is still warm, although for Vata and Kapha disorders a slightly warmer decoction may be used.

Enema treatment depends upon the innate potency of the herbs used in terms of their heating and cooling nature; i.e., cold temperature decoctions are not used for conditions that need a cooling effect. If the decoction is cold, it may create abdominal distention, constipation or bodily stiffness. If, on the other hand, the decoction is too hot, it may disturb Pitta, resulting in diarrhea and burning sensations in the body. The appropriate temperature for vasti decoctions, then, is warm or lukewarm.

Niruha Vasti Decoctions

Season: use seasonal guidelines

All decoctions make enough for one application.

> The following list of uncommon Ayurvedic ingredients used in the formulas set out below are defined here with their English names. Ask suppliers (Appendix G) to provide comparable herbs if these are not available.
>
> | Sanskrit | English |
> |----------|---------|
> | agnimantha | arnie leaves |
> | bilva | bael tree |
> | kashmari | comb teak leaves |
> | khadira | catechu tree |
> | kushta | costus root |
> | madana | emetic nut |
> | musta | nut grass |
> | palasha | flame tree |
> | trivrit | turpeth root |

Potent Dashamula Decoction

Body Type: Vata disorders

    2 c water
    1/4 c dashamula powder

If you do not have a double boiler, immerse a medium-size stainless steel pot containing two cups of water in a larger pot, 1/3 filled with water. Cover the large pot and bring the water to a boil. Add the dashamula powder to the smaller pot of water. Cover the large pot and simmer over low heat for 8 minutes until 1/2 of the decoction has evaporated. Remove from heat, keeping both pots together until the decoction becomes warm. Strain the decoction through a fine sieve, leaving the powdered sediment in the pot. Administer as enema while lukewarm. Reserve the powdered sediment for the warm bath that follows treatment.

Potent Gokshura Decoction

Body Type: Vata and Kapha disorders

    2 c water

    1 tsp agnimantha powder

    1 tsp kashmari powder

    2 tsp gokshura powder

    1 tsp bilva powder

    1/4 c castor oil

In a double boiler, bring the water to a boil and add powders. Cover and simmer over low heat for 5 minutes, or until 1/4 of the decoction has evaporated. Remove from heat and steep for 10 minutes; then strain through a fine sieve, retaining the sediment to use in the warm bath following treatment. Pour castor oil into the decoction directly before administering. The oil/decoction should be used while still warm.

Herbal Paste Decoction

Body Type: Vata and Kapha disorders

    1 tsp madana seeds

    1 tbs fennel seeds

    1 tbs ajwan seeds

    1 tsp bilva bark powder

    1 tsp calamus root powder

    1 tsp kushta powder

    1 tsp musta powder

    1 tsp pippali powder

    1 tbs rock salt (powdered)

    2 tbs honey

    1/2 c sesame oil

    2 c water

In a small cast-iron skillet, dry roast madana, fennel seeds, and ajwan over low heat for 5 minutes. Place in a suribachi and grind to a fine powder. Using the same skillet, dry roast herbal powders over low heat for 2 minutes. Combine with the ground seeds in a small stainless steel bowl. In a larger stainless steel bowl, combine honey and rock salt. Pour in sesame oil and add the roasted powders, mixing into a smooth, fluid paste. Using a double boiler, bring the water to a boil. Add paste, cover and simmer over low heat for 5 minutes until 1/4 of the paste/decoction has evaporated. Remove the double boiler from the heat and let the paste/

decoction become warm. Use a fine sieve to strain, retaining the powdered sediment in the sieve to be added to the warm bath water following treatment. Administer as enema while still warm.

Bilva Decoction

Body Type: Kapha disorders

    2 c water
    1 tbs bilva powder
    1 tbs trivrit powder
    1/2 tsp black pepper powder

In a double boiler, bring the water for the decoction to a boil. Add powders, cover and simmer over low heat for 8 minutes, or until 1/2 the decoction has evaporated. Remove from heat and let sit for 10 minutes. Strain through a fine sieve, retaining the powdered sediment to use in the warm bath following treatment. Administer the decoction while still warm.

Udumbara Decoction

Body Type: Pitta disorders

Note: Although the properties of this formula differ considerably from those used in niruha vasti, it may be used as an exception to the general rule for specific Pitta disorders, namely, diarrhea, rectal bleeding, and ulcerated colitis.

    1 c warm water
    1/4 c dried figs
    1/4 c pure ghee
    1/4 c sesame oil

In a small stainless steel bowl, soak figs in the warm water for 3 hours. Finely puree the figs in a hand food grinder with 1/2 cup of the soaking water to make into a thick juice. In the top of a double boiler, combine oil and ghee and warm on low heat for a few minutes. Stir the thick fig juice into the oil-ghee mixture and combine thoroughly. Administer as enema while still warm.

Licorice-Ghee Decoction

Body Type: Pitta disorders

    2 c water
    1/4 c licorice powder
    2 tbs pure ghee

Bring the water for the decoction to boil. Add licorice powder, cover and simmer over low heat for approximately 12 minutes, or until 3/4 of the decoction has evaporated. Remove from heat and strain the decoction through a fine sieve. The powdered sediment may be added to the warm bath following treatment. Combine the hot decoction with the ghee in a large cup. Cover and let sit for 10 minutes. Administer while still warm.

Fennel-Cucumber Decoction

Body Type: Pitta disorders

> 1 c milk
> 1 1/4 c water
> 1/2 c cucumber pieces (peeled and seeded)
> 1/2 tsp fennel powder
> 1/2 tsp atibala powder

In the top of a double boiler, combine milk and one cup of the water; bring to a boil over low heat. Using a hand food grinder, finely puree the cucumber, adding the remaining water to produce a juicy puree. Add the cucumber puree and herbal powders to the milk solution. Stir and simmer over low heat for 10 minutes. Remove from heat and let sit until lukewarm. Administer while still warm.

Sweet Oil Decoction

Body Type: all types

Note: Although this formula does not follow the norm for niruha vasti, it is used specifically in cases of diabetes and increases hemoglobin, protein and red blood corpuscles.

> 1/4 c honey
> 2 tsp rock salt (powdered)
> 1/2 c sesame oil
> 1/4 c dried castor root
> 2 c water

In a small stainless steel saucepan, warm oil; then stir in the honey and rock salt. In the top of a double boiler, bring the water to a boil, then add the castor roots. Cover and simmer on low heat for 8 minutes, or until 1/2 the water has evaporated. Remove the double boiler from heat and let sit for 10 minutes. Strain the decoction through a small colander. The roots may be thrown back on the earth. Pour decoction into the oil, honey and salt mixture. Stir thoroughly and administer while still warm.

HOME VASTI THERAPY

The following Home Vasti Therapy schedule is given for general maintenance of health, seasonal cleansing and mild Vata disorders. This schedule may also be used in place of the Yoga Vasti schedule.

Home Vasti Therapy Schedule

A series of 5 enemas: for mild conditions
1st day:	oil enema
2nd - 4th days:	decoction enema
5th day:	oil enema

Oil massage is recommended prior to vasti therapy. Observe the pancha karma healing diet and activity during treatment and for a period of one to two weeks following therapy.

HOME VASTI THERAPY: APPLICATION

The following decoctions may, in the case of mild disorders, be self-administered. They may also be used as a general seasonal cleansing routine. Follow the seasonal guidelines pertaining to specific conditions and observe the same dietary and activity regimen recommended for niruha vasti. The directions given on pg. 319 apply to the home enema therapy as well.

A comfortable alternative position to lying on your left side with your right leg propped up against your abdomen during the intake of the enema is to crouch on your elbows and knees on a clean bath towel spread on the floor. Keep your chest and head as close to the floor as possible and your hips up. This way you may be better able to retain the enema fluids.

One treatment per day over a period of three days may be administered.

Anuvasana Vasti Formulas

A double boiler should be used to prepare all enema decoctions. Use a regular stainless steel double boiler or construct the makeshift double boiler described on pg. 321.

Body Type: Vata, Pitta and Kapha disorders

All formulas make one application.

Triphala Oil Decoction

2 c water
1/4 c triphala powder
1/4 c sesame oil

In the top of a double boiler, bring the water to boil. Add the triphala powder, cover and simmer over low heat for 5 minutes, or until 1/4 of the decoction has evaporated. Strain through a fine sieve, retaining the sediment to add to the bath water following treatment. Add the sesame oil, cover and let sit for 10 minutes before using. Use while still warm.

Gotu Kola Oil Decoction

2 c water
1/4 c gotu kola powder
2 tbs sesame oil

Bring the water to a boil in the top of a double boiler. Add the gotu kola powder, cover and simmer over low heat for 5 minutes, or until 1/4 of the decoction has evaporated. Strain through a fine sieve, saving the sediment to add to the warm bath water following treatment. Add the sesame oil, cover and let sit for 10 minutes before using. Use while still warm.

Anuvasana Vasti Oils

Body Type: all types

For conditions requiring anuvasana treatment.

All formulas make one application.

Vata types:	use 1 cup of oil or unctuous substance per enema (maximum 9 enemas)
Pitta types:	use 1/2 cup of oil or unctuous substance per enema (maximum 5 enemas)
Kapha types:	use 1/4 cup of oil or unctuous substance per enema (maximum 2 enemas)

Note: Anuvasana vasti may be self-administered. Remember to observe the recommended healing diet during therapy.

Anuvasana Vasti Preparation

The oils or unctuous substances used are to be prepared in a double boiler.

Warm Sesame-Bala Oil

Conditions

Emaciation, exhaustion, nervous disorders, arthritis, bodily stiffness and pain, gout, lock jaw, breast pain and hemorrhoids

> 2 c water
>
> 1/4 c sesame oil
>
> 2 tbs bala powder

Heat the water in a double boiler and add oil. Add bala powder, cover and simmer on low heat for approximately 20 minutes, or until all the water has evaporated. Remove from heat and let sit for 10 minutes; then strain through a fine sieve, retaining the sediment for the warm bath taken after treatment. Administer while lukewarm.

Note: Substitutes for bala powder, used in the same quantity, are: bilva, fennel or purnarnava.

Licorice Medicated Oil

Conditions

Emaciation, exhaustion, nervous disorders, muscular atrophy, extreme bodily pain, breast pain, obstruction of urine, feces and semen, gout, stricture in urethra and lock jaw

> 2 c water
>
> 1/2 c sesame oil
>
> 2 tbs licorice powder

Heat water in double boiler and add oil. Add licorice powder, cover and simmer on low heat for approximately 20 minutes, or until all the water has evaporated. Remove from heat and let sit for 10 minutes; then strain through a fine sieve, retaining the sediment to add to the warm bath taken after treatment. Use while still warm.

Warm Ghee and Honey

Conditions

Emaciation, exhaustion, excessive bodily dryness, excessive bodily pain, muscular atrophy, obstruction of urine, feces and semen, arthritis and hemorrhoids

>   5 tbs ghee
>   3 tbs honey

Warm ghee in a double boiler. Remove from heat and add honey. Let sit for a few minutes until mixture becomes lukewarm. Administer while still warm.

Warm Sesame-Triphala Oil

Conditions

Nervous disorder, muscular atrophy, exhaustion, arthritis, physical pain, stricture in urethra, breast pain, hemorrhoids, gout and lockjaw

>   3 tbs sesame oil
>   1 tbs triphala powder

Place oil and powder in double boiler over low heat until oil is warm. Remove from heat and let sit for 10 minutes. Strain through a fine sieve, retaining the sediment to add to the warm bath following treatment. Administer while lukewarm.

VASTI REMEDIAL MENU

For complications during vasti treatment.
All formulas make one serving.

Khadira Paste Tea (Oral Remedy)

Conditions

Inadequate vasti, heart pains, chest pains, bodily pains

>   1 tsp honey
>   1/4 tsp rock salt (powdered)
>   1 tsp pure ghee
>   1/2 tsp khadira powder
>   1/2 tsp amalaki powder
>   2 c boiling water

In a small stainless steel bowl, mix honey and salt together. Add ghee and powders, mixing into a smooth paste. Pour boiling water into paste, cover and steep for 15 minutes. Pour the infusion carefully into a cup, leaving the sediment in the bowl. To be taken orally.

329

Herbal Castor Oil (Oral Remedy)

For persistent constipation after enema therapy.

1/2 tsp trivrit powder

1/2 tsp triphala powder

2 1/2 tbs castor oil

1/2 glass of fresh orange juice

In a small pottery bowl, mix oil and powders together. Serve orally, followed by the orange juice to wash away the repelling taste of the oil.

Amalaki, Pippali and Black Pepper Decoction

To be used when enema therapy has to be repeated.

2 c water

1 tbs amalaki powder

1 tsp pippali powder

1 tsp black pepper powder

Bring water to a boil in double boiler. Add powders, cover and simmer on medium heat for 8 minutes, or until 1/3 of the decoction has evaporated. Remove from heat and let sit until warm. Strain the decoction through a fine sieve, retaining the sediment to be added to the warm bath taken after treatment. Administer as enema while still warm.

Pippali and Rock Salt Tea (Oral Remedy)

For hiccoughs and coughing.

1 1/2 c boiling water

1/2 tsp pippali powder

1/2 tsp rock salt (powdered)

Pour boiling water into a large cup and add the pippali and salt. Cover and let steep for 15 minutes. Carefully pour the tea into another cup, leaving the sediment behind. Serve warm.

Warm Milk and Ghee (Oral Remedy)

For excessive therapy, exhaustion, emaciation.

1 c milk

1 tbs pure ghee

Warm milk in a small stainless steel saucepan. Remove from heat and add ghee. Cover and let sit for a few minutes before serving. A few pinches of nutmeg may also be added to this brew.

Wide-Awake Brew (Oral Remedy)

If unconscious during therapy.

    2 1/2 c water
    1/2 tsp trikatu powder
    1/2 tsp haritaki powder
    1/2 tsp palasha powder
    1/2 tsp chitraka powder
    5 drops of milk of the arka plant

Pour boiling water into a small stainless steel saucepan and add powders and arka milk (1/2 teaspoon rock salt may be used instead of milk of arka plant). Cover and steep for 15 minutes. Pour off the infusion, leaving the sediment in the saucepan. Have the subject drink two cups directly after regaining consciousness.

Sweet Corn Flour (Oral Remedy)

For diarrhea, mis-peristalsis.

    1 tbs corn flour
    1 tbs Sucanat
    1 tbs pure ghee

Dry roast flour in a small cast-iron skillet over low heat for a few minutes until it begins to turn golden brown. Mix in Sucanat and ghee. When ghee melts, remove from heat. Mix into a paste and take warm.

Corn Flour Mantha (Oral Remedy)

For mild constipation, vitiation of urine.

    3 c water
    1/4 tsp pippali powder
    1 tbs brown sugar
    1/4 c corn flour
    1 tbs pure ghee

Bring water to a boil in a medium-size stainless steel saucepan. Add pippali and sugar. Cover and let simmer on low heat for 20 minutes, or until 2/3 of the water has evaporated. In a small cast-iron skillet, dry roast the flour for a few minutes until it becomes golden brown. Add ghee to roasted flour and as soon as it begins to melt, remove the pan from heat. Mix ghee and flour into a paste, then add to the pippali/sugar decoction. Simmer for an additional 3 minutes, remove from heat. Stir until the paste dissolves completely. Let sit for 15 minutes before serving.

Triphala Tonic (Oral Remedy)

For insomnia, constipation.

> 3 c water
> 1/4 c brown basmati rice
> 1/4 c yoghurt
> 1 tsp triphala powder

In a small stainless steel saucepan, bring the water to a boil. Wash rice and add. Cover and simmer on low heat for 35 minutes, or until the rice is cooked. Stir in yoghurt; continue cooking, uncovered, for another 10 minutes. Remove from heat and let sit for 5 minutes. Add triphala powder and stir thoroughly. Take a few hours before bedtime.

Remedies for Strength

Season: all year
Body Type: all types

The following remedies are to be taken in the order given to alleviate extreme emaciation in both adults and children.

Salted Ghee

Two servings: adults
Four servings: children

> 1/4 c pure ghee
> 14 tsp powdered rock salt

Warm ghee in double boiler or small stainless steel saucepan. Mix in salt. Take in the morning before breakfast for 3 - 7 days.

Roasted Rice Gruel

Two servings: adults
Three servings: children

> 5 c water
> 1 c short grain brown rice
> 2 tbs ghee

Bring water to a boil in a large soup pot. Wash rice and dry roast it in a large cast-iron skillet over low heat for 15 minutes, or until the grains are golden brown. Use a wooden ladle to shift the rice around to prevent it from burning. Remove rice from skillet and place it in a bowl. Add ghee

332

to the heated skillet and let it melt over low heat for 5 minutes. Add to boiling water along with the rice. Cover and simmer on low heat for 2 hours. Remove from the heat and serve warm. Take with the following Sesame-Sugar Condiment as a mono-diet three times a day for 3 - 7 days.

Sesame-Sugar Condiment

Nine servings: adults

Eighteen servings: children

> 1 c sesame seeds
>
> 2 tbs brown sugar

Wash sesame seeds and dry roast in a large cast-iron skillet over low heat for 15 minutes, or until they are crisp but not burnt. Use a wooden ladle to shift the seeds around the pan to prevent them from sticking or burning. Remove seeds and add sugar to the heated skillet. Warm over low heat, then remove from skillet. Grind the seeds in a large suribachi, using a clockwise motion, until they are 3/4 ground. Place in a bowl, using a pastry brush or a clean cloth towel to brush all of the sesame powder into the bowl. Add the roasted sugar to the ground sesame seeds and blend the mixture together. Place in a clean, airtight glass jar and store in a cool, dry place. Condiment will remain fresh enough to use for one week. Sprinkle two tablespoons over each serving of roasted rice gruel.

Sweet Yoghurt

Two servings: adults

Four servings: children

> 2 c yoghurt
>
> 2 tbs Sucanat
>
> 12 strands of saffron

Blend all ingredients together in a stainless steel bowl and warm in a double boiler. Take after lunch for 3 - 7 days.

Milk-Ghee

Two servings: adults

Four servings: children

      2 c milk

      1 tbs pure ghee

Heat milk in a small stainless steel saucepan or in a double boiler. Add ghee. Remove from heat and let sit for a few minutes before drinking. Take one hour before bed for 3 - 7 days.

PART FOUR
Douching Therapy: Uttara Vasti
Home Therapy

As old as time itself, douching has been used primarily to refresh and cleanse the female's vaginal passages. Although douching may also occur through the penis to alleviate urinary disorders, and through the opening of the mouth of an ulcer to extract impurities and cleanse the ulcer, these practices are seldom used in modern day Ayurveda.

The process of douching is a simple application, which is palliative to many female disorders. Used over a short period of time, it can restore the healthy status of the uterus and alleviate vaginal disorders. As a natural form of birth control, douching may also be done directly after sexual intercourse. The vaginal passage and uterus may also be purified and mollified after menstruation by douching. Following menopause, occasional douching with special oils helps to revitalize the hormonal system, giving youthfulness and stamina to the body.

PREPARATION FOR UTTARA VASTI
Inappropriate Conditions
- During or immediately after the menstrual cycle
- Childhood
- During pregnancy (without the advice of an Ayurvedic physician)
- Vaginal bleeding or hemorrhaging
- Excess heat or cold weather
- Directly after eating
- Diarrhea
- After emesis
- After purgation
- After enema

Appropriate Conditions
- Vaginal infections
- Malodor
- Dryness or soreness of vaginal passage
- Stagnation in or disorders of the uterus

335

- Pre-menstrual syndrome
- Irregular or excess menstrual flow
- Four days after menstrual cycle
- Directly after sexual intercourse, as a birth control measure
- After menopause
- Venereal disease
- Sterility

Benefits

In addition to relieving the conditions listed above, this treatment has the added benefit of increasing ojas, replenishing the hormonal system and promoting fertility. This treatment also gives vibrant energy to the female organs.

Necessary Aids

- Vata and Kapha types: a small pottery bowl containing two table-spoons of warm sesame oil
- Pitta types: a small pottery bowl containing two tablespoons of lukewarm coconut oil
- 5 drops of appropriate essential oil for the bath, pgs. 397-399.
- Re-usable douche bag, with a douching nozzle
- Bathtub
- Clean cotton hand towel

UTTARA VASTI THERAPY: APPLICATION

Douching Treatment

- An oil massage or self massage is recommended before douching.
- Observe the sattvic diet on the douching days (see Chapter Eight).
- Spread a clean towel in the bathtub.
- Attach the nozzle to the douche bag and close the shut-off clip before pouring the douching solution in it.
- Smear the nozzle with an ample amount of oil or cocoa butter.
- Hang the douche bag containing the solution approximately three feet above where you will be lying.
- Undress and rest comfortably on your back with the legs apart and knees bent.
- Take a few deep breaths.

- Close your eyes and feel every limb in your body relaxing.
- Insert the nozzle into the vaginal passage.
- Squeeze your buttocks firmly together and lift the hips slightly off the ground.
- Some solution will spill in the process.
- As soon as the douche bag is empty, relax the hips, release the nozzle from the vaginal passage, and allow the douching solution to flow out gradually.
- Gently get up and remove the wet towel from the tub.
- Since the retention of decoction is so brief, you may immediately repeat the process.
- Afterwards, half-fill the bath, adding the drops of essential oil to the warm water.
- Allow yourself to sit and luxuriate in the bath until it cools.
- Dry yourself with the bath towel and gently massage your belly for a few minutes.
- Rest for a few hours after douching.

Uttara Vasti Formulas

Season: all year

Time: late morning or early evening

Duration of Treatment

> After menstrual cycle: a series of 3 douches on alternating days. If menstrual disorders or pre-menstrual symptoms exist, use prior to menstruation.

Preparation: the decoction or oil used to prepare the douching solution should be heated in a double-boiler. All formulas make one application.

Cleansing Douche

Body Type: all types

General Cleanser and Refresher

> 2 c water
>
> 1 tbs triphala powder
>
> 1 tbs aloe vera gel

Bring the water to a boil in a double boiler. Add triphala powder, cover and simmer on low heat for 3 minutes. Remove from heat and steep for 10 minutes. Strain the decoction through a fine sieve, retaining the sediment to add to your bath water. Stir in the aloe vera gel and administer while still warm.

Roseflower Douche

Body Type: Vata
Conditions
Scanty menstrual flow, sterility, vaginal dryness, uterine disorders

> 2 c water
> 1 tbs dried false unicorn leaves
> 1 tbs dried raspberry leaves
> 1 tsp dried red roseflower buds
> 1 tbs sesame oil

Bring water to a boil in a double boiler. Add dried leaves and buds. Cover and simmer on low heat for 5 minutes. Remove from heat and steep for 10 minutes. Strain, then add sesame oil. Keep the leaves and buds to add to your bath following the treatment.

Ashwagandha-Comfrey Douche

Body Type: Kapha
Conditions
Sterility, scanty sexual urges, stagnation in uterus, pre-menstrual pains or cramps, venereal diseases

> 2 c water
> 2 tsp ashwagandha powder
> 1 tsp comfrey powder
> 1 tbs aloe vera gel

Bring water to a boil in a double boiler. Add powders, cover and simmer on low heat for 5 minutes. Remove from heat and steep for 10 minutes. Strain the solution through a fine sieve, retaining the sediment for your bath following treatment. Stir in aloe vera gel and use while warm.

Shatavari-Saffron Douche

Body Type: Pitta
Conditions
Staleness and vaginal malodor, sterility, pre-menstrual pains or cramps, uterine disorders, toxicity in uterus, excessive sexual urges, excess vaginal heat, as a rejuvenant for older women

> 2 c water
> 1 tbs shatavari powder
> 1/2 tsp saffron (12 strands)
> 1 tbs coconut oil

Bring water to a boil in a double boiler. Add shatavari powder and saffron, cover and simmer on low heat for 5 minutes. Remove from heat and steep for 10 minutes. Strain through a fine sieve, retaining the sediment for your bath following treatment. Stir in the coconut oil and use while lukewarm.

Blessed Thistle Solution

Body Type: Pitta and Kapha

Conditions

Excessive menstrual flow, malodor or soreness in vaginal passage, uterine disorders

> 3 c water
> 1 tbs dried blessed thistle
> 1 tsp atibala powder
> 1 tsp dried passion flower
> 1 tsp dried hibiscus flower
> 1 tsp gum arabic powder
> 1/4 c boiling water

Bring 3 cups of water to a boil in a double boiler. Add dried herbs and atibala powder. Cover and steep for 10 minutes on low heat, or until 1/3 of the water has evaporated. Remove from heat and steep for 10 minutes. Strain through a colander, retaining the sediment for your bath following treatment. Mix gum arabic powder in the 1/4 cup of boiling water. Stir until it becomes slightly gel-like. Add to the decoction and use as a douche while lukewarm.

Sweet Lotus Solution

Body Type: all types

General cleanser and refresher.

> 2 c water
> 1 tbs lotus seed powder
> 1 tsp Sucanat
> 2 drops essential oil of fennel
> 1 tsp coconut oil

Bring water to a boil in a double boiler. Add lotus powder and Sucanat. Cover and simmer on low heat for 5 minutes. Remove from heat and steep for 10 minutes. Strain solution through a fine sieve, retaining the sediment for your bath water following treatment. Add coconut and fennel oils. Use while lukewarm.

Antibiotic Douche

Body Type: all types

Conditions

Vaginal infections, vaginal soreness, venereal diseases, uterus disorders, stagnation in uterus

> 3 c water
>
> 1 tbs echinacea powder
>
> 1 tsp comfrey powder
>
> 1 tsp dried lemon grass
>
> 1 tbs aloe vera gel
>
> 1 tbs coconut oil

Bring water to a boil in a double boiler. Add powders and dried herb, and simmer over low heat for 10 minutes, or until 1/3 of the water has evaporated. Remove from heat and allow to steep for 10 minutes. Strain the solution through a fine sieve, retaining the sediment for your bath after treatment. Add aloe vera gel and coconut oil. Use warm.

Rasa Douching Oil

Body Type: all types

For females over fifty.

> 2 c water
>
> 1/2 c coconut oil
>
> 1 tsp lavender rose flower buds
>
> 1 tsp saffron (24 strands)
>
> 1 tsp fennel seeds
>
> 1 tsp triphala powder
>
> 1/2 tsp Sucanat

Combine water and oil and bring to a boil in a double boiler. Add remaining ingredients, cover and simmer on low heat for 20 minutes, or until all the water has evaporated and approximately 1/2 cup of oil remains. Remove from heat and strain, retaining the sediment for your bath after treatment. Use lukewarm for douching.

SECTION V

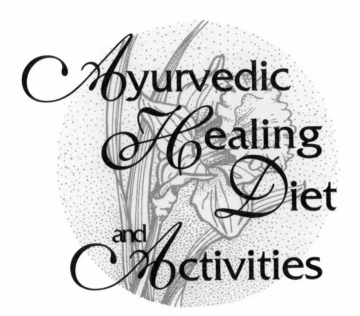

Ayurvedic
Healing
Diet
and
Activities

CHAPTER EIGHT
THE HEALING DIET

PART ONE
Food and Memory

*All the world seeks food. It is the life source
of all beings. Clarity, longevity, intelligence,
happiness, contentment, strength and knowledge are all rooted in food.*

—Charaka

Nourished by the elements, every tree, plant, shrub, herb, fruit and seed possesses the life-giving juice, *rasa*, the essence of which has been refined since the beginning of life. The word for food in Sanskrit, *annam*, means that which springs from the earth because of the nurturing rain water, the invigorating fire of the sun, and the massaging breath of the wind. In Vedic mythology, the first seed was said to have sprouted as a result of a strand of the creator's hair falling to earth. In fact, all life is born from the first seed of creation which contains the memory of all time. A wholesome seed is one which has not been tampered with or manipulated by human technology; only such a seed is capable of sprouting a happy plant.

Each food bears the intrinsic nature of its species. The asparagus fern, which grows within the calm shaded light of the forest, exudes the same gentle energy once it has been assimilated in our bodies. The coconut tree, which grows high up into the sky, bears fruit that is cosseted within husk and shell so that it remains cool, milky, and gelatinous. This food assuages the membranes of our tissues and mind. The ripened peach knows just when to let go of the branch of its mother tree so that we may feast on its succulent, sun-colored flesh.

Referred to as God itself in the Taittiriya Upanishad, food is much more than nutrition. In eating, we are assimilating God by churning the essences of the universe within our body, enabling us to recall our cognitive memories.

The universe's rasa is expressed through the six tastes, i.e., sweet, sour, salty, pungent, bitter and astringent. Each taste is imbued with the cosmic memory of its original seed from the time of the onset of creation. The sweet taste brings us virility, lavish love, abundant wealth and goodness, virtues that only the sweet taste can carry throughout the passage of all time. The sour taste imparts activity, courage and vivacity. Salty taste brings fortification and the ability to penetrate the most subtle cell of the body. Pungent taste gives us stimulation, invigoration and awakens our interest in pursuing life's challenges. Bitter taste gives us a reprieve so that we may peer deeply into our cognitive memories and extract negative forces stored within the organism. Working together with the bitter, the astringent taste discards damaged tissues and toxicity from the system while disciplining and restoring intelligence to the body and mind.

In Ayurveda, all food belongs to one of three categories. Good quality milk, ghee, wheat and fruits that are sweet and cooling are considered to be calm-inducing, *sattvic*, by nature. Stimulating and heat-producing foods, such as ginger, pepper and radish, are considered to be activating, *rajasic*, by nature. Heavy and debilitating foods, whether heat-producing or cold, such as excess garlic, alcohol, and ice cream, are considered to be mind dulling, *tamasic*, by nature. If we are to develop our capacity to be aware of our cognitive memories, an understanding of how certain foods affect our bodies and minds is essential.

THE FIRST FOOD

The Charaka Samhita identifies the first foods of the earth as rice and barley grains, mung beans, amalaki (gooseberry) fruit, rain water, rock-salt, honey, milk and ghee. Animals and birds such as the gray partridge and common quail, which inhabited the dry forests, served as supplements to this original diet.

Grains have been the primary sustenance of civilization from the beginning of time. Rice, regarded as the king of the grains, provides the system with the necessary complex carbohydrates if its bran layer remains intact. Wheat and barley are the most cooling grains, while millet, quinoa, buckwheat and rye are the most heat-producing. According to the Ayurvedic science of nutrition, all grains perform a necessary function, although we are advised to choose those which are most suitable to our individual constitution. The mung bean is considered to be the queen of the legumes. Beans provide the necessary protein as well as having a mildly astringent effect on the body. Like grains, all beans are beneficial to good health; however, the smaller the bean, the more nutritious it is.

Amalaki is one of the most ancient fruits on earth and contains five of the six universal tastes; only the salty taste is absent. A sour fruit with a sweet post-digestive taste, Amalaki is used extensively in Ayurvedic medicine because it is suitable for all three doshas and is an excellent rejuvenator and respirant. One of these fruits contains as much vitamin C as twenty oranges. Due to the heat resistant nature of the vitamins contained in the amalaki fruit, processing does not disturb its vitamin content, unlike so many other fruits.

Water is the most important element on earth. Without it, the ability to taste food would not exist. The first element to nurture the entire creation is sattvic cooling water. Ayurveda considers rain water to be the most vital elixir for achieving and maintaining good health.

Ayurvedic rock salt, called saindhava or sendha namak, contains all the necessary minerals for human well being. Hot and potent, yet more cooling than natural sea salt when taken into the body, rock salt may be used in small quantities even when other salts are prohibited. Rock salt contains very subtle properties which allow it to penetrate deeply into the minutest pores of the tissues and cells. Unlike most salts, it does not obstruct the channels of circulation, a necessary consideration during pancha karma therapy. Rock salt is digested by the system only after it is diffused throughout the organism. This salt is mined in its crystalline form, much like coal, from the dry, underground sea beds. In India, most of the rock salt comes from the Sindh Mountain regions of Pakistan. Rock salt is used in Ayurveda for many disorders stemming from all three doshas. Generally, however, it is best for Vata types; Pitta types are advised to use it moderately, and Kapha types minimally.

Considered the first food, grains, legumes, fruits, herbs, milk, ghee, honey and rock salt, then, are the substratum for the healing diet set out in this chapter.

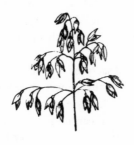

PART TWO
The Animal Is Not Our Food

From the earth came herbs (and) from herbs
came the seed that gave life to humans.
—Taittiriya Upanishad (11.1)

The Vedas, which preceded Ayurvedic knowledge, maintain that human food is primarily of plant origin, which, to some extent, is dependent upon the earth's minerals, supplemented by the natural foods provided by animals, i.e., milk and honey--in other words, foods obtained without slaughtering the animals themselves. Certain external parts of animals, birds and aquatic creatures have been used since the beginning of time to formulate medicines for alleviating various ailments. These include the tusks and teeth of the elephant, feathers of the peacock, antlers of the deer, musk drawn from the preputial gland of the musk deer, the dung of a healthy elephant, the urine of a healthy cow, venom of the snake, lac exuded by the lac insect, pearls from oysters, conch and cowrie shells, and coral from the reefs.

It is also known that animals have been sacrificed in ancient religious rites as atonement for the misdeeds of humans, or so that humans may capture, sacrifice and gain the intrinsic cosmic memories carried by the animal species. Later, in Ayurveda, animals were also sacrificed as medicine for humans suffering from debilitating diseases, such as amnesia, the loss of will to live, inertia, emaciation, anemia, severe vitiation of blood and semen, excruciating pain of the joints, organs, abdomen or veins. An animal's flesh is imbued with more consciousness than plant life and contains nature's intensely activating memory, in the form of rajas, the universal principle of mobility. Because of its active nature, animal flesh has been used therapeutically to build up a degenerating system while activating cellular memory in the human body. In this process, the impulses to live and to survive may be awakened.

In ancient practices, animal sacrifice for authentic human needs was conducted with harmonic accord, universal reverence, and sincere gratitude. We have distanced ourselves so far from the knowledgeable and reverent trading with nature practiced by the ancients that we can no longer barter with the lives of the animals for our survival because the most necessary faculty—our ability to remember cognitively—has become dramatically diminished. Through the loss of our

346

own cognitive memories, we are unable to cognize the sacred memories carried by the animals.

Essentially, the killing of animals today is tantamount to senseless slaughtering. Vedantans and Buddhists have used their influence to caution against killing animals for profit, food, or even medicinal use. Owing to the vast ecological corruption of the earth, mostly due to the human loss of cognitive memory, the animals too are losing their intrinsic, cosmic memories. As a result, even with the most harmonious sacrificial ceremony accompanying their demise, their flesh and provisions no longer render positive cures for human ailments.

The relationship of food and medicine to the bodily system of both animals and humans who eat in order to live is a dynamic exchange of energy and information. That which is carried within the cellular memory of the body is conditioned by the retention of each species' cognate form of memory. The cognitive memory carried by each human and the cosmic memory carried by every animal are both dependent upon the harmonic functioning of the individual or animal with nature. In abusing our own nature as a species, we have imposed irretrievable damage to the animals, the plants, and the earth as a whole.

The elephant carries the most stupendous memory, in both length and content, of any species on earth. This animal is the keeper of the knowledge of the earth's plants and herbs. The female elephant, a prime example of the animal species' memory, has been known to create phenomenal havoc in defense of her calves if they become endangered. In one instance, when an elephant calf was struck down by a train, the mother elephant retaliated by reducing the operating carriage of the train to scrap metal. Today, this same creature is being driven from its natural environment by the growing malaise of human ignorance and so-called human need. In the process, these divine and precious animals have begun to lose their memory. They have become disheveled and lost. In a recent study, many elephants are now being observed standing transfixed, incapable of defending, protecting, or avenging their young calves when in danger. This is a certain and foreboding sign that the elephant, an aggrieved species, is losing its intrinsic memory. If we lose the elephants, and all the cosmic memory they carry, we shall never be able to retain in the human faculty of mind or memory the knowledge of the herbs and plants and their sustaining and curative properties. Without the existence of the actual animal, its memory globules that make transference of thought and communication between all species possible, cannot sustain.

Likewise, the cow is considered by the Vedas to be the single most auspicious animal in the provision of animal-derived food. Called "go" in Sanskrit, this beneficent animal bears the same name as the holy scriptures and is reflected in the name of Lord Krishna, who was called Gopala, the one who protects both the sacred scriptures and the cows.

Ayurvedically, milk is considered the most complete food and the first sattvic food. Traditionally, it was collected well after the delivery of the cow's calf, so that it could be properly assimilated within the human system. From this wholesome

347

milk, the most healing unctuous substances for the human system are made, i.e., buttermilk, butter, yoghurt, and ghee. Because of the malaise and corruption so prevalent in today's animal husbandry, we are in serious danger of losing this first food of the earth. The artillery of poisons, chemicals, hormones, antibodies, and arsenic stimulants which are used in animal feed, as well as the cruel practice of imprisoning animals in stationary positions in over-crowded cells to wallow in their own excrement, are vicious and irretrievably damaging actions against the very animals who would happily contribute to our well-being. In the process, the intense pain suffered by the animals, as well as the pollutants in their feed, contaminate their flesh and seep into their milk. When this milk is consumed, the same pain and poison penetrate deeply into the tissues of the human body.

Thanks to the recent efforts of many independent farmers, it is possible to again obtain good quality milk and milk products. Many small, family-owned, organic milk farms have sprung up in the United States, where cows and goats are fed healthy feed, devoid of chemicals and poisons.

Butter, yoghurt and ghee, all made from organic quality milk, are considered to be highly nourishing foods that enhance health and replenish life. Milk, ghee, and butter are excellent for both Vata and Pitta disorders. Yoghurt is generally best used for Vata disorders, while Kapha disorders fare best with small quantities of goat's milk.

Ghee, considered to be the most vital of the dairy medicines, is associated with the element of love in the body. Its subtle action allows it to penetrate deep into tissues, making ghee an excellent vehicle for conveying herbal powders and medicines into the body. Ghee also imparts confidence and virility to the body. Sushruta regarded ghee as an intelligence building principle when used in the body, and Charaka praises its ability to promote both memory and the vital bodily essence, ojas. Ghee is made by boiling butter, thereby ridding it of the live enzymes that could encourage bacteria. The quality of the ghee depends on the quality of the butter, as well as on the method by which it is made and how it is stored. The older the ghee, the more medicinal it becomes.

In Ayurveda, honey is also used as a vehicle to carry medicines deeply into the bodily tissues. Because of its heat-producing potency, honey is excellent when used for both Kapha and Vata disorders. Although sweet in nature, it is also astringent, making it an effective medicine. Like milk, honey is a food derived from the animal kingdom. Unlike other animal derived foods, however, honey remains uncontaminated, due to the fiercely protective and precocious nature of the bees that produce it. Honey is a potent food, therefore, we need only a small quantity of it. Because it is not heat-stable and easily turns toxic when heated, honey should never be cooked.

PART THREE
Pancha Karma Healing Diet

A healing diet gladdens the heart, nourishes the body and revives memory.

— *Sushruta*

A healing diet nurtures the body and is, therefore, part of the strengthening routine, shamana. Containing the characteristics of both the brhmana and langhana regimes, the healing diet is administrated during and after pancha karma therapies. The Ayurvedic approach to diet is rooted in the need to cosset and mollify the body, mind, and spirit of the patient all within the appropriate seasons. During pancha karma therapy, a primary consideration is to stabilize the body's natural processes, to the extent possible, while it is being manipulated to let go of its excesses and wastes.

Prior to treatment, warm ginger tea may be served, if necessary, to encourage the patient to evacuate bodily wastes. Before abhyanga and snehana are administered, a linctus of sweet may also be given to the patient at breakfast to assuage any existing fears or anxieties. If snehana or svedana treatment involving the head is to be performed, three steps are taken the evening before therapy. First, a mild laxative such as castor root tea is administered along with warm ginger tea. Gargling with triphala decoction follows and, finally, a mild nasya treatment using water-diluted ginger juice is administered. These measures clear any obstruction remaining within the channels, ensure the doshas' equilibrium, and quiet the stomach.

During svedana treatment, agni and appetite are increased. To appease the patient, warm rice gruel and coriander tea are served during and after therapy. For its stabilizing effect, trikatu with ghee, along with a warm bath, are generally given to the patient following svedana therapy. The use of cold baths, drinks, and food which may shock the system are contra-indicated at this time, because the body needs time for its normal level of heat to be restored.

Unlike svedana therapy, vamana, virechana and vasti treatments diminish the agni. Thus, a warm rice gruel is usually served during the treatment period, followed by several days of rice porridge, mung bean soup, mixed vegetable soups and barley gruel, all accompanied by a small cup of warm water.

349

The length of time the post-therapy diet is to be observed depends upon the length of the treatment. If the total pancha karma treatment time takes a week, the post-dietary observations should also continue for a week. The healing diet used in pancha karma and its preparatory therapies are usually geared to the nature of the treatments, rather than to the individual prakriti. Since the nature of the healing diet is usually peaceful and nourishing, it accommodates all body types, restoring agni and allowing the body to adjust to its newly attuned state of freedom and revitalization.

Quantities of Food

To quote Charaka, "When one eats the proper measure of food, it is digested in a timely manner, thus promoting energy, healthy complexion, strength and longevity." The quantity of food eaten plays a significant role in maintaining our health. Generally, a person should eat enough food to satisfy the system, without experiencing a feeling of heaviness after eating. The ideal portion of solid food, recommended in Ayurveda, should be sufficient to fill one-half of the stomach volume, one-quarter to be filled with liquid, and the remaining quarter to remain empty to facilitate the digestive process. Another way of gauging the adequate amount of solid food to be taken at each meal, considered to be a fool-proof system, is to cup both hands together and measure the equivalent amount of food which would fill this "cup" to the brim. Likewise, a single cupped handful of liquid is equivalent to the ideal ration of liquid to be taken at each meal. Our hands are purposely designed to reflect the natural food capacity of our individual stomach.

Generally, for a person who is involved in exertive or laborious work, the quantity of food will need to be increased to accommodate the greater expenditure of energy. Similarly, for a person who is exerting very little energy throughout the day, the quantity of food will need to be reduced proportionately. The quantity of healing foods served during pancha karma is one third the normal size of a regular meal. Decreasing the amount of foods ingested during therapy allows the digestive system to re-organize itself by reducing its activities, while nourishing the body without unduly disturbing agni. Both the healing properties and the appropriate quantity of food allow apana and flatus to move downwards, while Kapha is reduced and agni is encouraged to rekindle.

Vital Unctuous Preparations

Sixty-four main unctuous preparations are used in pancha karma therapies. Among them are the substances prepared for therapies such as nasya, snehana, svedana, uttara and anuvasana vasti, virechana, karna purana, and gandusa. Several of these preparations are used for the healing diet during pancha karma as well and have a broad nomenclature, depending on what foodstuffs are used and in what proportions. For example, a thin gruel made from rice and ghee is called *mantha*; a decoction made from rice and ghee is called *peya*. When a mixture with four parts of water to one part rice is used it is called *vilepika*. When mung bean is added to vilepika, it is called *kichadi*. A thick rice porridge preparation is called *odana*; a thick gruel of rice, mung bean, black pepper and ghee is called *tarpana*. When a soup is made with six parts of water to one part barley, it is called *yavagu*; a bean soup made from horse gram and pigeon peas is called *yusha*; a spicy vegetable or herbal soup with or without buttermilk is called *khada*; when the milk whey or yoghurt, rock salt, sesame oil and urad bean are added to a khada, it is called *kambalika*. The bottom rice, after being cooked, is called *manda*. This portion of rice is especially fortifying for Vata types. A thick gruel made from any grain is called *krushara*. A sweet, fragrant liquid porridge made from milk and barley grits, cream of wheat, or tapioca is called *payasam*. A "shake" made from yoghurt, herbs, and spices, called *lassi,* is traditionally used to aid digestion. A sticky candy made from sugar cane juice is called *phanita*. A sweetener known as Sucanat may also be used instead of the sugar cane juice to make this preparation. Phanita may also be prepared as a syrup, commonly called a *sweet linctus*. A pudding made from milk, yoghurt or cream is called *utkarika*.

Cautionary Note

The healing diet may be used not only as a pancha karma dietary regimen but also as a cleansing and rejuvenating diet from time to time throughout the year. The seven day healing dietary routine may be observed at home during the appropriate cleansing seasons for Vata, Pitta, or Kapha disorders but should not be used as a mainstay regimen for long-term use, because it is designed as a periodic healing diet, especially for post-pancha karma use. The sattvic diet also should not be used as an all-year dietary regimen, since the body is made up of all five elements and needs the stimuli of all three gunas of sattva, rajas and tamas. Although sattvic foods comprise the greater part of the dietary recommendation for Pitta types and, to a large extent, work for the Vata types as well, some rajasic foods and, to a lesser extent, tamasic foods are also necessary to maintain the vital health of all bodily systems. Kapha types fare best when the greater portion of their diet is made up of rajasic food and, to a lesser extent, sattvic and tamasic foods.

For Internal and External Use

- Only organic or certified raw milk and dairy products. Pitta types may also use soya milk; Vata types may also use rice or almond milk. Do not combine cow's milk with salty, sour or acidic foods.
- Pure ghee made from milk, not from vegetable oil.
- Suitable oils for each type; do not use commercial brands or hydrogenated oil or combined mixtures of oils. Use only naturally processed oils available through health food stores.

- Pure spring, well or rain water.
- Natural brown sugar, jaggery or Sucanat wherever brown sugar is called for. Do not use white sugar or commercial brands of brown sugar.
- Natural raw honey.
- Ayurvedic rock salt. Sea salt may be substituted if rock salt is unavailable. Do not use commercial salt, iodized salt or salt substitutes.
- Spices and herbs that are not shelf-old and have not been irradiated—Ayurvedic herbs are not irradiated.
- Fresh fruits that have not been waxed or sprayed with chemical pesticides.
- Dried fruits that have not been sulfurized or treated with processed sugars or chemicals.
- Organic vegetables, grains and legumes.
- *Avoid* pre-packaged foods (even from health food stores), and excessive use of fermented products such as soya sauce, liquid amino acids and soya byproducts, except for tofu and soya milk.

It is recommended that the necessary ingredients be purchased from natural health food stores and/or through Ayurvedic resources, some of which are listed in Appendix G.

POST-THERAPY HEALING DIET SCHEDULE

This schedule is to be observed for the same length of time after treatment as the length of therapy itself, i.e., if the pancha karma treatment or treatments last for seven days, the healing diet which follows should be observed for seven days after the treatment has ended.

Day	Morning (8-9 am)	Late Afternoon (4-6 pm)
1	Peya	Peya
2	Peya (no salt/oil)	Vilepika (no salt/oil)
3	Vilepika	Tarpana Mantha
4	Yusha	Yavagu/Kichadi
5	Vegetable Yusha	Odana
6	Thick Kichadi	Odana
7	Khada/Payasam	Resume normal diet

Note: The appropriate seasonal diet for each body type is discussed in my previous book, *Ayurveda: A Life of Balance.*

Note:
1. If desired, a third meal may be given between noon and 1 p.m. by repeating the same meal given in the morning. If the length of therapy exceeds seven days, repeat the dietary recommendations sequentially from days four through seven until the end of the dietary period.
2. Although a normal diet is to be resumed afterwards, be careful not to use any excessively oily, spicy, cold, stale or unhealthy foods for two months following therapy.
3. After virechana therapy, tarpana should be given on the third day instead of vilepika.
4. Peya, vilepika and/or kichadi may also be served exclusively during pancha karma therapy. The quantity of food served during and after therapy should be one-third of the person's normal intake.

POST-THERAPY HEALING DIET

Season: use pancha karma seasonal guidelines

Body Type: all types

Bala Peya-Rice Decoction

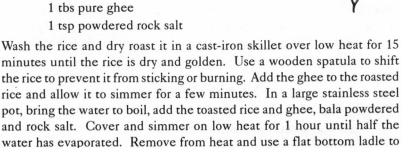

Four servings:
>   1 gal water
>   1 c short grain brown rice
>   1 tbs bala powder
>   1 tbs pure ghee
>   1 tsp powdered rock salt

Wash the rice and dry roast it in a cast-iron skillet over low heat for 15 minutes until the rice is dry and golden. Use a wooden spatula to shift the rice to prevent it from sticking or burning. Add the ghee to the roasted rice and allow it to simmer for a few minutes. In a large stainless steel pot, bring the water to boil, add the toasted rice and ghee, bala powdered and rock salt. Cover and simmer on low heat for 1 hour until half the water has evaporated. Remove from heat and use a flat bottom ladle to mash the rice into a thick decoction. Serve the pureed rice peya while still warm.

Note: Plain peya may also be made without the addition of bala powder.

Peya (without oil and salt)

Four servings:

>2 qt water
>1 c short grain brown rice

Bring the water to boil in a large stainless steel pot. Wash the rice and dry roast in a cast-iron skillet over low heat for 15 minutes until it is dry and golden. Use a wooden ladle to shift the rice to prevent it from sticking or burning. Add the roasted rice to the boiling water. Cover and simmer on medium heat for 45 minutes until the rice becomes soft. Use a flat bottom ladle to puree the soft rice into a gruel. Serve while still warm.

Basmati Rice Mantha - Thin Rice Gruel

Two servings:

>5 c water
>1 c white basmati rice
>1 tsp pure ghee
>1/2 tsp powdered rock salt
>1/2 tsp cumin seeds
>1/2 tsp ajwan seeds

Bring the water to boil in a stainless steel pot. Wash the rice and add to the boiling water. Cover and simmer over low heat for 20 minutes. In a small cast-iron skillet, heat the ghee and roast the seeds for a few minutes until they are golden brown. Pour the ghee and seed mixture into the rice gruel, along with the salt. Stir briefly and continue cooking the rice for an additional 20 minutes until the rice kernels are completely broken down. Remove from heat and allow to cool for 10 minutes before serving.

Vilepika - Rice Gruel

Four servings:

>2 c medium short grain brown rice
>1 tbs pure ghee
>6 c water
>1 tsp powdered rock salt
>1 tsp cumin seeds
>1 tsp coriander seeds

Wash the rice and dry roast it in a large cast-iron skillet for 15 minutes over low heat until the rice is dry and golden. Use a wooden spatula to shift the rice to prevent it from burning and sticking. Add half of the ghee to the roasted rice and allow it to simmer for a few minutes. Bring the water to boil in a medium size stainless steel pot and add the toasted rice, ghee and salt to it. Cover and simmer over low heat for 1 hour, until half the water has evaporated. Remove from heat and let the covered pot sit undisturbed. In a small skillet, heat the remaining ghee over low heat. Slightly crush the seeds in a small mortar and pestle. Add to the heated ghee. As soon as the seeds turn golden brown, stir the ghee and seed mixture into the cooked rice gruel. Serve while still warm.

Vilepika (without oil and salt)

4 servings:

>   2 c medium grain brown rice
>   6 c water
>   1 tsp cumin seeds
>   1 tsp coriander seeds

Wash the rice and dry roast it in a large cast-iron skillet for 15 minutes over low heat until it is dry and golden. Use a wooden spatula to shift the rice to prevent it from sticking or burning. In a medium size stainless steel pot, bring the water to boil. Add the roasted rice, cover, and simmer on low heat for 45 minutes. Dry roast the seeds in a small skillet for a few minutes. Use a small mortar and pestle to crush them slightly, then add to the cooked rice gruel. Continue cooking for another 15 minutes. Remove from heat and allow the pot to sit undisturbed for 10 minutes before serving the gruel.

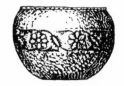

Amalaki Mantha - Fruit Decoction

Two servings:

      6 c water

      1 c pitted dates

      1/2 c raisins

      1 tbs amalaki powder

      2 tbs Sucanat

      1/2 tsp rock salt

Bring the water to a boil in a stainless steel pot. Add the dates, raisins, amalaki powder, Sucanat and salt. Cover and simmer on low heat for 40 minutes, until the dates and raisins are soft. Remove from heat and use a flat bottomed ladle to puree the cooked fruit. Allow the decoction to sit for 10 minutes before serving.

Grape Mantha - Fruit Decoction

Two servings:

      5 c water

      1 c grape juice

      1 c fresh pomegranate fruit

      1/4 tsp grated fresh ginger

      1 tsp pure ghee

      1/4 tsp powdered rock salt

      2 tbs honey

Combine the water and juice and bring to a boil in a stainless steel pot. Add the pomegranate fruit and salt. Cover and allow to simmer on low heat for 10 minutes. In a small cast-iron skillet, heat the ghee over low heat and add the minced ginger. Saute the ginger for a few minutes until it turns slightly brown. Add the ghee and ginger to the fruit decoction. Allow the decoction to cook for an additional 20 minutes. Remove from heat and allow to sit for 25 minutes before adding the honey. Serve immediately.

Rice and Mung Tarpana - Rice Porridge

For post-virechana use.

Two servings:

>   4 c water
>   1 c basmati brown rice
>   1/4 c whole mung beans
>   1/4 tsp pippali powder
>   1/4 tsp black pepper powder
>   1/4 tsp powdered rock salt
>   1 tsp pure ghee
>   1 tbs brown sugar

Bring the water to a boil and add the rice, mung, pippali, black pepper and salt. Cover and simmer on medium heat for 25 minutes. In a small cast-iron skillet, warm the ghee and add the sugar. Allow to sit over low heat for a few minutes until mixture begins to bubble. Add the mixture to the rice and mung tarpana. Continue to cook for another 30 minutes on low heat, until the tarpana becomes a thick porridge. Remove from heat and allow it to sit for 15 minutes before serving.

Pigeon Pea Yusha - Bean Soup

Two servings:

>   1/2 c dried pigeon peas
>   1/2 c urad beans
>   10 c water
>   1 tsp powdered rock salt
>   1 tbs pure ghee
>   1/2 tsp black cumin seeds
>   1 tsp coriander seeds
>   1/2 tsp black peppercorns
>   1 tsp fresh lemon juice

Wash the pigeon peas and urad beans and soak them for 5 hours in sufficient water to cover them. Bring 10 cups of fresh water to boil in a large heavy soup pot. Strain the soaked peas and beans and add to the boiling water, along with the salt. Cover and simmer on medium heat for 40 minutes. Use a small mortar and pestle and crush the seeds and peppercorns. In a small cast-iron skillet, heat the ghee and add the crushed seeds. Allow the seeds to fry for a few minutes, then add to the soup mixture. Continue cooking the soup for an additional 20 minutes until the peas and beans are soft and crumbly. Remove from heat and let sit undisturbed for 10 minutes, then stir in the lemon juice. Serve immediately.

Mung Yusha - Bean Soup

Two servings:

> 8 c water
> 1 c yellow split mung bean
> 1/4 tsp turmeric powder
> 1 tsp powdered rock salt
> 1 tbs sunflower oil
> 1/2 tsp cumin seeds
> 1/2 tsp caraway seeds
> 1/2 tsp grated fresh ginger
> 1 tsp minced fresh cilantro

Bring the water to boil in a large heavy soup pot. Wash the beans and add to the boiling water, along with the salt and turmeric powder. Cover and simmer on medium heat for 25 minutes. Use a suribachi or mortar and pestle to grind the seeds to a fine powder. In a small cast-iron skillet, heat the oil. Add the powdered seeds, along with the grated ginger and fresh cilantro. Stir and let sizzle over low heat for two minutes, then add to the soup. Cover and continue cooking for an additional 15 minutes, until the beans have lost their shape. Remove from heat and let sit for 10 minutes before serving.

Yavagu - Barley Soup

Two servings:

> 8 c water
> 1 c milk
> 1 c pearl barley
> 1/4 short grain brown rice
> 1 tsp powdered rock salt
> 1/2 tsp cardamom seeds
> 1/4 tsp coriander seeds
> 1/2 tsp ajwan seeds
> 1 tbs pure ghee
> 1 tsp minced fresh mint

Combine the water and milk in a large heavy soup pot and bring to a boil. Wash the barley and rice and add to the boiling water, along with the salt. Cover and simmer over medium heat for 35 minutes. In a small cast-iron skillet, dry roast the seeds over low heat for 3 minutes. Use a suribachi to grind the roasted seeds to a coarse powder. Using the same skillet warm the ghee and pour it, along with the powdered seeds, into the barley and rice soup. Cover and cook for an additional 20 minutes over low heat, until the barley grains are very soft. Remove from heat and add the minced mint. Cover and let to sit for 15 minutes before serving.

Carrot Yavagu - Barley and Carrot Soup

Three servings:

  10 c water
  1 c hulled barley
  1 c carrots, cut into 1-inch cubes
  1 tsp powdered rock salt
  1/2 tsp black peppercorns
  1/2 tsp cumin seeds
  1/2 tsp coriander seeds
  1 tsp sunflower oil
  1/2 tsp minced fresh basil

Scrub wash the carrots before cubing; do not peel. Bring the water to a boil in a large heavy soup pot. Wash the hulled barley and add to the boiling water, along with the carrots and salt. Cover and allow to simmer over medium heat for 45 minutes. In a small cast-iron skillet, dry roast the seeds and peppercorns over low heat for 3 minutes, then grind to a fine powder using a mortar and pestle or a suribachi. Heat the oil in the same skillet. Remove from heat and add the minced basil. Cover and allow the basil oil to sit for 15 minutes, then add to the soup, along with the roasted powdered seeds. Continue cooking over low heat for an additional 15 minutes. Remove from heat let sit for 15 minutes before serving.

Okra Yusha - Vegetable Soup
Two servings:

      1 tsp dried tamarind

      8 c water

      1/2 c yellow split mung bean

      2 c thinly sliced okra

      1 tbs pure ghee

      1 tsp powdered rock salt

      1/4 tsp turmeric powder

      1/2 tsp cumin powder

      1/ tsp ginger powder

      1/4 tsp pippali powder

In a small bowl, soak the tamarind in 1/2 c hot water for 5 hours. In a large, heavy soup pot, bring the water to a boil. Wash the mung beans and add to the boiling water, along with the okra and salt. Cover and simmer for 45 minutes over medium heat. In a small cast-iron skillet, heat the ghee, add the powders, and immediately add to the soup mixture. Use a small spoon to mash the soaked tamarind into a pulp. Pour the pulp, along with the soaking water and tamarind roughage, into the soup. Allow the soup to cook for an additional 15 minutes. Remove from heat and let sit for 10 minutes. Remove the tamarind roughage before serving.

Note: Asparagus, string beans, carrots, lotus roots, zucchini and crook neck squash may also be used instead of okra, in the same quantity. Or, to provide variety, one-third cup of each of these vegetables may be used.

Kichadi - Rice and Bean Mixture
Kichadi may also be served as a mono-diet after therapy. It is an excellent diet following vasti and virechana therapies.

Four servings:

      8 c water

      1 1/2 c white basmati rice

      1/2 c yellow split mung bean

      1 tsp powdered rock salt

      1/2 tsp ajwan seeds

      1/2 tsp coriander seeds

      1/2 tsp cumin seeds

      2 tbs pure ghee

Bring the water to boil in a large stainless steel pot. Wash the rice and beans and add to the boiling water, along with the salt. Cover and simmer on medium-low heat for 25 minutes. In a small cast-iron skillet, roast the seeds for a few minutes over low heat, until they are golden brown. Grind them into coarse pieces, using a mortar and pestle or a suribachi. Heat the ghee in the same skillet and add the crushed seeds. Sizzle for 2 minutes, then pour into the rice and beans mixture. Cover and continue cooking on low heat for another 10 minutes. Remove from heat and let the kichadi sit for 10 minutes before serving.

Thick Kichadi - Rice and Bean Mixture

Four servings:

> 1 tbs dried tamarind
> 10 c water
> 1 1/2 c brown basmati rice
> 1/2 c whole mung bean
> 1 tsp powdered rock salt
> 1 tsp cumin seeds
> 1 tsp coriander seeds
> 1/2 tsp black peppercorns
> 2 tbs pure ghee

Soak the tamarind in 1/2 cup of hot water for 5 hours. Bring the 10 cups of water to a boil. Wash the rice and beans and add to the boiling water along with the salt. Cover and simmer over medium-low heat for 40 minutes. Roast the seeds and peppercorns in a small cast-iron skillet over low heat for a few minutes until they crackle, then crush them into coarse bits, using a mortar and pestle. Heat the ghee in the same skillet, then add the crushed seeds and immediately pour into the rice and bean mixture. Use a small spoon to mash the tamarind into a pulp and add, along with the soaking water and roughage, to the rice and bean mixture. Stir, cover, and continue cooking on low heat for an additional 15 minutes, until the kichadi becomes a thick porridge. Remove from heat and let cool for 15 minutes. Remove the tamarind roughage from the kichadi before serving.

Odana - Thick Porridge

Two servings:

> 4 c water
> 1 c milk
> 1 1/2 c arborio rice
> 1/2 tsp cinnamon powder
> 1/2 tsp ground black pepper
> 1/4 tsp turmeric powder
> 2 tbs brown sugar
> 12 strands of saffron
> 5 drops of essential oil of orange
> 1 tbs pure ghee

Combine the water and milk in a large, heavy stainless steel pot and bring to a boil. Wash the rice and add to the boiling water along, with the powders, ground pepper, and sugar. Cover and simmer over medium heat for 30 minutes. Dilute the saffron in two tablespoons of water, letting it sit for a few minutes before adding to the porridge, along with the essential oil. Stir, cover, and continue to cook over low heat for an additional 15 minutes. Warm the ghee in a small skillet and add to the porridge. Remove from heat and let sit for 15 minutes before serving.

Note: An equal quantity of short grain rice or sweet rice may be substituted for arborio rice.

Khada - Buttermilk and Vegetable Soup

Four servings:

> 10 c water
> 1 c carrot
> 1 c asparagus
> 1 c yam
> 1 tsp powdered rock salt
> 1 tsp chitraka powder
> 2 c buttermilk
> 1 tsp fennel seeds
> 1 tsp cumin seeds
> 1 tsp coriander seeds
> 1 tbs sesame oil

Bring the water to a boil in a large heavy soup pot. Scrub the carrots and cut on a slant into 1/4-inch thick pieces. Wash the asparagus and cut on a

362

slant into 1-inch pieces. Scrub the yam and cut into 1/2-inch cubes. Add the yam and carrots to the boiling water. Cover and simmer for 15 minutes over medium heat. Add the asparagus pieces along with the chitraka powder and salt. Use a small mortar and pestle to coarsely crush the seeds. Heat a small cast-iron skillet, pour in the oil and let it become warm. Add the crushed seeds and sizzle for 2 minutes. Stir into the soup, along with the buttermilk. Continue cooking over low heat for another 10 minutes, stirring occasionally to prevent the buttermilk from separating. Remove from heat and serve while still warm.

Tapioca Payasam - A Sweet Milky Decoction

Four servings:

> 1 c tapioca (small beads)
> 2 c cold water
> 1 c milk
> 1/2 tsp cinnamon powder
> 1/2 tsp cardamom powder
> 1/4 tsp fennel powder
> 12 strands of saffron
> 1 tbs pure ghee
> 2 tbs brown sugar
> 5 drops of essential oil of vanilla

Soak the tapioca in two cups of cold water for 20 minutes. Bring the milk to a boil over low heat. Add the tapioca, along with its soaking water, to the boiling milk. Stir in the powdered ingredients. Soak the saffron in two tablespoons of water for a few minutes, then add to the tapioca mixture. Warm the ghee over low heat, then add, along with the sugar and essential oil. Cook uncovered over low heat for 30 minutes, stirring frequently to prevent the tapioca from sticking together. Remove from heat and let sit for 10 minutes before serving.

Note: An equal amount of cream of wheat or fine barley grits may be substituted for the tapioca.

Sattvic Diet for Pitta and Vata Types

The sattvic diet is considered a brhmana routine, a regimen used to restore bulk, energy, and vitality to the body. It may be taken occasionally throughout the year and is especially beneficial when taken during the mild seasonal cleansing activities and through the seasonal junctions. For cleansing routines which exceed a three-day period, and after the intense pancha karma treatments, the post pancha karma healing diet is recommended. Most suited to the Pitta and Vata types, the sattvic diet is also excellent for maintaining a cooling balance in the body during the summer and fall seasons.

The sattvic diet contains foods that are sweet and calming in nature, essential energies for both Vata and Pitta types. Because these two types are also dynamically opposed to each other in many instances, appropriate substitutes or additional ingredients are noted in each Sattvic Diet recipe in order to address the particular needs of each type. These substitutes and/or additions may not necessarily be sattvic in nature, but they are healing for their respective types. The same procedures and quantities are to be used of substituted foods as those indicated in the original recipes. When an ingredient is to be added, the quantity and the timing for introducing it are noted at the end of the recipe.

To summarize, then, the sattvic diet is used for cleansing routines and occasional use (except where otherwise indicated).

Season: all year

Body types: Pitta and Vata, except where otherwise indicated

Conditions

Pitta disorders, Vata disorders, post-vasti therapy, post-virechana therapy

Basmati Rice Kichadi

Four servings:

    6 c water
    1 1/2 c white basmati rice
    1/2 c yellow split mung bean

1/2 tsp powdered rock salt

1 tsp cumin seeds

1 tbs pure ghee

Bring the water to a boil in a large stainless steel pot. Wash the rice and beans and add to the boiling water, along with the salt. Cover and simmer on low heat for 20 minutes. In a small cast-iron skillet, heat the ghee and add the cumin seeds. When the seeds turn golden brown, pour the mixture into the kichadi. Stir, cover, and continue to simmer for an additional 5 minutes over low heat. Serve while still warm.

Note: Both Vata and Pitta types may substitute equal amounts of bulgur, cous cous or jasmine rice for the white basmati rice. Vata types may also add a pinch of asafoetida along with the salt.

Saffron Rice

Two servings:

4 c water

1 c white basmati rice

1 tbs pure ghee

1/2 tsp coriander powder

1/2 tsp atibala powder

1/4 c milk

12 strands of saffron

1 tsp date sugar

Bring the water to a boil in a medium-size stainless steel pot. Wash the rice and, in a large cast-iron skillet, dry roast it over low heat for 12-15 minutes, shifting it with a wooden spoon to prevent sticking and burning. When the rice is dry and golden, remove it from the skillet. Warm the ghee in the same skillet and add the roasted rice while maintaining a low flame. When the ghee begins to sizzle, add the rice and ghee mixture, along with the coriander and atibala powders, to the boiling water. Pour the milk into the ghee-lined skillet, add the saffron and sugar, and let sit for 2 minutes on low heat, then add to the boiling rice. Cover and simmer for 25 minutes over low heat. Serve warm or cool.

Note: Both Vata and Pitta types may substitute equal amounts of bulgur, cous cous or jasmine rice for the white basmati rice.

Cracked Wheat-Coconut Pilaf

Two servings:

> 2 1/2 c water
> 1 c cracked wheat
> 1/2 tsp powdered rock salt
> 1/4 c grated fresh coconut
> 1 tbs coconut oil
> 1 tsp ajwan
> 1/2 tsp fennel seeds
> 1/4 c snow peas

Bring the water to a boil in a stainless steel saucepan. Heat a large cast-iron skillet and dry roast the cracked wheat for approximately 15 minutes over low heat, stirring occasionally with a wooden spoon to prevent it from sticking or burning. Add the roasted wheat to the boiling water, along with the salt. Using the same skillet, dry roast the grated coconut in the same way. When the coconut is slightly brown, add it to the wheat mixture. Heat the oil in the same skillet and add the seeds; when they turn golden brown, add them to the wheat mixture. Cover and let cook for 20 minutes over medium-low heat. Add the snow peas, stir, cover and continue cooking on low heat for an additional 10 minutes. Serve warm.

Note: Vata types may add 1/2 teaspoon cardamom seeds and 1/2 teaspoon coursely ground black pepper. Follow the same procedure as for the fennel and ajwan seeds.

Mango Soup

Two servings:

> 6 c water
> 2 c sliced ripe mango
> 1 tsp sunflower oil
> 1/2 tsp cardamom powder
> 1/2 tsp coriander powder
> 1 tsp lemon juice
> 1/2 tsp powdered rock salt
> 3 tbs kudzu starch
> 1/2 c yoghurt

Bring the water to a boil in heavy soup pot and add the mango slices. In a small cast-iron skillet, heat the oil over low heat and add the powdered spices. After a few minutes, add to the soup, along with the salt and lemon juice, rinsing the skillet in the boiling mango water. Dilute the kudzu starch in 1/2 cup of cold water and add to the soup, stirring until the starch turns clear. Cover and simmer on low heat for 25 minutes, stirring occasionally. Remove from the heat and let sit for 5 minutes. Using a flat bottom ladle, puree the mango pieces, then blend the yoghurt into the soup. Let the soup cool, uncovered, for 15 minutes before serving.

Note: For both Vata and Pitta types, equal amounts of fresh ripe peaches, nectarines, plums, sweet strawberries, raspberries or melon may be used instead of mango. Vata types may use bananas, avocado, orange or grapefruit slices instead of mango. Pitta types may also use grapes, sweet orange slices, sweet pineapples or apples instead of mango. Both types may add a tablespoon of minced fresh mint for extra flavor.

Coconut Milk Soup

Two servings:

>   4 c water
>   1 c coconut milk (see directions on pg. 488, Appendix E)
>   1/2 tsp powdered rock salt
>   6 fresh neem (curry) leaves
>   1 tbs pure ghee
>   1 c grated fresh coconut (see directions on pg. 488)
>   1 tsp coriander seeds
>   1 tsp cumin seeds
>   1/2 tsp minced fresh ginger

Bring the water to a boil in a heavy soup pot. Add the coconut milk, salt, and neem leaves. Heat the ghee in a cast-iron skillet over low heat and add the grated coconut, stirring occasionally until the coconut turns slightly brown. Add to the boiling coconut milk mixture. Using the same ghee-lined skillet, roast the seeds for a few minutes until they begin to crackle. In a small suribachi, grind the seeds to a fine powder and add to the soup, along with the ginger. Cover and simmer on medium heat for 15 minutes. Serve warm or cold.

Note: Vata types may add 1/2 teaspoon of tamarind paste to the soup when adding the spices.

Barley-Carrot Pilaf

Two servings:

> 2 c water
>
> 1 c barley grits
>
> 1 c finely cubed carrots
>
> 1/2 tsp powdered rock salt
>
> 1 tbs sunflower oil
>
> 2 tbs sesame seed
>
> 1 tsp coriander seeds
>
> 1/2 tsp cardamom seeds
>
> 1/2 tsp black cumin seed
>
> 1 tsp lime juice

Bring the water to a boil in a stainless steel pot. Wash the grits and add to the boiling water, along with the carrots and salt. In a small cast-iron skillet, heat the oil. Wash the sesame seeds and roast them in the heated oil for 10 minutes over low heat, shifting them with a wooden spoon to prevent burning. Add to the barley mixture. Using the same skillet, roast the spice seeds for a few minutes until they begin to crackle. Remove from heat and, using a mortar and pestle, bruise them slightly, then add to the barley mixture. Cover the pot and simmer on medium-low heat for 25 minutes. Stir in the lime juice. Remove from heat and let sit, covered, for 5 minutes before serving.

Note: Vata types may substitute an equal quantity of cracked wheat or cracked oats for the barley grits. They may also add 2 cloves of minced garlic to the mixture along with the spice seeds. Pitta types may substitute an equal amount of sunflower seeds for the sesame seeds, following the same procedures.

Barley-Yam Soup

Two servings:

> 6 c water
>
> 1 c pearl barley
>
> 1 tbs pure ghee
>
> 1/2 tsp powdered rock salt
>
> 1 large yam
>
> 1 tbs minced cilantro
>
> 1/2 tsp ground black pepper
>
> 1/4 tsp turmeric powder

Bring the water to a boil in a heavy soup pot. Wash the barley and add to the boiling water, along with the salt. Scrub wash the yam, cut it into 1-inch cubes, and add to the barley water. Warm the ghee in a cast-iron skillet over low heat and add the cilantro, black pepper, and turmeric. When the mixture begins to sizzle, add to the barley water. Rinse the skillet in the barley water, making sure all of its contents are transferred to the soup water. Cover and simmer over medium heat for 40 minutes. Serve warm.

Note: Vata types may substitute equal quantities of short grain brown rice or cracked wheat for the barley, and fresh parsley for the cilantro.

Wheat-Date Porridge

Two servings:

> 6 c water
> 1 c whole wheat kernels
> 1/4 c raisins
> 1/4 c pitted dates
> 1/2 tsp orange zest
> 1/2 tsp cinnamon powder
> 1/2 tsp cardamom powder
> 1 c milk
> 2 tbs brown sugar
> 5 drops essential oil of vanilla

Bring the water to a boil in a heavy stainless steel pot. Wash the wheat kernels and add to the boiling water, along with the raisins, dates, orange zest and spice powders. Stir, cover, and let simmer over medium-low heat for 1 hour. Then add the milk, sugar, and vanilla essence. Stir, cover, and continue to cook on low heat for an additional 30 minutes. Add water, if necessary, to prevent the porridge from sticking. Serve warm or cool.

Note: Pitta types may use an equal amount of soya milk instead of cow's milk. Vata types may use rice or almond milk instead of cow's milk. As noted at the beginning of the chapter, these substitutions may be observed throughout all the food recipes requiring cow's milk.

Rice-Mung Porridge

Two servings:

> 4 c water
>
> 1 c short grain brown rice
>
> 1/2 c whole mung beans
>
> 1/2 tsp powdered rock salt
>
> 1 tbs pure ghee
>
> 1 tbs cumin seed
>
> 1/2 c yoghurt

Bring the water to a boil in a heavy stainless steel pot. Wash the rice and beans and add to the boiling water, along with the salt. Heat the ghee in a small cast-iron skillet over low heat and add the cumin seeds. When the seeds turn golden brown, add to the rice and beans. Rinse the pan with the porridge to ensure that all the ghee is transferred. Cover and cook over medium-low heat for 45 minutes. Stir in the yoghurt and continue to cook, uncovered, over low heat for an additional 10 minutes. Serve warm or cool.

Note: Vata types may include 1/2 teaspoon of tamarind paste when adding the rice and beans to the boiling water. Pitta types may substitute equal amounts of cream for the yoghurt and omit the salt or omit the yoghurt and retain the salt.

Asparagus and Soya Crumble

Two servings:

> 1 c water
>
> 1 lb fresh asparagus
>
> 1/2 c soya bean flour
>
> 1/2 tsp powdered rock salt
>
> 1 tbs butter
>
> 1/2 tsp black peppercorns
>
> 1 tsp coriander seeds

Bring the water to a boil in a large stainless steel skillet. Wash the asparagus, snip off the hard ends, and add to the boiling water. Cover and steam boil for 5 minutes over medium heat. Remove asparagus and retain cooking water. Heat a cast-iron skillet and roast the flour for a few minutes until golden. Add the asparagus cooking water, along with the salt, to the roasted flour in the skillet and, if necessary, a small amount of water to form a soft dough. Cover the skillet and cook the dough over medium-low heat for 10 minutes until it becomes cake-like. Remove from heat and let cool. Warm the butter in a small skillet. Use a mortar and pestle to coarse-grind the peppercorns and coriander seeds, then add to the heated butter. When the mixture begins to sizzle, pour it over asparagus. Crumble the soya cake over the asparagus and serve while still warm.

Note: Vata types may use an equal quantity of beets, carrots, crook neck squash or zucchini, scrubbed and sliced into 1/4-inch rounds, green beans or okra instead of asparagus. Pitta types may use an equal quantity of broccoli, Brussels sprouts, cauliflower, green beans, okra, crook neck squash or zucchini, scrubbed and cut in 1-inch pieces, instead of asparagus.

Lotus String Beans

Two servings:
>1 1/2 c water
>1 lb string beans
>1 medium size fresh lotus root
>1 tsp sesame oil
>1/2 c soya milk
>1/4 tsp turmeric powder
>1 tbs maple syrup
>1 tbs kudzu starch
>1/2 tsp powdered rock salt

Bring the water to a boil in a stainless steel skillet. Wash the string beans, nip off the ends, and add to the boiling water. Steam boil over medium heat for 5 minutes; remove from cooking water. Scrub the lotus root and slice into 1/4-inch thin circles. Heat the oil in a small cast-iron skillet over low heat and add the lotus slices. Brown on each side and remove them from the skillet. Add soya milk to the unwashed skillet and bring to a boil over medium heat. Stir in turmeric powder and maple syrup. Dilute the kudzu starch in the string bean cooking water, then add to the soya milk. Stir until the mixture becomes smooth and gel-like. Remove from heat and add salt. Arrange the string beans and lotus slices on a platter and pour the sauce over them before serving.

Fruit Lassi

Four servings:

> 1/2 c dates
> 1 c water
> 2 c milk
> 1 c yoghurt
> 1 tbs brown sugar
> 1/4 tsp minced fresh mint

Wash dates and puree, using a hand food grinder. Combine water, milk, yoghurt, sugar and mint in a mixing bowl and whip with an egg beater until mixture froths. Stir in the pureed dates and serve immediately.

Note: Dried mango, pineapple, peaches, and figs, as well as raisins, may also be used to make lassi for both Vata and Pitta types. If fresh fruits are used, the cow's milk and yoghurt should be replaced with three cups soya milk for Pitta types, and the same quantity almond milk for Vata types.

Essential oils note: A few drops of one of the following essential oils may also be used in the lassi mixture for both types: peppermint, saffron, coriander, licorice, lavender, lemon, orange, fennel, chamomile, vanilla, lemon grass, raspberry, rose or sandalwood. Vata types may also use almond, ginger or cardamom essence.

Herbal powders note: 1/2 teaspoon of an herbal powder, such as triphala, bhringaraja, atibala, gotu kola, maha bala, shatavari, cinnamon, coriander or cardamom may also be added for both types.

Vermicelli Payasam

Four servings:

> 2 c water
> 1 c cream
> 1 lb vermicelli (thread-like whole wheat noodles)
> 3 c milk
> 1/2 tsp cardamom powder
> 1/4 tsp turmeric powder
> 12 strands of saffron
> 2 tbs honey
> 5 drops of essential oil of sandalwood

Bring the water to a boil in a medium-size stainless steel pot. Add the vermicelli and cook over medium heat for 3 minutes, stirring to prevent it from sticking together. Then add the cream and milk, along with the powders. Stir, cover, and simmer on low heat for 5 minutes. Soak the saffron in two tablespoons of water for a few minutes, then add to the payasam, along with its soaking water. Remove beverage from heat and keep it covered while it cools. Then add honey and essential oil.

Sattvic Teas

Season: all year

Body Type: Pitta and Vata
Kapha use occasionally

Fennel-Lavender Tea

Two servings:
>3 c water
>1/2 tsp fennel seeds
>1/2 tsp dried lavender leaves

Bring the water to a boil in a small stainless steel saucepan. In a small skillet, dry roast fennel seeds for a few minutes until they are golden in color. Add to the boiling water, along with the lavender leaves. Cover and remove from heat. Let the infusion sit for 5 minutes; then strain. Serve warm or cold.

Note: For both Vata and Pitta types, the same quantity of milk may be used instead of water; or equal portions of water and milk may be used. Vata types may substitute 1/2 teaspoon minced fresh ginger for the fennel seeds.

Coconut-Peppermint Tea

Two servings:
>3 c coconut milk or water
>1 tbs dried coconut
>3 drops essential oil of peppermint

Bring the milk or water to a boil. In a small skillet, dry roast coconut for a few minutes until it begins to turn slightly brown. Add to the boiling liquid, along with the essential oils. Cover and remove from heat. Let infusion sit for 15 minutes before serving. This tea may be served either strained or unstrained.

Saffron-Lime Tea

Two servings:

> 3 c water
>
> 12 strands of saffron
>
> 1 tsp fresh lime juice
>
> 1 tsp brown sugar

Bring the water to a boil in a small stainless steel saucepan. Add the saffron, lime juice and sugar. Cover and remove from the heat. Let sit for 5 minutes before serving.

Lotus-Walnut Tea

Two servings:

> 3 c water
>
> 5 pieces dried lotus root
>
> 1 tsp walnut pieces

Bring the water to a boil in a small stainless steel saucepan. Add the lotus root and walnuts and boil on low heat for 3 minutes. Remove from heat. Cover and let sit for 5 minutes, before straining. Serve warm or cool.

Coriander-Bala Tea

Two servings:

> 3 c water
>
> 1/2 tsp coriander powder
>
> 1/2 tsp bala powder

Bring the water to a boil in a small stainless steel saucepan. Add the powders, cover, and remove from heat. Let sit for 3 minutes before serving.

Note: Vata types may substitute ginger powder for the coriander.

Shatavari Tea

Two servings:

> 3 c water
>
> 1/2 tsp shatavari powder
>
> 1 tsp maple syrup

Bring the water to a boil in a small stainless steel saucepan. Add the shatavari powder. Cover, remove from heat, and let sit for 5 minutes. Then add the maple syrup. Serve warm or cool.

Rose-Raspberry Tea

Two servings:

> 3 c water
>
> 1 tsp dried organic rosebuds
>
> 1 tsp dried raspberry leaves

Bring the water to a boil in a small stainless steel saucepan. Add the rosebuds and raspberry leaves. Cover, remove from heat, and let sit for 7 minutes before straining. Serve warm or cool.

Note: Vata types may add a teaspoon of lemon juice to the tea directly before serving it.

Licorice-Aloe Tea

Two servings:

> 3 c water
>
> 1 tsp dried licorice root
>
> 1 tbs aloe vera gel

Bring the water to a boil. Add the licorice root to the boiling water and simmer over low heat for 7 minutes. Remove from heat, strain, cover, and let sit for 3 minutes. Then add the aloe vera gel. Stir and serve lukewarm or cool.

Note: Vata types may substitute 3 or 4 star anise seeds for the aloe vera gel, adding them with the licorice root to the boiling water.

Fresh Mint-Orange Tea

Two servings:

> 3 c water
>
> 10 fresh mint leaves
>
> 1/4 tsp orange zest

Bring the water to a boil in a small stainless steel saucepan. Slightly bruise (tear) the leaves and add to the boiling water, along with the orange zest. Cover, remove from heat, and let sit for 5 minutes before straining. Serve warm or cool.

Comfrey-Lemon Tea

Two servings:

>   3 c water
>   1 tsp dried comfrey leaves
>   3 drops of essential oil of lemon

Bring the water to a boil in a small stainless steel saucepan. Add the comfrey leaves. Remove from heat and add the essential oil. Cover and let sit for 5 minutes before serving.

Note: Both Vata and Pitta types may substitute dried peppermint leaves for the comfrey.

Kudzu-Cumin-Chamomile Tea

Two servings:

>   3 c water
>   1/2 tsp cumin seeds
>   1 tsp dried chamomile buds
>   1 tsp kudzu starch
>   1 tsp Sucanat

Bring the water to a boil in a small stainless steel saucepan. Dry roast the cumin seeds in a small skillet for a few minutes until they are golden brown. Add to the boiling water, along with the chamomile buds. Remove from heat, and let sit for 5 minutes, then strain. In a small bowl, dilute the kudzu in a 1/4 cup of cold water. Reheat the tea and add the kudzu mixture. Stir until the tea becomes gel-like and clear. Add the Sucanat, remove from heat, and serve while still warm.

Note: Vata types may use 1 teaspoon of cardamom pods instead of the chamomile buds.

Note for the Bath: The seeds, leaves and buds remaining from the teas may be added to your bath water. Or you may reverently return them to the earth from whence they came.

PART FIVE
Energizing Diet for Kapha Types

The energizing Kapha healing diet is also considered part of the shamana regimen. However, it is associated with the langhana routine in that it is light, reducing and invigorating in nature rather than the brhmana routine used in the sattvic diet. Like the sattvic diet used by Pitta and Vata types, which adds bulk, this diet may be used by Kapha types occasionally throughout the year, while the post pancha karma healing diet may be used during the main seasonal cleansing routines, and after the intensive pancha karma treatments. Kapha types may also use this dietary regimen during seasonal junctions, as well as through the late winter and early spring.

Season: all year/occasional use

Body Type: Kapha

Conditions
Kapha disorders

Millet Kichadi

Four servings:

> 5 c water
> 1 1/2 c millet
> 1/2 c yellow split mung beans
> 1/4 tsp powdered rock salt
> 5 fresh or dried neem leaves
> 1 tsp corn oil
> 1 tsp cumin seeds

Bring the water a to boil in a large stainless steel pot. Wash the millet and beans thoroughly and add them to the boiling water, along with the salt and neem leaves. Cover and simmer on low heat for 25 minutes. In a small cast-iron skillet, heat the oil and add the cumin seeds. When the seeds turn golden brown, pour into the kichadi. Stir, cover, and continue cooking for another 10 minutes. Serve while the kichadi is still warm.

Spicy Buckwheat Pilaf

Two servings:

      2 1/2 c water
      1 c buckwheat kernels
      1/2 tsp powdered rock salt
      2 celery stalks
      2 scallion stalks
      2 small carrots
      1 tsp sunflower oil
      1/2 tsp cayenne powder
      1/2 tsp ajwan seeds
      1/2 tsp black peppercorns
      1/2 tsp white peppercorns

Bring two cups of water to a boil in a medium size saucepan. Wash the buckwheat and dry roast it in a cast-iron skillet over low heat for 15 minutes, shifting it with a wooden spoon to prevent burning. Add the roasted grain to the boiling water, along with the salt. Cover and simmer over low heat for 15 minutes. Wash the celery and slice thinly. Wash the scallions, snip a small piece off their root ends, and slice thinly, keeping the two vegetables separate. Scrub wash the carrots and slice into 1/4-inch thin pieces. Pour the remaining water into a skillet and bring it to a boil. Add the celery and carrots. Cover and steam boil over medium heat for 3-4 minutes. Strain the vegetables and retain the cooking water. Add oil to the same skillet and saute the scallions for a few minutes, then add to the cooking buckwheat, along with the cayenne powder. Roast spice seeds in oil-lined skillet over low heat until they begin to crackle. Remove from heat and grind coarsely in a suribachi. Add the ground seeds, along with the carrots and celery, to the buckwheat mixture. Cook the pilaf for an additional 5 minutes, then remove from the heat. Toss the vegetable cooking water into the mixture. Remove immediately from the pot and place in a serving bowl. Serve warm.

Note: An equal quantity of barley, millet, and occasionally long grain brown rice may be used instead of the buckwheat.

Barley-Parsley Soup

Two servings:

      6 c water
      1 c pearl barley
      1/4 tsp powdered rock salt

1 tsp corn oil

1 c shredded red cabbage

1/2 c diced onions

1/2 c minced fresh parsley

1/2 tsp dried dill

1/2 tsp black pepper powder

1/4 tsp turmeric powder

1/4 tsp coriander powder

Bring the water to a boil in a heavy soup pot. Wash the barley and add to the boiling water, along with the salt. Cover and simmer on medium heat for 30 minutes. In a large cast-iron skillet, heat the oil and saute the onions over medium heat for a few minutes until they become soft, then add the cabbage and parsley. Stir, cover, and saute the vegetable mixture on medium heat for 3 minutes. Remove from heat and add to the cooking barley. Combine the spice powders and dill, then dry roast them in the oil-lined skillet over low heat for 1 minute. Add to the soup by rinsing the skillet in the soup mixture. Cover and continue cooking for an additional 20 minutes, before removing from heat. Serve the soup warm.

Chana Dhal - Pea Soup

Four servings:

6 c water

1 1/2 c yellow split peas

1/4 tsp powdered rock salt

1/2 tsp sunflower oil

1/2 tsp minced fresh ginger

1/2 tsp minced fresh green chilies

1/2 tsp pure ghee

1 tsp cumin seeds

Bring the water to a boil in a large heavy soup pot. Cover and simmer on medium heat for 15 minutes. Wash the beans and add to the boiling water, along with the salt. Heat the oil in a small cast-iron skillet over low heat. Saute the ginger and chilies for 2 minutes and add to the beans by rinsing the skillet in the soup water. Warm the ghee in the same skillet and add the cumin seeds. When they turn brown, add to the soup. Cover and continue simmering over low heat for an additional 15 minutes before removing from heat. Serve warm.

Note: An equal quantity of red lentils and green split peas may be used instead of yellow split peas.

Three Grain Gruel

Use only in the spring to reduce excess fat.

Three servings:

      8 c water
      1/2 c dried corn
      1/4 tsp powdered rock salt
      1/2 c hulled barley
      1/2 c millet
      1/2 tsp black pepper powder
      1/2 tsp coriander powder

Bring water to a boil in a large heavy soup pot. Wash the grains separately and add the corn to the boiling water along with the salt. Cover and simmer over medium heat for 1 hour, then add barley, millet, pepper, and coriander. Continue cooking for another 45 minutes, then remove from heat. Let the gruel sit undisturbed for 15 minutes before serving.

Note: For weight reduction, use this gruel as a mono-diet, followed by 1/2 cup of the Triphala-Buttermilk preparation for 7 days.

Triphala-Buttermilk

Use only in the spring to reduce excess fat.

Three servings:

      1 c buttermilk
      1 tsp triphala powder
      1 tbs honey

Warm the buttermilk in a double boiler. Remove from heat and stir in triphala powder. Let sit, covered, for 5 minutes, then add honey. Take as a dessert following the Three Grain Gruel for 7 consecutive days.

Cumin-Lemon Millet

Two servings:

      3 c water
      1 c millet
      1/2 tsp powdered rock salt
      1 tsp sunflower oil
      1 tsp cumin seeds
      1 tsp fresh lemon juice

Bring the water to a boil in a medium-size stainless steel pot. Wash the millet thoroughly and add to the boiling water, along with the salt. Cover and simmer on low heat for 20 minutes. Heat the oil in a small cast-iron skillet and roast the cumin seeds for a few minutes until they are golden brown. Add to the cooking millet, along with the lemon juice. Continue cooking for 10 minutes, then remove from heat. Serve warm.

Note: An equal quantity of barley, corn grits or bulgur may be used occasionally instead of millet.

Asparagus and Corn Crumble

Two servings:

      1 c water
      1 lb asparagus
      1/2 c corn flour
      1/4 tsp powdered rock salt
      1 tsp sunflower oil
      1/4 c diced red bell peppers
      1/2 tsp minced fresh garlic
      1/2 tsp minced fresh ginger
      1/2 tsp cayenne powder
      1/2 tsp black pepper powder

Bring the water to a boil in stainless steel skillet. Wash the asparagus, snip off the hard ends, then add to the boiling water. Cover and steam boil for 5 minutes over medium heat. Remove the asparagus and retain the cooking water. In a small cast-iron skillet, dry roast flour over low heat for a few minutes until it turns golden brown. Transfer it to a mixing bowl. Pour oil into the same skillet and saute red pepper, garlic, and ginger over low heat for 3 minutes. Stir in cayenne, black pepper, and roasted flour. Add the asparagus cooking water and blend into a soft dough. Add a little more water if necessary. Cover the skillet and "bake" the dough over low heat for 10 minutes until, it becomes firm and cake-like. Remove from heat and let cool, then crumble it over the cooked asparagus.

Note: An equal amount of broccoli, string beans, carrots, collards, kale, mustard greens or daikon radish, cut as desired, may be used instead of asparagus.

Brussels Sprouts in Cream Sauce

Two servings:

 1 1/2 c water
 1 lb Brussels sprouts
 1/2 c soya milk
 1/4 tsp black pepper powder
 1/4 tsp turmeric
 1/4 tsp dried dill
 1/4 tsp powdered rock salt
 1 tsp kudzu starch
 1 tsp sunflower oil

Bring the water to a boil in a large stainless steel skillet. Wash the Brussels sprouts and add to the boiling water. Steam boil the sprouts over medium heat for 5 minutes. Remove sprouts from cooking water. Add soya milk to the cooking water, along with black pepper, turmeric, dill and salt; simmer over low heat. Dilute the starch in two tablespoons of cold water and stir into the soya milk mixture; continue stirring until it begins to turn clear and gel-like. Remove from heat. Heat the oil in a cast-iron skillet over medium heat. Saute the cooked Brussels sprouts for 3 minutes. Pour the kudzu sauce over the sprouts and remove from heat. Serve immediately.

Note: An equal amount of cabbage, mushrooms, peas or spinach, cut as desired, may be used instead of the Brussels sprouts.

Fruit Shake

Four servings:

 1/2 c fresh pitted cranberries
 1/2 c fresh pitted cherries
 1 c water
 1 c soya milk
 1/4 tsp orange zest
 1 tsp honey

Wash the fruits and puree them in a hand food grinder. Combine the water, milk, orange zest and honey in a mixing bowl and whip with an egg beater until frothy. Stir in the pureed fruits and serve immediately.

Note: Equal amounts of fresh or dried apples, apricots, mango, peaches, persimmon, and pears as well as fresh raspberries, blueberries, and blackberries, may be used instead of the cranberries and cherries.

Stimulating Teas

Season: all year

Body Type: Kapha

Vata and Pitta (occasional use where indicated)

White Pepper-Orange Tea

Two servings:

3 c water

1 tsp white peppercorns

1/2 tsp dried orange peel

1/4 tsp fresh ginger juice

Bring the water to a boil in a small stainless steel saucepan. In a small cast-iron skillet, dry roast the peppercorns over low heat for a few minutes until they turn slightly brown. Add to the boiling water, along with the orange peel and ginger juice. Remove from heat, cover the saucepan and let sit for 10 minutes. Then strain and serve warm.

Note: Vata may also use.

Dandelion Tea

Two servings:

3 c water

1 tsp dried dandelion leaves

Bring the water to a boil in a small stainless steel saucepan. Add dandelion leaves. Cover the pot and remove from heat. Let tea to steep for 10 minutes, then strain and serve.

Note: Pitta may also use.

Gotu Kola Tea

Two servings:

3 c water

1 tsp gotu kola powder

Bring water to a boil in a small stainless steel saucepan. Add powder to the boiling water and remove from heat. Cover and steep for 7 minutes. Serve strained or unstrained.

Note: All types may use.

Ginger-Eucalyptus Tea

Two servings:

> 3 c water
> 1/2 tsp minced fresh ginger
> 3 drops of essential oil of eucalyptus
> 1 tsp honey

Bring the water to a boil in a small stainless steel saucepan. Add the ginger and essential oil, then remove from heat. Cover and allow to steep for 10 minutes, then strain and stir in honey. Serve warm or cool.

Note: Vata may also use.

Cinnamon-Cardamom Tea

Two servings:

> 3 c water
> 3" piece of cinnamon stick
> 10 green cardamom pods

Bring the water to a boil in a small stainless steel saucepan. Add the cinnamon and cardamom and remove from heat. Cover and steep for 10 minutes, then strain and serve warm.

Note: Vata may also use.

Cherry Bark Tea

Two servings:

> 3 c water
> 1 tbs cherry bark pieces
> 5 strands of saffron

Bring the water to a boil in a small stainless steel saucepan. Add cherry bark and saffron. Cover and simmer over low heat for 3 minutes. Remove from heat and let sit for 5 minutes, then strain. Serve warm or cool.

Note: Pitta may also use.

Rosemary-Sage Tea

Two servings:

>   3 c water
>
>   1 tsp fresh rosemary
>
>   7 fresh sage leaves

Bring the water to a boil in a small stainless steel saucepan. Slightly bruise the rosemary and sage by rubbing them firmly in your hands. Add to the boiling water. Cover and simmer for 2 minutes on low heat. Remove from heat and steep for 10 minutes. Strain and serve warm.

Red Clover-Raspberry Tea

Two servings:

>   3 c water
>
>   1 tsp dried organic red clover buds
>
>   1 tsp dried raspberry leaves

Bring the water to a boil in a small stainless steel saucepan. Add buds and leaves and remove the saucepan from the heat. Cover and steep for 10 minutes, then strain and serve warm.

Note: Vata may also use.

Peppermint-Raisin Tea

Two servings:

>   3 c water
>
>   1 tsp dried peppermint leaves
>
>   1 tbs raisins

Bring the water to a boil in a small stainless steel saucepan. Add peppermint and raisins. Simmer over low heat for 3 minutes. Remove from heat, cover and let sit for 5 minutes. Strain and serve warm.

Note: Vata may also use.

Bhringaraja Tea

Two servings:

    3 c water

    1 tsp bhringaraja powder

Bring water to a boil in a small stainless steel saucepan. Add powder and remove from heat. Cover and let sit for 10 minutes. Serve strained or unstrained.

Note: All types may use.

Sweet Jasmine Tea

Two servings:

    3 c water

    1 tbs organic dried jasmine flowers

    1 tsp honey

Bring the water to a boil in a small stainless steel saucepan. Add the flowers and remove from the heat. Cover and steep for 10 minutes, then strain. Stir in honey and serve warm or cool.

Note: The seeds, leaves and buds strained from the teas may be added to your bath water. Or they may be reverently returned to the earth from whence they came.

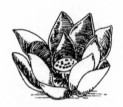

CHAPTER NINE

THE HEALING ACTIVITIES

PART ONE
During and After Pancha Karma

Rejoice at your inner powers for they are the
makers of wholeness and holiness in you.
— *Hippocrates*

During pancha karma treatments, when the body is being skillfully manipulated in the interest of relieving its noxious excesses, maintaining homeostasis in the body is essential. Pancha karma's preliminary treatments, such as snehana and svedana, serve to mollify the mind and body. At the same time, the healing diet acts as a palliative to the organism. However, achieving total harmony is possible only when the subject is fully present and prepared to receive therapy and is willing to allow the body to release its negative forces.

CALMING ACTIVITIES

Allow Yourself

Give yourself to the process without fear and trepidation. Abandon yourself to Mother Nature and allow her forces to empty you. Trust that she will also replenish you. In succumbing completely to the natural forces of the universe, you will be allaying your agitation in the process.

387

Choose Carefully

The choice of therapist also plays a vital role in your having the confidence necessary to permit the universe to guide you. The criteria for choosing your care-giver are that he/she is well-schooled in the art of pancha karma, experienced in its practice, and provides treatment in a warm and properly-equipped place where you feel comfortable and may be supported in your time of need. Although the practitioner may be a qualified general physician, it is very important to keep in mind that he/she may not be adequately versed in the field of Ayurveda or pancha karma.

Ayurvedic physicians are generally qualified to practice pancha karma. In India there are also many excellent pancha karma therapists who are not Ayurvedic physicians but are profoundly skilled in the art of the cleansing therapies. Moreover, they often have far more experience in these practices than many Ayurvedic physicians whose modern approaches are becoming more prescriptive than supportive in nature. Use your own sense of cognition to pre-screen and select the right care-giver for you. To help you with your choice, you may wish to invite the assistance of someone close to you who is healthy and whom you trust. Be wary of the advertising media. As pancha karma services become better known, they are likely to become adroitly advertised. It behooves you, therefore, to look behind the glossy publicity sent to lure you, and to assume responsibility for your choices. Also, remain alert to your cognitive ability throughout your period of receiving treatment. It may prove to be your best source of information about your condition and how best to attend to it.

Gather Information

Once you have chosen a care-giver, look to gain as much information as possible about the treatment you are contemplating. Keep notes on what is being proposed to you and how you are expected to function throughout the period of therapy. Query the practitioner about each and every detail of your program and about the negative and positive factors that may ensue as a result of therapy. Knowing as much as you can about the practitioner's intentions and the therapy itself enables you to maintain a calm disposition throughout the course of treatment. By being relaxed in this way, you are better able to maintain the necessary alertness without feeling overly vigilant and "on guard."

The primary requirement in any form of therapy, wholistic or otherwise, is a clear sense of awareness, which is not impinged upon by fears, distrust, criticism and paranoia, while your body, mind, and spirit are being emptied of their non-essentials.

Trust Yourself

Stripped to the core by the processes of pancha karma therapy, you are advised to wear thoughts of trust, not only in the therapy and its facilitator, but in the grace of the Lord. Trust, when it is not blind, is the most healing of emotions, and is foremost if any therapy is to be successful. Often, when the mind is immersed in details, clarity can sometimes perish, thus clouding the feeling of trust. Therefore, it becomes necessary to look to and live for a while within the luminosity of your own cognitive being. Review the ideas presented earlier in this book about listening to your own fine whispers of the cognitive truth. Learn ways of divining with nature so that her response clarifies any existing confusion. As my teacher Dayananda Saraswati would say, "Sit in yourself." As my dear colleague Beverley would say, "Just watch the thoughts." Regarding any confusions, the yoga adept Dr. Rao would say, "Do nothing."

In India, the homeland of this exquisite art of life, one learns quickly to trust the infinite wisdom of the Lord and eventually the self. Amid the chaos of erratic activity and the cacophony of mind-boggling noises, stupendous calm and gusto combined exist in the humans who live there. As one taxi driver said, "There are only four essentials to living: good horn, good brakes, good nerves and good luck." Put another way, the horn signifies our intentions; the brakes are our ability to stop and contemplate; nerves are the essential fibres of our courage and choices, and, finally, luck is simply the grace of the Lord.

General Observations
- Do not speak loudly
- Do not laugh loudly
- Do not overeat
- Observe your natural bodily urges
- Walk or travel sparingly
- Do not sit excessively
- Do not participate in feelings of anger, fear, or anxiety
- Do not expose yourself to extreme heat, cold, wind or dust
- Avoid sexual activity
- Avoid a coarse, dry diet
- Avoid staying up late at night
- Avoid sleeping during the day
- Remain prayerful and observant
- Allow the body, mind, and spirit to rest in the bosom of the universe

Note: These observances should also be maintained during the preliminary treatments of abhyanga, snehana and svedana.

PART TWO

Daily Rituals

Early Rising

In the Vedas, it is said that forty-eight minutes before sunrise is the most auspicious time of day. Thus, the age-old recommendation to rise and greet the day at this time. Beginning your day with the rising of the sun allows the body to release its waste early, which at once calms the mind. The sages tell us that early rising is the single, most effective action to be observed in order to maintain good health and longevity.

The first activity recommended upon rising is to drink water kept overnight in a copper vessel. This measure helps to prevent constipation and encourages efficient peristaltic movement of the large intestine. The copper water may also be used to clear the nasal passages by inhaling approximately one tablespoon into each nostril. This insufflation helps to maintain excellence in sight and intellect. Copper water is contra-indicated for those who are ill or excessively overweight. It is also not to be used after emesis or purgation therapy, during recuperation from bodily injury or by those who are prone to hiccoughs.

Cleansing the Teeth

Of the body's ten sacred apertures, through which we interphase with the entire cosmos, nine are related to the physical body: eyes, nose, ears (each possessing two openings) and the mouth, urinary passage and rectum. The most important gateway of the human body, the mouth, is tended to first. The ancients were renowned for the excellent health of their teeth and gums. As Dr. Harry Campbell said, "If civilization means cleanliness, good character, and long life, the ancient Indians were more civilized than modern people who have learned to drink 'bed' coffee and tea without cleaning their teeth." Traditionally, brushes made from freshly broken twigs of trees, such as the neem, khadira or licorice, were splayed at the ends and used to cleanse the teeth and massage the gums daily. Due to the natural bitterness, astringency, and freshness of the twig brushes, they served as an excellent oral antiseptic, as well. The use of twig brushes is contra-indicated for people suffering from indigestion, nausea, breathing difficulties, bronchitis, fever, facial paralysis, inflammation of the mouth, heart disease, and from diseases of the eyes, ears and head.

390

Cleansing the Tongue

The tongue, our organ of taste, is one of the main bodily indicators used in Ayurvedic diagnosis because it reveals the telltale signs of both mild and serious health conditions. For example, a pale, whitish tongue accompanies a decrease in red blood cells and/or an anemic condition. A yellowish tongue indicates a bilious disorder in the liver or gall bladder. A bluish tongue indicates heart disorder. A thick white coating on the tongue signals excess mucus in the system, a yellowish or greenish coating indicates a Pitta or bilious disorder, and a dryish, grayish coating indicates excess Vata or a colonic disorder. A dehydrated tongue is a sign of decreased bodily plasma. When the tongue is coated, respiration becomes shallow as a result of prana being impinged in the body.

Traditionally, tongue cleaners made from a thin, smooth flexible foil of gold, silver, or copper, or the thin bark of the twigs used for tooth brushes, approximately 1 foot in length and 1/2 inch wide, arched and held by both hands, were used to scrape the tongue. Gold was used primarily by those with Vata constitutions, while silver was used by Pitta types and copper by Kapha types. The bark of the twig was used by all types. Today, both bamboo and stainless steel tongue scrapers are available and may be used by all three types. Four or five scrapings of the tongue every morning constitute a daily routine. The mouth should be rinsed with cold water afterwards.

Gargling

Gargling is the next procedure observed in the early morning ritual of cleansing the mouth. First, cold water is used to remove excess Kapha from the mouth, followed by a simple gargling solution consisting of herbs such as triphala and licorice powder or essential oils such as musta, cypress, or peppermint. Generally, on a fortnightly basis, a sesame oil and water solution is used or one ounce of sesame seeds are chewed. This measure adds vitality, moisture, and "sneha" to the oral cavity. (See gargling procedures and decoctions in Chapter Five.)

Cleansing the Nasal Passages

The nasal passages are cleansed next. A few drops of medicated oil or sesame oil are inserted into each nostril. After cleaning your hands and clipping your nails, you may also dip your little finger into warm sesame oil and insert it into each nostril, gently twisting the finger to apply. Be careful not to remove the hairs from the nostril; in the Charaka Samhita, it is said that the removal of these hairs may cause impairment of the vision.

Medicated powders called "snuff" were also highly recommended by Charaka. He claimed that snuff performed the functions of both nourishment and purification of the nasal passages. Cleansing the nasal passages maintains clarity of the sense organs, prevents the organs of sight and smell from becoming impaired, safeguards against premature baldness and graying of the hair, and encourages abundant head hair growth. A simple form of nasya therapy, the daily insufflation of oils or powders in the nostrils also nourishes the cranial joints, sinews and tendons, while adding mellowness to the voice. (See also nasal cleansing procedures and formulas under nasya, Chapter Five.)

Caring for the Eyes

Revealing light, the eyes are our most delicate sense organ. They may be cleansed daily by washing them with cool water, or with a triphala decoction containing one quarter teaspoon of triphala powder in a glass of warm water, which is allowed to sit for a half hour before being strained through a very fine sieve. The decoction is poured into an old-fashioned eye-glass which is then cupped over each eye, the head bent back slightly. Blink the eyelids to allow the decoction to wash the eye for a minute or so; then release the eye-glass. A small bit of white antimony paste may also be applied with a lead or zinc pencil on the inner edge of the lower lid. This removes irritations, burning sensations, hyper-secretion, painful tearing of the eyes, and also protects the eyes from glare, wind and dust. Do not use antimony paste directly after meals or during any illness or exhaustion. (For serious eye disorders, refer to akshitarpana procedures in Chapter Five.)

Caring for the Ears

The ears are cared for by dipping the tip of the little finger into a small amount of warm sesame oil, inserting the finger into the ear and rotating it around the aperture. A few drops of oil may also be poured directly into the ear channels. Caring for the ears in this way keeps the mind and body balanced, while maintaining healthy audibility. (For disorders of the ears, see karna purana procedures, Chapter Five.)

Your Daily Bath

After the sense organs have been cleansed and stimulated, the bath is the single most vital daily sadhana for maintaining cleanliness and longevity. Once or twice a week, the entire body may be dry-brushed with a natural bristle brush before taking the bath.

Baths are invigorating, cleansing, palliative to body and mind, and serve as a release for all negative energies. The body is made pliable and is refreshed by bathing. Traditionally, the right hand was reserved for the auspicious function of service to the self and the universe, while the left hand was used for cleansing the lower body's aperture, as well as tending to routine cleansing details. A bath is recommended at both the beginning and ending of the day. Vata and Kapha types may take warm baths, while Pitta types benefit from lukewarm or cool baths.

After the body has been thoroughly cleansed, it should be anointed with chemical-free creams or natural oils such as coconut or sesame, and garbed with clean clothing of natural fibers. The colors of our clothes influence our energies. Earth colors such as ivory, rust, brown, tan, beige, burgundy and dark green are very healing and grounding to Vata types. Bright riveting colors such as red, orange, jade, turquoise, royal blue, purple, yellow and pink are stimulating and positive colors for the Kapha types; Vata types may also wear these colors occasionally to enhance invigoration. Mellow colors such as lavender, sky blue, white, pale yellow and pale pink accent the Pitta type and help to tone their intense energies. Each type may also be adorned with appropriate gems and natural scents. (For this information, see seasonal cleansing therapies for each type in Chapter Three.)

Trimming the Hair and Nails

As a general maintenance procedure, the hair, beard and nails should be trimmed twice a month, preferably during the waxing period of the moon. As well as being clipped, the nails should be scrubbed and buffed with a small amount of sesame oil or a natural nail cream. The cuticles should never be clipped. Use the blunt end of a nail file to gently push them back. Never use nail polishes. Proper care of your hair and nails promotes health, virility, cleanliness and beauty. Massage the hands and feet regularly as part of your bodily care program.

A Wholesome Diet

Strength is the seat of health and therefore it should be maintained by all means.

—*Charaka*

Referring to both diet and exercise, Charaka advises the use of wholesome food and activity in our daily life. The meal is the most sacred gift the universe provides. It is, therefore, necessary to maintain the land that grows our food so that we and all other species may flourish. Safeguarding this dear and precious earth from the contamination of chemical wastes and inorganic pollutants is the birth responsibility of each human. Only when the earth is rich and healthy and the pastures are flourishing once more, can a good seed, the source of our food, be sustained. Be alert without being fearful of the quality of the seeds you plant and the foods you purchase. Refrain from using foods that are chemically treated, genetically manipulated, irradiated or otherwise tampered with. Refrain also from eating animals and their products that are heavily polluted with pesticides, hormones, and artilleries of other drugs.

Because we become what we eat, we must remain cognizant of the quality of our food. By refusing to use the poisonous fodder so often referred to as food and in our efforts to rejuvenate clean wholesome foods, we will be able, once again, to repast in the resplendence of real food.

Sadhana of the Hands

In the Vedas, the hands and feet are referred to as the "organs of action." By using our organs of action, we engage in the moment-to-moment remembering of the five elements of our nature. Our hands are vital extensions that enable us to touch and be in touch with creation.

A timeless sadhana, eating food with our hands allows us to harmonize with nature. The mere touching of food with the fingertips stimulates the five elements. Each finger is an extension of one of the five elements.

Ayurveda encourages us to use our body as the ruler and measuring cup for all our needs. We are born with all the tools needed to exercise our gifts for sadhanas, including those needed to feel and measure foods as we prepare them.

Your hands should partake fully in all food preparation. Knead your energy into the dough, massage your hands with the grains, and roll the rice balls between your palms. Allow the universal energy to enter and transmute your own energy. Mash potatoes and yams with your hands. Tear leafy greens gently with your fingers. When the hands must have a medium, use the grinding stone, mortar and pestle or the hand grinder for grinding; the suribachi for the positive energy provided by clockwise motion. This is sadhana. The closer to nature each utensil or apparatus, the more connected and therefore healing the prepared food will be to the energy of the cosmos.

A hand filled with sadhana is a hand that will heal yourself and others. It is charged with the prana of the five elements, which when used harmoniously, is in constant exchange with nature. In keeping with this principle, you need to become comfortable using your hands and eyes for all measuring. In Sanskrit, the term *anjali* refers to the volume that can be held by your two hands cupped together. Two anjalis of food from your own hands are designed by nature to fill your own stomach. When you are cooking for others, use two anjalis for each adult and one anjali for each child. Likewise gauge your spices or accents with your own pinch. Like your handful, it is tailored to provide a suitable amount for your own personal body needs. The Sanskrit term *angula* refers to the distance between the joints of each finger. This unit of measure is cosmically designed to gauge spices and herbs, such as cinnamon sticks and ginger.

Amount in your cupped hands	=	equivalent of 1 cup
Size of your pinch	=	equivalent of 1/16 teaspoon
Liquid in your palm	=	equivalent of 1 tablespoon
Length of your finger joint (1 angula)	=	equivalent of 3/4 inch

394

Sadhana means your participation with everything. Use only those tools that are absolutely necessary. As soon as possible, give up using measuring cups and spoons, as well as useless kitchen paraphernalia. These adjuncts are distracting and interrupt your direct energetic exchange with the food.

It may be difficult at first to take this conscious step, to trust the accuracy of your own physical-spiritual apparatus. With time, you will become comfortable enough to return to the original and most natural system of measurement. I urge you to translate all the conventional measurements in this book. Use your own personalized measures based on your limbs, hands, and fingers. Exercise this sadhana at your own pace.

General Mealtime Observances

The Vedas recommend certain simple observances during mealtime. These are as follows:

- Offer a small amount of the food to the home fires before eating.
- Offer a prayer of gratitude.
- Clear the breath passage of the right nostril before eating.
- Sit facing east when eating.
- Drink a half cup of warm water before meals, if agni is generally low.
- Observe silence while eating.
- Chew your foods properly, savoring each mouthful.
- Do not eat too quickly or too slowly.
- Eat a sufficient quantity of food that satisfies you without over-eating.
- Stroll forty yards or so after eating.
- Allow three hours for digestion before taking another meal.
- Do not sleep immediately after eating.
- Do not engage in sexual activities immediately after eating.

Note: Since the home fire has sadly become extinct, you may light a small fire with pine kindling (also called fat wood) in a large earthen crock pot and offer into it a small amount of the food before each meal. The ashes from the crock pot should be returned to the earth daily.

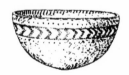

Gentle Exercises

Wholesome physical exercise helps the symmetrical growth of limbs and muscles while improving digestion and complexion. It reconstitutes energy making the body light, firm and compact, while safeguarding against inertia and inducing cheerfulness.
—*Sushruta*

Every step we take, every motion we make, not only massages the limbs but influences the patterns of energy in the universe. A mere gesture demonstrates the exchange of energy and information with the cosmic forces. Every creature and plant uses energy harmoniously, following the rhythms of the wind and rain, the force of the sun and the vibrations of the soil. We do not yet, it seems, truly understand harmony in the motion of our bodies. An ancient saying in India is that a woman should imitate the walk of an elephant if she is to learn absolute grace and sensual divinity in her movements.

The postures proposed for human exercise, a classic tradition of all ancient cultures, were mostly named after the animals and trees. In yoga, for example, the peacock, locust, scorpion, fish, tortoise, frog, crocodile, swan, heron, horse, dog, lion, camel, snake, as well as the lotus flower and even the fluid state of the human embryo, named garbha-pinda, are terms used to demonstrate the various postures. The names, movement and energy of each animal or vegetation are invoked so that we may attain their cosmic memories within our own organisms, thus influencing and remembering our sacred dance with the universes.

Our daily movement should be directed to the gathering of strength while we dispense the various necessary activities. When our activities are carried out wisely, they conserve strength, while encouraging stamina and the release of excess energy.

Ayurveda defines human strength in three ways: the individual strength or vulnerability inherited at birth; the strength which is influenced by the seasons (we are generally stronger in the winter than in the summer, and those living in temperate climates are usually stronger than those living in a tropical climate); and, thirdly, the strength which is acquired by one's own efforts, i.e., by practicing disciplines such as yoga, tai-chi, sports, walking, recreational activities, wholesome nutrition and other wholesome observances of daily life. The latter type of strength is based on the premise that each person is wholly responsible for the care-taking of his/her own health.

Gentle physical activities hasten the removal of bodily wastes and the repair of bodily tissues, enlivening the cells. Cognitive memory impulses are then heightened, and the feelings of joy and invigoration travel with rapidity throughout the organism. Well-paced and consistent, physical exercise promotes stamina, regulates the digestive fire and increases longevity. During activity, more air is inhaled into the lungs, and the rate of purification of the blood increases. The heart, working faster, pumps the purified blood through the entire organism. As a result, the tissue and bodily wastes, as well as ama, are excreted at an accelerated rate, which, in turn, facilitates the production of new tissues.

Through ample, but not excessive, physical exercise, sweat is produced, which invigorates the skin and encourages decongestion in lungs, kidneys, liver and spleen. Both Charaka and Sushruta caution against excessive activities, and intense or stressful exercises, which include highly competitive sports. When physical activities are excessive, the rate at which blood races through the body sends frantic impulses to the organs and tissues, which, in turn, dangerously propel the excretion of live tissues along with bodily wastes. As a result, the states of emaciation, amnesia, and undue fatigue are certain to occur. Moreover, the cellular intelligence of the body responds in fear, due to tissue deprivation. At the same time, excess endorphin and adrenaline produced by the brain dull the mind and senses, as well as the internal language of the body. Strenuous activity also depletes life-sustaining ojas. Physical disorders such as consumption, hemorrhaging, excess thirst, aversion to foods, nausea, fevers, asthma, physical accidents and delusions may occur as a result of physical strain. Exercising is contra-indicated directly after meals, sexual activities, and during illness.

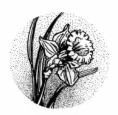

Nurturing Sadhanas for Each Body Type

Vata: Spring, summer, and autumn are considered to be moderately vulnerable seasons for Vata. Vata's natural times of weakness, and, therefore, its most vulnerable periods, are in the rainy season (early fall) and late winter, as mentioned earlier. It is important that Vata types observe a schedule of gentle care and wholesome sadhanas throughout the year. The following nurturing sadhanas are recommended for use during the more vulnerable seasons.

- Ayurvedic massage with sandalwood oil, sesame oil, aguru oil, kesare oil
- Gentle exercise—yoga, pranayama, meditations, strolling, and so on
- Padabhyanga (Ayurvedic foot massage)
- Warm baths with essential oils such as jasmine, rose, cinnamon, cardamom, and musk
- Gentle body brushing. Three times per week, before bath, apply natural moisturizers and cream to your skin
- Special care with the daily cleansing of the orifices—head, nose, mouth and ears, as well as the excretory orifices
- Gentle physical activity throughout the year
- Swimming in lakes, rivers, and streams in the summer (with quick dips in the autumn)
- Receiving the rays of the full moon for a few hours in the spring, summer, and autumn
- Walks in flower gardens during the spring, summer, and autumn
- Family sadhanas, with small, quiet group activities such as cooking, grinding grains and seeds, making masalas, home pickling, and so on
- Seasonal enema therapy, supervised by an Ayurvedic practitioner
- Sexual activity—mild throughout the year, with more emphasis on foreplay
- Aroma therapy, with essential oils such as musk, geranium, cardamom, jasmine, rose, kesare cinnamon, nutmeg, and vanilla; the natural fragrance of seasonal flowers also helps to restore Vata
- Warm and colorful clothing of natural fibers, vivid or earth colors, and naturally scented
- Warm and moist living space
- Healing gems and metals, i.e., amethyst, beryl, yellow sapphire, lapis lazuli, opal, garnet, topaz, coral, ruby, gold

Pitta: Autumn, late winter, and to some extent the early winter are considered to be moderately vulnerable seasons for Pitta. Pitta's natural time of weakness occurs in the autumn, Pitta's most vulnerable time. During both periods, but even more so in autumn, Pitta types are urged to maintain balance through the following wholesome, routine sadhanas.

- Ayurvedic massage with sandalwood oil, coconut oil, aguru oil, and kesare oil
- Baths, both lukewarm and cool, with essential oils such as jasmine, rose, coriander, and spearmint
- Daily body brushing before baths
- Special care with the cleansing of the orifices—head, nose, mouth and ears, as well as the excretory orifices
- Active exercise—yoga, athletic sports, and so on
- Padabhyanga (Ayurvedic foot massage)
- Swimming in lakes, rivers, and streams in autumn
- Receiving the rays of the full moon for a few hours every week in autumn and early winter
- Group sadhanas—community planning, group activities with the visual arts, painting, drawing, and so on
- Seasonal purgation therapy, supervised by an Ayurvedic practitioner
- Special care with daily cleaning of the home and a wholesome diet; the use of astringent, bitter, and cooling herbs is vital during autumn
- Sexual activity—active in late winter, moderate in early winter, and sparingly for the rest of year
- Aroma therapy with essential oils such as jasmine, rose, peppermint, licorice, coriander, vetiver, honeysuckle, sandalwood, and fennel
- Warm and light clothing—natural fibers and naturally fragrant; colors: violet, white, light blue, purple
- Dry and cool living space
- Healing gems and metals—pearl, coral, amethyst, moonstone, emerald, clear quartz, silver, and white gold

Kapha: Late winter, and to some extent, the early fall and early winter are considered a moderately vulnerable time for Kapha. The spring is Kapha's most vulnerable time, and therefore Kapha's natural time of weakness. During these times, and especially in the spring season, Kapha types are urged to maintain balance through the following wholesome sadhanas.

- Ayurvedic massage with aguru and kesare oil
- Active exercise—yoga, athletic sports, walking and so on
- Padabhyanga (Ayurvedic foot massage)
- Warm baths with essential oils such as sage and patchouli
- Daily body brushing before baths
- Family sadhanas—cooking, spice grinding, seed and grain grinding, masala making, and so on. In spring, the use of pungent, bitter, and astringent herbs is vital
- Seasonal emesis therapy, supervised by an Ayurvedic practitioner
- Special care with daily cleansing of the orifices—head, nose, mouth, and ears, as well as the excretory orifices
- Sexual activity—active in both phases of winter, moderate for rest of year
- Aroma therapy with essential oils such as sage, eucalyptus, wintergreen, patchouli, camphor, cardamom and allspice, during the late winter and spring
- Warm and dry living spaces
- Colorful and warm clothing of natural fibers
- Healing gems and metals—opal, ruby, beryl, emerald, garnet, lapis lazuli, gold, and copper

Note: For the cooking sadhanas, refer to my previous book, *Ayurveda: A Life of Balance*.

PART THREE
Ablutions for the Practitioner

The art of medicine consists of amusing the patient, while nature cures the disease.

—Voltaire

There are certain universal rites of conduct which are necessary for the practitioner and attendants to perform before beginning the treatment of a patient. Clearing your energy field is a vital preliminary measure to summoning your healing nature. The most effective means to clear the field is to be actively engaged in the ongoing process of observing a harmonious and disciplined life, free from indulgences and crisis. A healer must be able to summon the spirit of brightness, goodness, simplicity, honesty, cleanliness, purity, compassion and humility in his/her own life before being able to help others to heal. In Vedic thought, this is the prerequisite for participating in helping the sick and the infirm.

A daily application of wholesome sadhanas, which include baths, prayers, the use of simple natural clothing, wholesome meals and exercise, and sharing in family activities, are a necessary component of a Vedic practitioner's spiritual life. To paraphrase Jack Kornfield, it is difficult to sit and meditate after a day of lying and stealing. A spiritual life which is not grounded in reverence for other beings is not a genuine spiritual life. Further, without the benefit of a truly spiritual life, the effectiveness of one's healing powers is decidedly limited.

Another important prerequisite for becoming a true Ayurvedic practitioner is a firm knowledge of the Ayurvedas, preferably gained under the tutelage of an accomplished master. The lifelong homage to one's master and to the lineage which precedes him/her is vital to the preservation of the wisdom gained. It is also essential for practitioners to have the support of their peers so that information can be shared; one's strength and dharma reinforced and resolved through collaboration.

The daily application of this Ayurvedic wisdom allows it to grow, mature and become resplendent, but it can only flourish when your heart is replete with gratitude for all that you receive.

Cleansing Ablutions for the Practitioner

- Rise a half hour before sunrise.
- Take your bath and observe the cleansing routines for the mouth, tongue, teeth, eyes, ears and nose. (See Daily Rituals, Chapter Nine.)
- Facing the sun and allowing the cool morning air to wash over you, observe your prayers. A traditional Vedic prayer to garner the healing energies of the universe is offered on pg. 408.
- Do mild stretches or observe yoga postures and pranayama (yogic breathing exercises).
- Take a wholesome breakfast at least two hours before tending to your first patient.
- Wear a clean simple cotton garment suited to your work. (See practitioner's smock recommended design, Appendix D.)
- Wear a clean silk undershirt. Silk protects your energy from being wasted and acts as a screen to filter out negative energies.
- Wash your hands after attending to each patient.
- Take a break in the middle of the day. Leave the treatment area and if possible take a brief bath and change your clothing.
- Offer a prayer to Lord Surya, the Sun, for your protection. One such Vedic prayer is The Twelve Names of the Sun, pg. 411.
- Take a light lunch and allow yourself at least one hour before returning to your patients.
- At the end of the day, leave all patient care details behind, and seek to refresh yourself. You may wish to bathe again and change into comfortable clothes made of natural fibers, or you may choose to take a walk, a swim and so on.
- Offer your prayers again at sunset, before taking your evening meal.
- Observe a relaxing time afterwards with friends or family.
- Observe a brief period of pranayama, activating the left breath, along with light stretches to induce calmness.
- Observe a period of meditation, allowing all the stress to dissipate, all thoughts to leave the mind, and trusting the universe to replenish your vital energies.
- Retire to bed before midnight.

PART FOUR

Ablutions for the Subject

Expressions of gratitude and honesty enable the healing energies of the universe to permeate your being. Gratitude for being given the sacred staff of life, gratitude to the good earth for providing abundantly when you learn how to receive her gifts, and gratitude to those whom you conscript to help you heal are all essential parts of the expression of healing. Disease forces us to come to terms with ourselves; but, before healing can occur, complete honesty must prevail. Time must be invoked to sift through the years of cumulative pain, from the very first compromise to the most recent denial of the cognitive self, with the fervent wish to reconcile the self and rid it of its disease.

Keeping a daily journal is an excellent sadhana during this time, for it helps to empty the pain as clarity is gained. The cognitive voice or your inner guide, silenced for so long, must once more be awakened so that you may heal.

Cleansing Ablutions for the Subject

- Try to rise with the sun every morning.
- Open the windows and allow the cool morning air into your life.
- Take your bath and observe the cleansing routines for mouth, tongue, teeth, eyes, ears and nose. (See Daily Rituals, Chapter Nine.)
- Sit facing the sun and offer a prayer for the guidance and clarity of both yourself and your health care practitioner. Pray for courage and complete healing. A traditional Vedic prayer for healing is the Triyambikam Mantra on pg. 409.
- Do some mild stretches or yoga postures and pranayama (yogic breathing exercises).
- Observe the dietary regimen suitable for your body type and condition.
- Wear clean, simple clothing made of natural fibers, preferably cotton. Do not wear silk clothing.
- Entrust yourself to the care of your health practitioner while maintaining a calm and observing spirit.
- Release all anger and fear before entering the treatment room.

- Invoke the universal spirit to walk with you in your time of healing.
- Do not be afraid to question or clarify anything which comes to mind during your treatment, even if it may appear inappropriate.
- After you return home, follow the recommendations given by your health care practitioner.
- Wear a clean, comfortable cotton garment and observe a period of meditation a few hours after your evening meal.
- Empty your mind by allowing the thoughts to dissolve, including the anxiety-ridden thoughts. If the thoughts persist, observe them and allow them to enter in and out of the mind. Try not to feed on them by becoming fearful, anxious, and so on.
- Ask the universe to help you regain your health. Leave your burdens in the bosom of the universe before going to sleep.

Note: These ablutions should also be observed when therapies are applied at home.

PART FIVE

Ablutions for the Mind and Heart

What is essential is invisible to the eye.
It is only with the heart that one can truly see.
—Antoine Saint-Exupery,
The Little Prince

COSMIC GLOBULES

In cleansing body, mind and heart we are signaling our intentions to replenish our natural energies which are connected to the universe. In turn, the cosmos sends its healing agents to our aid. The expression of our intentions is one of the most powerful ways that the human can interphase with the universe. When our intent is clear, and it is of a positive nature, it serves to help us heal and grow.

Prayers, as an expression of our intention, are the most powerful vehicle of communication that the human possesses. Thus, prayer is a numinous ablution necessary not only as a prelude to body/mind cleansing, but also as a primary sadhana in our daily lives. As we utter the sacred words inherent in all prayers, cosmic forces gather around to form a vibratory field of immense protection. At once, we are cast into a timeless spell, while being enhanced by the reflection of our own emotion in the form of cosmic globules.

Functioning through the vibratory space of the cosmos, cosmic globules are tiny spherical bodies similar to air bubbles and imperceptible to normal human vision. They are as susceptible to negative forces as they are to positive ones. Once an intention is expressed, the universe is its receptor, which, in turn, responds through vibrations in the form of these cosmic globules. This means that when there is an angry confrontation between two people, the vibrations of those expressions or intentions are received by the globules. In congregate force, they arrive at the scene of the activity and enhance whatever situation is occurring. They envelop the entire situation, thus providing a spell-binding force which enhances whatever emotions are being played out in that situation. The synergy of our own personal emotions, combined with the forces of the globules, leaves us almost incapable of redressing negative emotions once they are displayed. This is why it is so important that we work through our emotions completely before they rush headlong into negative expressions.

Generally, there is a long period of grace granted to us after we have experienced negative thoughts regarding ourselves or others. During that time, we have the opportunity to review our intentions. As soon as we are ready to act, the cosmos unleashes its forces to assist us. The nature of this assistance is determined by the quality of our intentions. It is wise to assume that all so-called accidents are due, at least in part, to the nature of our energies and how they are expressed. The globule forces of the universe can only enhance situations that already pre-exist. Since what exists is partly the result of our intentions, it behooves us to be aware of them and, if necessary, to alter them.

SEVEN DAILY TRANSITIONS

Each and every day has seven sacred phases, which, when observed, bring complete peace to body, mind and spirit. These phases provide us with the necessary transitions that help us maintain excellent health. To perform certain ablutions, or actions, at the appropriate times of day, therefore, enables us to facilitate this beautiful process.

As we rise from sleep, we observe the cleansing of our body and the elimination of bodily wastes. The next action is to offer prayers to the universe. There are three distinct intentions expressed within a prayer, namely: praying for the wellness of all beings, offering gratitude to the Lord for being alive and, finally, seeking wisdom and clarity to help us as we make our way through life.

The third action is to eat wholesome meals in order to sustain our energy and vitality. The fourth action is to work, to apply ourselves to the development of the mind and the natural progress of the universe. The fifth action is to play, to revel in the universe's beauty, to appreciate the flowers, streams, light and love cast within nature, to exercise and to dance with the universe.

The sixth action is contemplation. Different from prayer, contemplation is the simple action of being within the self and allowing it to remain empty of thoughts: to bask in the silence of the sacred. It is the most valuable sadhana for replenishing our internal nature with nature itself, a time for the self to understand its own primal nature of oneness with and in all. The final phase or action of the day is to rest, to sleep, so that the organism may be re-charged from nature's abundant well of life.

THE POWER OF PRAYER

When energy flows, overflows, without any
motivation, it becomes delight. That is the moment
when you have started pouring into God. And
the moment you start to pour into God, God starts
pouring into you. It happens simultaneously.
  —William Blake

A prayer is the invocation of our divinity and expresses an honest intention to the omniscient Lord, often in the form of a request for relief from pain. By praying, we are able to invite self cognition through the effort of turning back to the universe for answers. Prayers invoke our cosmic nature; while praying, we at once feel the support of the Lord, whether or not the results are immediately apparent. Inner luminosity is rekindled, and the cognitive memory of our indelible journeys in the universe once more comes to light.

Our own divinity is often compared to shrines of precious gems sitting in the center of each being. Honest intentions expressed in the form of prayers avail us of the wealth of our endless spirit source. As I. E. Taimni said, "This does not mean that precious stones begin to fly through the air and fall at our feet." Rather, we are able to reach the sacred epicenter of our divine being, a space more dear and precious than all the gems in the heavens.

The following Vedic prayers are offered to address one's personal healing. The proper intonation of these Sanskrit prayers is necessary, since every syllable holds a numinous sound, which, when uttered correctly, invokes the proper universal response.

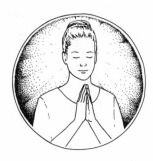

Prayer Before Pancha Karma Treatment

I call upon the following gods to protect me—Brahma, Rudra, Indra, Prithivi, Chandra, Surya, Vayu and Agni—as well as upon the group of medicines which are being used as rejuvenators, upon the *rishis*, or sages, and upon the nectars of the gods. So, too, may all other medicines chosen for me be the best.

Brahma:	The creator, golden in color, has four faces, representing the four directions of the universe.
Rudra:	The dissolver of the universe, has three eyes and is yellow and bright like the sun. He is smeared with holy ashes and has a pleasant countenance.
Indra:	Lord of the Firmament.
Prithivi:	Lord of the Earth.
Chandra:	Lord of the Moon.
Surya:	Lord of the Sun.
Vayu:	Lord of the Air.
Agni:	Lord of the Fire.

Morning Prayer

To garner the healing energies of the universe.

Na tatra suryo bhati na chandratarakam
Nema vidyuto bhanti kuto'yamagnih
Tameva bhantamanubhati sarvam
Tasya bhasa sarvamidam vibhati

Om Shanti Shanti Shanti

There the sun does not shine
Nor the moon or the stars
There this lightning does not shine
Nor does the fire
Only by the shining light of That (Supreme Being)
All else shines in various ways

Prayer for Healing

*Tryambakam yajamahe sugandhim
pushti vardhanam
Urvarukamiva bandhanan mrityor
mukshiya ma amritat
Om Shanti Shanti Shanti*

We worship the fragrant three-eyed One (Rudra) who
confers ever increasing prosperity; let us be saved from
the hold of death, like the cucumber freed from its
vine; let us not turn away from liberation.

Prayer for Clarity and Self Cognition

*Om Purnamadah purnamidam purnat
purnamudachyate
purnasya purnamadaya
purnamevavashishyate
Om Shanti Shanti Shanti*

That is whole; this is whole
from the whole, this whole came.
Remove this whole from that whole,
what remains is still whole

Prayer for Success and Auspicious Beginnings

Oh Lord Ganesha with the broken tusk, with the
magnificent body, effulgent as a thousand suns.
The one who is adorned in white
and is the glow of the moon.
I meditate upon thy ever smiling countenance.
Protect me oh Lord from danger.
May all obstacles be removed from my life.
May all my beginnings be auspicious.
Om Shanti Shanti Shanti

Prayer for the Removal of all Obstacles

Shuklambaradharam vishnum
shashivarnam chaturbhujam
prasanna vadanam dhyayet
sarva vighnopashantaye

Om Shanti Shanti Shanti

For the removal of all obstacles,
may one salute Ganapati
Who wears white clothes and is all pervasive
Whose color is of the moon
Who has four arms, and whose countenance is pleasing.

Sunrise and Sunset Prayer

Prayer for Clarity, Intelligence and the Spirit of Gratitude.

The Twelve Names of the Sun

Om Mitraya namah	Salutations to my Friend.
Om Ravaye namah	Salutations to the twelve Suns.
Om Suryaya namah	Salutations to the Wise One.
Om Bhanave namah	Salutations to the Source of Perception.
Om Khagaya namah	Salutations to the Celestial Ganges.
Om Pushne namah	Salutations to the One who makes the paths of Dark and Light.
Om Hiranya garbhaya namah	Salutations to the One born of Consciousness.
Om Marichaye namah	Salutations to the Radiant One.
Om Adityaya namah	Salutations to the Mother of the twelve Suns.
Om Savitre namah	Salutations to the Ever-generating One.
Om Arkaya namah	Salutations to the Fire.
Om Bhaskaraya nama:	Salutations to the Power of Reflection.

Om Shanti Shanti Shanti

Prayer of Gratitude

Brahmarpanam brahma havih
Brahmagnau brahmana hutam
Brahmaiva tena gantavyam
Brahmakarma samadhina
Om Shanti Shanti Shanti

Brahman is the offering.
Brahman is the oblation.
Poured out by Brahman into the fire of Brahman,
Brahman is to be attained by the one
who recognizes everything as Brahman.

(Brahman refers to the Absolute One, Pure
Consciousness.)

A Prayer for the Wellbeing of the Universe

Svasti prajabhyah paripalayantam
Nyayena margena mahim mahisah
Gobrahmanebhyah subhamastu nityam
Lokasamasta sukhino bhavantu
Kale varsatu parjanyah prthivi sasyasalini
Deso yam ksobarahitah brahmanah
santu nirbhayah
Om Shanti Shanti Shanti

May everyone be prosperous. May the peacemakers
righteously rule the Earth. Let the animals and people
of wisdom be protected at all times. May all be happy.
May the rains come at the proper time. May the Earth
produce grains. May the world be free from famine.
May the people of contemplation have no cause for fear.

412

THE PRACTICE OF JAPA FOR A SILENT MIND

The silence you experience between each thought is your own fullness, the same fullness that is pure consciousness.

—Swami Dayananda Saraswati

Japa, the repetition of a meaningful word or phrase, is a beneficial practice for everyone and is especially so for Vata and Pitta types. The Sanskrit word, japa, means that which puts an end to the cycles of births and deaths, or the attainment of complete peace through silence. The observance of japa destroys all of the mind's impurities.

An ancient Vedic practice for quieting the mind, japa gives the reigns of control to the mind which, in turn, guards the thoughts. When we are concerned with our dreams and our disappointments, fears and commitments, what to eat, what to wear, where to go, how much we have, how much more we need, we are thinking, thinking, and thinking; and the mind becomes thick with thoughts.

Japa is an action that draws the mind to a single point. Using a rosary or *japa mala*, which usually has 108 beads, involves turning one bead at a time while repeating a specific mantra (a Vedic phrase or verse, each word charged with numinous power). Repetition of the mantra generates a deep vibration that is in accord with the heart; eventually all unwanted, extraneous thoughts are silenced. Being at peace with one's self is to be quiet. Peace is silence, silence of the mind. Peace is being able to quietly thin the mind of its erratic secretions.

In the preliminary stages of japa practice, the mantra is repeated audibly and within the same time intervals. Japa is not a series of continuous thoughts. Rather, the mantra is meant to replace all existing thoughts by becoming the only presiding thought. The beginning and ending of each mantra denotes the beginning and end of each thought, each with its own separate crisp beginning and end. In between each mantra is silence. By repeating the mantra, we gain the silence between the mantras. This silence is pure consciousness. It is you, in fact, before thoughts and activities are superimposed upon you. This silence is peace, and maintaining this silence is meditation.

At the beginning and for some time, other thoughts will come while repeating the mantra. Always go back to the sound of the mantra. Do not worry about the thoughts. Allow the thoughts to flow in and out by going back to the sound of the mantra. The thoughts will resolve themselves into the silence if you do not concentrate on them. Otherwise, you will become caught up in them.

One very excellent mantra that is practiced by students of the Vedas is "Om namah shivaya," reflecting the eternal sound of the Lord's name. You may use any mantra as long as it has some deep spiritual meaning for you, for only then will the crowded thoughts begin to thin and dissolve.

Each bead of the rosary is held until you complete the mantra; then the fingers move on to the next bead, and the same mantra is repeated. In this way you continue until all of the beads have been turned. There is usually an extra "marker" bead to indicate that you have finished one rotation.

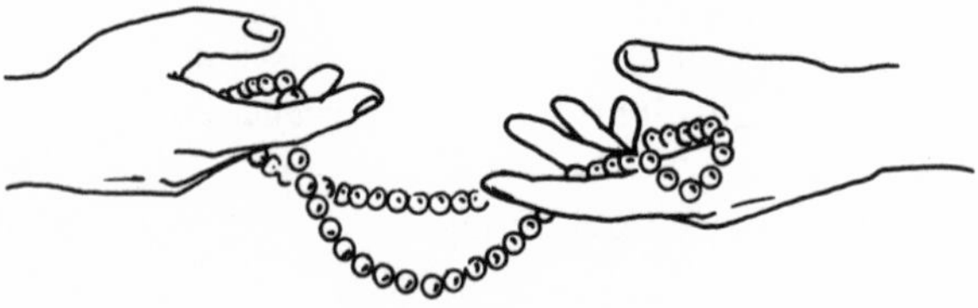

Figure 46: Japa

PART SIX
Pranayama: Breathing Practices

The divine fire blazes forth in full splendor when the mind is drawn to concentrate on meditation.

—Patanjali

The ancient Vedic seers culled an elaborate system of breathing practices to discipline the mind. These breathing practices, known as *pranayama*, are in keeping with the harmonic rhythm of the universe. Prana is the life-force that holds body, mind and spirit together. We obtain prana from the atmosphere and our food. Whereas the lungs play the major role in the respiratory process, prana is transported by every cell in the body. The colon, for example, is said to produce certain volatile fatty acids which, like oxygen, food and water, are carriers of prana. The good health of the entire organism determines how much prana we can absorb into the body.

Pranayama is essential to our well-being, because it controls the breath and respiration that are life itself. By practicing pranayama properly, one quickly feels many changes in attitudes and feelings. A deep inner calm and control over life's events are experienced. It is necessary, however, to remember not to approach contemplation or meditation mechanically.

Practice breathing from the solar plexis area by lying on your back with one hand on the stomach. At the beginning, exaggerate the inhalation slightly by deliberately pushing out your stomach and lengthening your exhalation so that it lasts two or three times longer than your inhalation. Too often when we begin to do breathing exercises, there is a tendency to breathe into the upper chest area only and to push our shoulders upward. Inhalation has nothing to do with sniffing air into the nostrils. In fact, it is best to ignore the nostrils completely and focus your attention on your solar plexus area. Concentrate on the sound of the incoming breath and not on the breathing. The sound will pull the breath along. Then exhale by concentrating on the sound of the exhalation leaving the body and traveling slowly, very slowly, upward, outward, holding the sound like a tenor holds a note, releasing it in a crescendo, from loud to soft to very soft to loud again. After practicing for a short time, you will find that the breath flows naturally without effort.

415

Morning Pranayama

Sit in the upright yoga mudra position, the lotus position, or any similar position that is comfortable for you (Fig. 48). Inhale through the left nostril by blocking the right nostril with your right thumb (Fig. 47). Then exhale through the right nostril by blocking your left nostril with your right ring and little fingers. Then inhale through the right nostril and exhale through the left. Continue for approximately 5 minutes, always inhaling through the same nostril you just exhaled from.

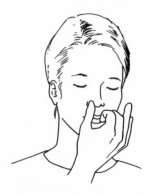

Figure 47: Nostril Breathing

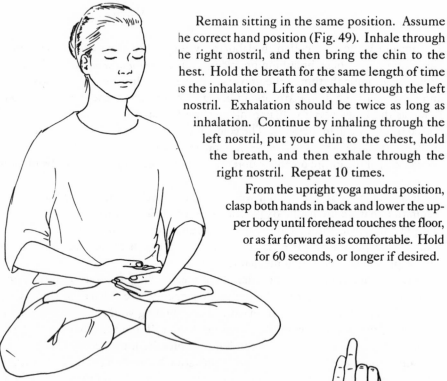

Remain sitting in the same position. Assume he correct hand position (Fig. 49). Inhale through he right nostril, and then bring the chin to the hest. Hold the breath for the same length of time ıs the inhalation. Lift and exhale through the left nostril. Exhalation should be twice as long as inhalation. Continue by inhaling through the left nostril, put your chin to the chest, hold the breath, and then exhale through the right nostril. Repeat 10 times.

From the upright yoga mudra position, clasp both hands in back and lower the upper body until forehead touches the floor, or as far forward as is comfortable. Hold for 60 seconds, or longer if desired.

Figure 48: Yoga Mudra Position

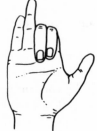

Figure 49: Hand Mudra

PART SEVEN

Observances
During Home Application Treatment

To be enlightened is to be intimate with all things.

—Dogen

Communal Spirit

Ayurveda was born during a time when the spirit of communal activity flourished, a time when many hands made light the work to be done. In reclaiming this ancient art, we are also calling back into our lives the gathering and celebration of hands working together. Although a skilled healer existed in each person, it was the women who reaped, thrashed and hulled the grains and beans necessary to make the healing poultices, while the young girls dried the leaves, roots, barks, flowers and seeds used in the medicines. It was the young boys who collected the grasses, dung, mud and water necessary to facilitate the healing therapies. While the men built the sweat lodges, furnaces, pits and trenches necessary to accommodate the therapies. It was the village elders who tended to the fires necessary for making medicines and producing warmth.

When the seasonal cleansing time of year dawned, sacred oblations were offered to the fire by the local priests. Mantras resounded in the crisp air of springtime and autumn. The elephants, cows, camels and mules readily released their earth-cleansing dung, which was then used to daub the sveda pits and lodges, and to incinerate medicines and reduce them into powders.

The hawks soared clockwise in the skies; the crows kept a reverent distance; the deer forsook the tall grasses bordering the villages and retreated to the forests. The pearls were perfected and ready to be plucked from the oysters. The peacock shed a few of its tail feathers; the musk deer released its sac of musk oil on the ground; the bees filled the honey combs to the brim; and the insects completed their construction of "galls" on the trees. Human activity was once more about to flourish and all of nature succumbed willingly, leaving behind the essentials which were converted into medicines. An old Indian proverb says, "It takes a village to raise a child." Even today, it still takes a whole community to heal a member. Let us not continue to extract the application of these treatments from the bosom of the community, leaving it scattered and uninvolved. A community functions as a result of its people, not its physicians, priests, politicians and merchants. As we pull together, the activities we birth together will be a thousand times more resplendent than the ones performed alone.

Practicing Home Therapies

Most of the preparatory treatments within the abhyanga, snehana and svedana groups may also be applied at home, with the help of friends or family members. Follow the procedures carefully, observing the seasonal guidelines and conditions within the therapies marked for home use. The most auspicious days to begin your home practices are Sunday and Monday.

- Choose a clean, sunny, well-ventilated, sparsely furnished room which is fairly dry and cool and has hardwood flooring. If possible, maintain this room only for the use of your healing programs and the observance of meditation and prayers.
- Before beginning a home program of treatments, call your community health members and invite their participation.
- Schedule a small gathering on a weekly or bi-weekly basis to join hands and minds in the practice of the healing treatments.
- Begin your activities by gathering all the necessary ingredients and· equipment you may need for your treatment of choice. The best day of the week to do this is on Saturday.
- Start by practicing to prepare the formulas and recipes needed for the treatment.
- Then administer a few trial treatments, taking turns among yourselves in giving and receiving them.
- If available, invite your local Ayurvedic practitioner to conduct a few classes in the elementary techniques of massage, oelation, poultice application and fomentation. The best days of the week to receive these instructions are on Thursdays and Fridays. Remember to collect a suitable donation from your members to compensate your learned guest for his/her sharing of this knowledge.
- Although there may not be an Ayurvedic practitioner readily available in your community, there are many wholistic health caretakers who are beginning to incorporate the Ayurvedic approach

within their existing practices. These practitioners may also be called upon to assist you with your home group practice.

- Attend as many Ayurvedic instructional classes as you can in the interest of attaining a firm grasp on the principles of this remarkable healing art.

PART EIGHT
The Forgotten Dharma - Sexuality

I am Happiness, untethered and free
No other happiness exists apart from me.
Love is not towards others,
Nor can I love myself,
For I am Love
          —Advaita Makaranda (v. 24)

Sadhana of Sexual Union

Dharmas are the unwritten codes of proper conduct inherent in all life. India is weaned on the tradition of dharma handed down from the rishis, seers of ancient time. These universal values, belonging to all humans, protect us with resplendent grace when we are guided in all activities by the spirit of goodness, wholesomeness, honesty, compassion, cleanliness, reverence to nature and devotion to the Lord.

All life seeks union in many ways. Cohesion within ourselves and with nature is foremost; the sharing of thoughts and activities with others in the form of friendship is also important to our existence. One of the deepest sharings that all creatures experience at some time or another is the sadhana of sex. Even the renunciate, who has sublimated the normal physical urges of sexuality, seeks to form a union, not with another person but with God. The yoga of life is union, and the cosmic intention in human sexual activity is the bonding of two people who henceforth walk as one in the universe.

A primal dance of nature, sexual union is a necessary means of replenishing both male and female energies, although the yogins have sublimated and gone beyond this physical dharma. Practiced within the universal dharma, or wholesome activity considerate of others, the male feeds the female with his juice. This nourishment is then transformed into life-supportive essence, safeguarding the procreative energies of the female while she matures into the prime of motherhood. The vital life-sustaining essence, called ojas, as well as the supreme life-protecting warmth, called tejas, can only become enhanced between the couple after a long period of practicing this cosmic dance. Just as a mother feeds her baby with her own milk, over a period of time the male feeds his female partner with the essential, cosmic nutrients of his sperm. When preserved within a monogamous union, both ovum and sperm, continuously replenished, gain progressive strength until they join to become a new life. From this bonding, the future seed sprouts with prowess and brilliance, seasoned by the esteem and love infused within the threads of the sacred material spun over a long and integral period of relationship.

When the new life makes its way from the watery domain of its mother's womb into the world, its entire genetic composition is influenced and shaped by the intention and actions of the parents long before cohabitation and, quite decisively, during the time of union between sperm and ovum.

The wisdom and esteem of the human self warn against the indiscriminate and lawless indulgence of sexual intercourse. Practiced without dharma, life-forming nectar turns to poison. Life springing from a union of that nature is generally plagued with uneasiness and sorrow. When the potentially blissful dance of sex is reduced to a blistering tedium, devoid of esteem, dignity and universal rhythm, chaos and sorrow for all involved are certain to follow. Disregarding the rhythmic vibrations of nature and indulging in sexual misconduct are certain to incur the loss of love, happiness, the decline of faith and the perishing of trust, all of which are vital to human affairs.

Our intentions are an essential prelude to all activities, especially sexual interchange. Practiced as an entirely physical action, without allegiance to the dharmas, sexual involvement becomes emotionally and physically depleting and deprecating. A sure way to transmute ojas and tejas into poison, indiscriminate sexual practices are primal violations against love, happiness, the essences of self. To quote an old Indian saying, when sex is performed without proper intention and regard for human esteem, "At once, one crumbles as a dry, sapless, worm-eaten and decayed piece of wood at the merest touch." If not physically the case, it certainly is true for the spirit. In violating this privileged spirit, our ability to truly love becomes diminished and, after some time, we chance losing it completely.

The Hindu pantheon of gods and goddesses imbided in the stupendous sharing of sexuality and love, all in accord with universal values. The tradition of sexual interplay, primarily for producing the continuance of life and insuring a future, though procreating, has been observed as a sacred duty of all species. Foreplay and the various other activities involved in the happy dance of sexual intercourse and its aftermath have always been a beautiful and enriching part of this numinous duty.

All the other days are considered harmonically inauspicious times to conceive children. Negative results may ensue in the physical, emotional and spiritual health of both parents and child when conception occurs outside of these well-aspected times.

Sexual Dharmas

When sexual cohabitation occurs during the harmonically auspicious time culled from the ancient science of Vedic astrology, health, wealth, virility, vitality and spiritual virtues abound in human life and its issuances. The opposite results hold true when sexual activities are performed during the poorly aspected times of year. Disregarding the timely and necessary conditions for sexual activity creates chaos, disease, unhappiness and poverty.

Auspicious Time and Conditions for Cohabitation

- Primarily during the early and late winter periods, with the following days being the most auspicious: 8th, 14th, 15th day of both the light and dark phases of the moon.
- During the spring, rainy season (early fall), and autumn, sexual intercourse should occur only on the three auspicious days cited above of both the light and dark phases of the moon.
- After a purifactory bath in a cool, clean, sheltered place.
- After prayers are observed and honorable intentions declared.
- Early evening is considered the best time for sexual interludes.

Posture During Sex

Certain positions are considered disharmonious during sexual activity. These postures create disequilibrium and often times disease. When a woman assumes the prone position during sex, the Vata dosha becomes aggravated. When she lies on her right side during sexual activity, the Kapha dosha becomes displaced and, in turn, obstructs the opening of the uterus. When she lies on her left side, the Pitta dosha becomes constrained, resulting in excess internal heat, which, in turn, incinerates the sperm and ovum.

The best posture is considered to be for the woman to lie comfortably on her back in a relaxed position. The prone posture is considered the best position for a man during sexual activity.

Progeny of Son or Daughter?

Harmonic timing and circumstances relating to sexual activity has nothing whatsoever to do with social conventions and religious dogma. True cognizance of nature's rhythms, which are steeped in harmony and allowance, is required to fully understand why timing and intentions are so vital to wholesome sexual activity. Far from the denial and suffocating strictures of neo-religious social dictates regarding sexuality, harmonic sexual relationship is an expression of the universe itself.

According to the Ayurvedas, to conceive a son sexual intercourse should be convened on the 4th, 6th, 8th, 10th or 12th day following the first day of the woman's menstrual cycle. For instance if the menstrual cycle began on the 5th of the month, the 4th day from the beginning of the cycle will fall on the 9th day of the month, the first auspicious day for cohabitation to produce a son. The 10th, 12th, 14th and 16th day of that particular month will be the remaining auspicious days pertaining to that particular menstrual cycle.

To conceive a daughter, sexual intercourse should occur on the 5th, 9th and 11th days following the first day of the woman's menstrual cycle. Note that the 7th day is considered inauspicious.

Inauspicious Time and Conditions for Cohabitation
- During dawn, dusk, midnight or daylight
- On the evening or day of the anniversary of a parent's death
- On the evening or day of the full moon
- On holy days
- During the astrological passages of a planet from one sign of the zodiac to another (consult your astrologer for details)
- During the summer season
- Without the observance of prayers or clarification of intentions
- Before taking a bath and in unclean circumstances
- Excessive sexual activity (over-indulgence may lead to physical pain and diseases, i.e., asthma, fever, jaundice, convulsions and venereal diseases)
- Sexual intercourse on the 1st, 2nd and 3rd days of a woman's menstrual cycle; conception during this time poses a serious threat to the child's life

423

AFTERWORD

Daily Deity Rules

$\mathcal{T}$he sun, moon, planets, stars and asterisms all serve to guide human activity to its harmonic end. Each day is ruled by an auspicious deity and yields natural support for activities of a certain nature. Sunday, ruled by the Sun, *Surya*, is a good day for celebrations and community efforts. The sadhanas of grinding the grain and seeds were done on this day in the past. This is also an excellent day to prepare the formulas for home treatments. It is a day to offer prayer and gratitude to Mother Earth, a day for women to celebrate their womanhood. It is also a good day for traveling, feeding friends and family, and for resolving disputes. Activities such as selling products and other income-related activities, quarreling, entering a new home, and undertaking heavy work, are all contra-indicated on this auspicious day.

Monday, ruled by *Shiva*, the cosmic teacher of wisdom and the destroyer of evil in the universe, is an excellent day to begin work-related activities, a new career, agricultural planting and gardening work, legal suits, and to initiate all financially related matters. Considered the most invigorating of days, Monday is also a very good day to enter a new home, make marital arrangements, practice sports, bet on the races and so on. It is a day when all negative influences can be easily dispelled; therefore, medical help is best sought on this day. If ill, Monday

425

is the day recommended for taking a healing bath. This is also a good day to begin home application therapies. Very few activities are contra-indicated on a Monday except arguments.

Tuesday is ruled by Mars, *Mangala*, who grants the easy attainment of success on that day. Considered a good day for putting one's courage and strength to the test and to defeat enemies, it is a also a good time for bonding with friends and good people. Tuesday is an auspicious day for activities relating to cows and bulls. It is also a good time for traveling, especially in connection with work-related matters and proposals of marriage. Tuesday is also a good day to listen to music and to provide community relief work. Activities contra-indicated on Tuesday are sexual coitus, activities involving the use of weaponry or fire, rituals to bring the rain and the deliberation of legal disputes. This day may create a natural surge of worries and loneliness.

Ruled by Mercury, *Buddhi*, Wednesday is a good day for both the successful expression of artistic work, and the acquisition of wealth. It is an excellent day for rulers and politicians and a good day to begin a romance. Sexual intercourse on this day should be directed only to the conception of a child; otherwise, a loss of love may result. It is an excellent day to wage war against evil deeds and doers. The contra-indications for this day are the beginning of new undertakings, sexual coitus (without pregnancy in mind), and quarreling in the work place. Special caution must be exercised on Wednesday concerning the exchange of words since the day is charged with a natural volatility.

Thursday, ruled by Jupiter, *Guru*, is an excellent day for financial undertakings, efforts to recover wealth or lost articles, and the acquisition of food grains. It is also an auspicious time for delivering speeches, pursuing an important position, and to defend oneself against attack. Activities relating to functions and festivals are well aspected for this day.

Guru also means teacher and signifies the universal regard for the carriers of knowledge. Thursday, then, is the day to offer gratitude and compensation to your teachers, even if the offering is a simple word of thanks. There is, presently, a scarcity of regard for and gratitude to those who carry the knowledge we so desperately need in our lives. Becoming too familiar with those who are sent to help you may result in a lost opportunity for learning. A good teacher is the most valuable gift the universe has to give. It is enough to show a simple reverence towards those who are learned and living among you, while maintaining a quiet dignity and a respectful distance.

Traveling is strongly contra-indicated for Thursdays. Caution is also advised in the commencement of a new undertaking on this day. Also, the emotions of grief and loss of courage may impinge on this day.

Friday is ruled by Venus, *Shukra*, and brings great success, especially for women. Pleasant occurrences such as easy friendships and effortless gains frequent this day. Prayers may be offered at this time for the rains to come. It is a good day to begin educational ventures, or to purchase vehicles. Charitable work and auspicious deeds also flourish on a Friday. It is also a good day to invite a teacher to your home. Friday, brightly lit with happiness, is a good time to pray for healing energies. Serious illness may also be treated on this day. A good day for advancement in the armed forces, Friday also lends itself well to travel.

Saturday, ruled by Saturn, *Shani*, is the day to resolve legal matters unless they involve family members. It is also a day that supports financial gains and career advancement, as well as being an influential time to combat negative forces. Saturday is a good day to gather or purchase your food staples, especially those to be used for your home treatment. It is also a good day for recruiting the help of your community against the sale of poisonous food and medicines, although caution will be necessary if children are involved. Saturday is an excellent day for traveling and for the acquisition of wealth and food grains. An excellent day for sexual activities and the acquiring of horses, Saturday is definitely the time for expressing courage, goodwill and increased effort. This day is also well aspected for digging into the earth for wells and to create pits for sveda therapies. The contra-indications are for new undertakings. Alertness is needed concerning old enemies and caution must be exerted not to acquire new ones. The mood of Saturday is generally worrisome, especially in family-related matters. Anger may also prevail on this day, although if awareness is maintained, the positive signs of comfort and courage can override any negative emotions.

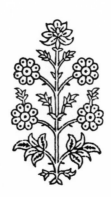

Om: Sound of the Lord

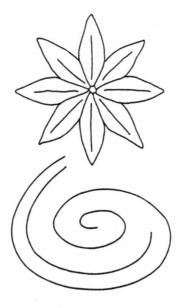

Please join me in the closing of this book with the chanting of the universal sound, *Om*, boundless source of silence, issuing forth all sounds, unfolding the Supreme Being's primal energy, and holding the cumulative total of all divinity. Om, the manifestation of the creative impulse of the cosmos, the resonance of totality comprising the infinite first syllable "ah" compelling creation; the substantial syllable "ou" bringing forth preservation; the final syllable "mm" resolving the creation into infinite dissolution, followed by the ultimate silence out of which all sound comes, is sustained, and falls back into.

To begin and end every endeavor with Om is to acknowledge the unseen Source, the divine Hand in everything we do.

Om Shanti Shanti Shanti

SECTION VI

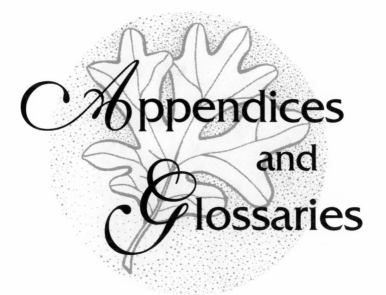

Appendices
and
Glossaries

AYURVEDIC PHARMACOLOGY

Energetics of Ayurvedic Substances

THE MAGICO-SPIRITUAL NATURE OF PLANTS

Deeply rooted in the earth's energy, plants carry the memory of all time. The knowledge of the medicinal properties of plants in Ayurveda has been culled from the wisdom handed down from the ancient sages. Infinite numbers of plants and herbs have been energetically evaluated by the ancient seers, who defined their medicinal value and rendered them into dried herbs, powders, tinctures, oils and so on.

As mentioned earlier, the cosmic memory of all plants is carried by the elephants, the most supreme elephant considered to be Gaja. While the elephants remain an alive species, they continue to bless us by "preserving" that function of our memory which retains plant knowledge. This so called preservation occurs on an energetic level whereby the pervasive vibrations of the elephants' innate wisdom of plant life and medicines are subtly transmitted into the memory functions of all other species. This transmission happens in the same way the moon may reflect on the surface of a lake, the moon symbolizing the elephant's memory and the lake representing the human memory receptor. If the moon were removed, there could be no reflection of it in the lake. Likewise, if the elephants were eradicated from the earth, humans could no longer sustain the knowledge of plant medicine in their memory bank.

Each member of every species bears certain distinct psychic features and plants are no exception. Hindu mythology is replete with the sacred and magical origins of plants and animals. To give a few examples, the lotus plant, considered the cradle of the universe, unfolding from formlessness into resplendent glory, is used plentifully in Ayurvedic medicine. The lotus plant is said to be endowed with cosmic memory of the universe's beginnings in the primordial waters. Its flower is said to have sprung from the navel of Lord Vishnu himself. To imbibe lotus medicine is to have every cell and tissue of the body revel in the luminous nature of the lotus itself.

Ashwagandha, the plant named after the power and smell of the horse, is said to impart its intrinsic nature of vitality and prowess to the human body when taken.

Known for its virility, ashwagandha is thought to arouse the memory of potency in every cell of the body.

Similarly, the pomegranate plant and its fruit carry the cosmic memory of prosperity and fertility. Traditionally this fruit is used to purge envy, jealousy and other negative vibrations from the body, allowing it to prosper and bask in the abundant light of the self.

The sesame seed is said to have appeared first when a sweat droplet from Lord Vishnu's body fell to the earth and sprouted into the sesame plant. Soon, the plant put forth beautiful white trumpet shaped blossoms. When eaten, sesame seeds are said to invoke the memory of rejuvenation, giving "sneha," lavish love, to the cells and tissues.

Ginger carries the force of the earth's fire deeply into the tissues of the body. Along with this heated memory, ginger, also called the universal medicine, is thought to awaken the body's memory of the universe's original fire when all manifestation transformed into life. Similarly, the black pepper, named after the sun, imparts solar vibration throughout the organism, allowing the body to resonate with light and heat.

In this way, plants are said to contain much more than their stationary appearance would suggest; they impart the significant memories which sustain all life. The energy and nature of a number of plants used in the pancha karma treatments are discussed in detail below.

Description of a Few Plants Used in Vamana Therapy

Apamarga

Known as the prickly chaff plant in English, apamarga is used extensively in pancha karma, the leaves, flowers, seeds and root being used in emesis therapy. Pungent and bitter in taste with a heating potency, apamarga is used to alleviate hemorrhoids, hiccoughs, and abdominal disorders, as well.

Arka

Also known as sadapushpi and akda in India, where it grows profusely, and belonging to the caltrops family, this plant is used extensively in pancha karma. Its roots, leaves and flowers are used in emesis therapy. The "milk" of the plant is known for its sharp potency, and a few drops are sometimes used in purgative decoction as an alkalizer. The flowering buds sprout off the base of the leaves and bloom into umbrella-shaped flowers. The fruits are white and red in color with an inner cottony texture. Arka is pungent and bitter and has a heating potency. It is used both as an emetic and purgative and to ward off tumors, ulcers, skin diseases and abdominal disorders.

Ela

Known as cardamom in English, these green or black pods and seeds are famous in both the Vedic kitchen as well as in the Ayurvedic pharmacy. Cardamom is aromatic, sweet, pungent, and heating in nature. It is used extensively in the pancha karma's nasya, svedana and the vamana therapies, and also as a digestant, heart tonic, and to alleviate urinary disorders.

Karanja

Known as Indian beech in English, this plant is used extensively in pancha karma. Karanja is pungent and bitter in taste with a heating potency. The leaves, bark, seeds and root are included in emetic medicine and are also used to ward off nervous tension, phlegmatic disorders, parasites from the body, skin diseases, ulcers and hemorrhoids.

Madana

The fruit of the madana tree, originally found growing in the Himalayas, is well known for its extensive use in vamana therapy and has been discussed in great detail by the great Ayurvedic trio, Charaka, Sushruta and Vagbhatta. This tree has as many names as there are languages in India. In English, it is known as the emetic nut or bushy gardenia. Approximately fifteen feet in height, this very thorny tree has large white and yellow leaves and flowers. Its fruits, madana phala, are kidney-shaped and, in taste, are sweet, bitter and astringent. They are collected in the spring and summer seasons while not yet ripe, wrapped in kush grass and then buried under cow dung, barley grain, mung or urad legumes for eight days until the fruit is soft and ripe. They are then placed in the sun to dry.

In one of Charaka's formulas, madana pippali, one seed of the fruit is removed and ground with honey and sesame butter. This paste is then dried and used as an emetic in vamana therapy. Madana, because of its sweet and bitter taste, is also used for alleviating skin disorders, abdominal distension, swellings, tumors, ulcers and to facilitate the expulsion of flatus from the body.

Madhuka

Also known as *yastimadhu* in Sanskrit and licorice in English, this creeper is used in a number of Ayurvedic remedies. Both its root and bark are used as a supplementary ingredient in emesis therapy and as a main herb in purgation therapy. Sweet in taste with a cold potency, licorice is also used to alleviate thirst, toxicity, fatigue, nervous tension and blood disorders.

Musta (*nagar musta*)

The musta weed, known as nut grass or coco grass in English, has a wiry rhizome-root system from which thin tubers sprout. In many countries, this healing plant is mistaken for a useless weed and eradicated.

Bitter, pungent and astringent in taste with a cold potency, musta is used in Ayurveda to alleviate fevers, restore circulation and menstrual regularity, and stimulate digestion. It is also used as a diuretic and to alleviate skin diseases, burning sensations, and internal bleeding. Musta serves as a supplement to emetic medicines as well.

Nimba

Also known as neem, the leaves of this big tree are renowned for their bitterness. Nimba is both bitter and pungent in taste with a cold potency. Both leaves and roots are used extensively in Ayurveda. The leaves are used in emesis therapy and to rectify blood disorders, skin diseases and agni disorders.

In India the twigs of the nimba tree are still used as disposable toothbrushes. Due to its natural antiseptic quality, neem is an excellent medicine for the prevention of tooth decay and gum disorders. Neem powder is also used as a natural pesticide. The neem plant has recently been imported into Florida from India for cultivation.

Pippali

Commonly called long pepper, and native to India and Java, the unripe peppers are gathered and stored to ripen before use. Pippali is a primary ingredient in Ayurvedic medicine to alleviate Kapha disorders. It is pungent, volatile and fiery in taste with a heating potency. Used as a digestant and a carminative in Vedic cooking, pippali is also extensively used in Ayurveda to relieve disorders of the spleen, asthma, diabetes and bronchitis. It is also a natural emetic.

Sveta bimba

Known as the ivy gourd in English, the fruits, leaves, bark and root of this plant are used in pancha karma. Commonly referred to as bimbi in India, the ivy gourd comes in two varieties: one is bitter and the other sweet. Both plants have a cooling potency. The fruit of the sweet variety is used for blood disorders, swellings, anemia, fevers, and in emesis therapy. The fruit of the bitter variety is used to relieve Kapha disorders such as cold, cough, mucus, and lethargy.

Vacha

Also known as sweet flag, myrtle flag or calamus, this branched rhizome is a perennial renowned for its medicinal uses in Ayurveda. The roots are reddish, hairy and usually clustered together. Aromatic in nature, vacha root is bitter and pungent

436

in taste with a heating potency. The Sanskrit word "vacha" means "speech." True to its name, vacha is used as a brain tonic and to improve the capacity of speech. Used extensively in both emesis and purgation therapy, vacha is also effectively used to remove digestive and mental disorders, heart diseases, constipation, uterine disorders and infections.

Vidanga

Also known as embelia and viranga, this creeper bears white flowers and black berries. The berries, used extensively in Ayurveda, are pungent and heating. Vidanga is used to reduce obesity and phlegmatic disorders, to stimulate digestion, to build immunity and destroy internal parasites such as fungus, yeast, bacteria and worms, and, combined with pippali, as an oral contraceptive.

Description of a Few Plants Used in Virechana Therapy

Badri

Known as the jujube tree in English, badri is a small evergreen tree with thin scraggly branches and sharp thorns, bearing clusters of tiny star-shaped yellow flowers and red oval leaves. A grove of these trees, high up in the Himalayas, was chosen in ancient times as a sacred site for the saint Narayana, the incarnation of Lord Vishnu; today Badrinath, a Hindu pilgrimage site, still stands sequestered in the glory of this same badri grove.

The berries of this tree are used to make sherbet or jams, and the berry juice is used in purgation therapy.

Castor (*eranda*)

Of African origin, the eranda or castor plant as it is called in English, is now cultivated in India and in many tropical countries. This sharply purgative plant grows both as an annual herb and a perennial tree and is used to alleviate many diseases. The castor plant is sweet, pungent and heating in nature. The seeds and oil are used primarily in Ayurvedic medicine for purgative therapy; to relieve nervous disorders, pain and heart diseases; and to destroy internal parasites. The roots of the castor plant are used to cure inflammatory conditions, fever, asthma, and anal disorders. The leaves are used in Kapha conditions such as asthma, cough, cold, and phlegmatic disorders. The flowers are used to cure glandular tumors, and the fruits are used to rekindle digestive fire and to restore the appetite.

Lotus (*kamala*)

The Sanskrit word kamala means desirous, excellent and rosy. In Hindu mythology, the lotus, to use the English name, is considered to be the cradle of the universe. It symbolizes the universe unfolding from formlessness into full glory. When the universe is in its dissolved state, Lord Vishnu floats on the water with a lotus flower blooming from his navel. Brahma, the Creator, emerges from the lotus and creates the world. The consort of Vishnu, the goddess Lakshmi, appears standing on a pink lotus, lotus-eyed and wearing lotus garlands. Often portrayed in ancient Vedic mythology as the sun and the lotus, Lord Vishnu and the goddess Lakshmi are symbols of the eternal love that interlaces the entire universe.

Native to the ponds and lakes of Kashmir, China and Japan, the lotus plant decorates the ponds surrounding the temples in India with its exquisite blue, white, pink and red flowers.

The lotus flower is considered to be the most magnificent flower on earth. Deeply rooted in mud, the lotus flower is framed by large waxy leaves, often used in India as disposable plates for food served during religious ceremonies.

The roots, flowers, leaves, stamens and seeds are all used extensively in Ayurvedic medicine, including its pancha karma therapies. The lotus is sweet, astringent and cooling in nature and is used as a nutritive tonic, an aphrodisiac and to calm nervous disorders. The seeds are used as a tonic for the heart.

Palasha

Commonly called "Flame of the Forest", the palasha tree is regarded as sacred in India. Its bright red and orange parrot-shaped flowers are used to make the dye powders that devotees of Lord Vishnu and Lord Shiva rub on their foreheads. The Latin name for this tree, butea monosperma, is after the Earl of Bute, a patron of botany, and the Sanskrit word, *palasha*, means both beauty and leaf.

The palasha tree has been the topic of many exotic and esoteric stories. Legend has it that the tree came to life on earth when a falcon's feather dipped in Soma, the nectar of the gods made from the qualities of the moon, fell to earth and became the seed for the palasha tree.

The wood, fruit, leaves, flowers, seeds and bark are all used in pancha karma therapies, the wood, bark and leaves for the earth sveda therapies, and the fruit, leaves and seeds for purgation.

The palasha tree provides the raw material for the red, astringent gum used in tanning leathers. The lacquer produced from the lac insects which inhabit the tree is used in dyes and as a sealing wax. Its leaves are still used in India to make disposable plates and as fodder for cattle, while its roots are used to make rope.

Pomegranate (*dadima*)

The English word commonly used for dadima, pomegranate, is derived from the French word *pomme garnete*, meaning seeded apple. In the Vedas, the pomegranate is a symbol of fertility and prosperity. Due to its astringent, sweet and cooling nature, the Prophet Mohammad is said to have advised his disciples to purge their envy by eating this fruit. Legends reveal that the pomegranate has always been used to ward off evil spirits.

Reddish orange flowers with crumpled petals bloom at the end of the stiff, slender branches of the pomegranate tree. Grown in both evergreen and deciduous varieties, the pomegranate is a short bushy tree. The size of large macintosh apples, the fruit has a hard skin that splits open or "laughs," once ripened, to reveal a cluster of carmine red fleshy seeds, the edible part of the fruit.

Medicinally, every part of the pomegranate tree is used in Ayurveda. Its fruit is used as a blood cleanser and tonic, while the root bark is used to dispel internal parasites. Pomegranate juice is used for purgation therapy and to promote digestion, while the fruit rind is used as a mucus membrane anti-inflammatory.

Sesame (*tila*)

The Sanskrit word "tila" means a small particle, while the word "sesame" comes from the Arabic "sesam," meaning herbs. The sesame plant is believed to have been first cultivated in the Indus Valley; and, during Vedic times, sesame was the only seed oil used. In Hindu mythology, the sesame seed is said to have germinated from a drop of Lord Vishnu's sweat as it fell to the earth.

A tall, erect annual, the sesame plant bears lovely white trumpet-shaped flowers. The fruit is a two-celled pod bearing flat pear-shaped seeds, white, buff or black in color. When the fruits are ripe, the pods burst open and the seeds are scattered. Renowned for its use in Ayurvedic medicine, the seeds and oil are used extensively in virechana, vamana and vasti therapies. The sesame seed is used as a base for many herbs and substances to treat a variety of Vata ailments. Although best for Vata types, it may be used medicinally by all types. Heralded as one of the first foods of the universe, sesame is sattvic in nature and induces a peaceful state of mind.

Trikatu (*ginger, black pepper, and long pepper*)

Like triphala, trikatu is an ancient Ayurvedic formula consisting of equal portions of three pungent spices: ginger, black pepper and long pepper. Unlike triphala, trikatu is highly heat producing.

This ancient trilogy, known as the three pungent spices, is one hundred times more potent in its combined form than any one of its three ingredients. Used in both virechana and vamana therapies, trikatu is also the main formula used to restore digestive disorders and to eradicate the presence of ama from the body. Trikatu is an expectorant, decongestant, and a stimulant; as such, it is also used to alleviate conditions of coldness, mucus and stagnation in the body.

Each of the three spices is stimulating and heat producing. Together, they form a potent synergy for restoring many Vata and Kapha ailments.

Ginger *(ardraka)*: Ginger, known in its dry form as *sunthi* and in its fresh form as ardraka in Sanskrit, carries the forces of the earth's fire. In the Vedas it is called "vishvabhesaja," the universal medicine. Although heating, pungent and sweet in nature, ginger is considered a sattvic or peace-producing food.

Native to Southeast Asia, ginger is a perennial creeper with a thick tuberous rhizome producing an erect annual stem. At the end of the stem, greenish purple flowers bloom. The root is a powerful cardiac tonic as well as a digestive stimulant. Used with lime juice and honey, it provides excellent relief for anorexia; used with lime juice and rock salt, it promotes digestion. Ginger is also used for colds, flus, indigestion, nausea, laryngitis, arthritis, constipation, hemorrhoids, and headaches, as well as in purgation therapy. Although it is best for Vata and Kapha disorders, it may be used medicinally by all types.

Black pepper *(maricha)*: Named after the sun in Sanskrit, maricha contains potent solar energy. A powerful digestive stimulant, it burns up ama and rekindles agni. Like the sun, black pepper is rajasic or energy-producing in nature.

A perennial climbing shrub, the black pepper plant bears small white flowers and tiny yellow berries that turn red as they mature. Native to South India, they thrive in the humid shade. Their vines are often found climbing the trunks of the coconut tree.

Black pepper is used to alleviate chronic indigestion, obesity, congestion, coldness in the body, bronchitis, sinusitis, intestinal parasites and toxins in the colon. Although it is best for Vata and Kapha disorders, it may be used medicinally by all types.

Long pepper *(pippali)*: The third component of the trikatu formula, pippali activates the subtle fire (tejas) inherent in black pepper and ginger.

Native to India and Java, these peppers are gathered while green and allowed to dry to preserve maximum heat potency. When dried, the peppers are gray in color with a mild aroma and fiery taste. Pippali is used as a carminative, a stimulant and a digestant, as well as an emetic for Vata and Kapha disorders.

Triphala *(amalaki, bibhitaki, and haritaki)*

Triphala, used extensively in Ayurveda, is the combination of three ancient medicinal fruits belonging to the myrobalam family: amalaki, haritaki, and bibhitaki. These three fruits are reduced to a powder, called triphala, or prepared as a rejuvenating jam. Triphala is among the most ancient and common of the Ayurvedic remedies.

Together the synergy of these three potent myrobalam fruits provides a harmonic remedy of infinite prowess for a thousand human disorders. Among other things, triphala strengthens the stomach and intestinal tract, restores the immune system, safeguards the tissues and organs, strengthens the brain, heart, nerves and liver, improves appetite, reduces internal heat and quenches thirst, neutralizes ama, alleviates urinary disorders such as diabetes, and is a superb rejuvenative tonic. Triphala is used in virechana therapy to produce mild purgation and is excellent for all types.

Amalaki: Native to India, the fruit of the amalaki tree consists of five segments, representing the five elements in Hindu mythology. The amalaki tree is said to be the first tree of the universe. Its fruits are large and pulpy and become black when dried. Although the entire tree is used, in Ayurvedic medicine the fruit is considered to be the most important part of the plant.

Amalaki is sweet, sour, pungent, bitter and astringent, yet cooling in nature. Independently, it is used as a nutritive tonic, blood cleanser and for restoring normalcy to the tissues. Although amalaki is dominantly sour, it is good for all types.

Bibhitaki: The third sister in the myrobalam family of trees, bibhitaki grows primarily in arid regions. A big, prolific tree, its fruits are large, round and pulpy with astringent and sweet tastes. Bibhitaki has a heating potency and is used for eye diseases, hair loss, bronchial asthma, constipation, skin diseases and as an anti-inflammatory and expectorant. Bibhitaki may be used by all types.

Haritaki: Mentioned repeatedly in Ayurvedic texts, haritaki fruits are borne on a large tree with thick leaves and yellow flowers. They are pear-shaped and brownish black in color. Considered a sister to the amalaki tree, haritaki grows in both cold and hot climates. The variety grown in temperate climates is used more extensively in Ayurveda. This fruit is esteemed by Vedic and Buddhist seers alike, the Buddha often portrayed holding the haritaki fruit in his right hand.

When used independently, haritaki promotes longevity, heals disorders of the heart, opens bodily channels, and increases prana. It is also used to alleviate grief, depression, cancer conditions, eye disorders, skin diseases, rheumatism and diabetes. Like amalaki, haritaki is heating in potency and contains five of the six tastes; only the salty taste is absent. Good for all types, it may be taken in the summer and autumn with a small amount of brown sugar, in the early fall with a small amount of rock salt, in early winter with a small amount of ginger powder, in late winter with a few pinches of pippali powder, and in the spring with a small amount of honey.

Trivrit

The root of the trivrit plant is known best for its extensive use in Ayurvedic purgative therapy. Like the madana fruit used in emesis therapy, trivrit has also been mentioned by Charaka and Sushruta, as well as Vagbhatta.

There are two types of trivrit plant, a black variety and a red variety. In Ayurvedic medicine the root of the red trivrit plant is preferred.

441

Trivrit is sweet, astringent and dry in nature and is used in purgation therapy to alleviate Pitta and Kapha conditions such as skin diseases, fever, mental disorders, gynecological disorders, stomatitis, anorexia and bronchial asthma.

Description of a Few Herbs Used in Vasti Therapy

Aloe (*kumari*)

Cool, calm and beautiful are the meanings of the Sanskrit word, kumari. Also known as aloe vera, this plant is native to the dry, sunny terrains of Southeastern and Northern Africa, Spain, Indonesia, India, the Caribbean and, more recently, Australia and the Southwestern United States. The aloe has been used medicinally for millennia by the Indians, Chinese, Greek, and Egyptians.

Bitter, sweet and astringent in taste, aloe vera is used to restore normal health by altering existing nutritive and excretory processes. Considered an excellent blood cleanser, this plant is also used as a mild laxative, as a liver and spleen tonic, to regulate the intestines' peristaltic movements, to promote digestion and to relieve abdominal distension by promoting downward movement of wind. Aloe vera alleviates all three doshas and is also effectively used in reducing Pitta disorders such as fevers, skin diseases, burns, ulcers and oedema. Aloe vera works especially on the pituitary glands, thyroid and ovaries.

As an overall rejuvenative, aloe vera calms the tissues and body and softens and smoothes the complexion. Used in both douching and enema formulas, aloe vera is soothing to the intestinal and vaginal passages. It removes parasites from the colon and, along with other ingredients in enema therapy, acts as a cure for intestinal tuberculosis, convulsions and epilepsy. Externally, aloe vera may be used to heal wounds and burns and as a conditioner for hair and scalp.

Ajwan

A strong digestive, respiratory and nerve stimulant, ajwan, commonly known as wild celery seed, is used mainly for high Vata conditions such as intestinal gas, intestinal spasms, and nervous disorders. Ajwan is also excellent for Kapha disorders such as colds, flus, asthma, bronchitis, laryngitis, oedema, sinus congestion and kidney malfunction. It clears out deep-seated ama and revitalizes metabolic functioning. Also used as one of many ingredients in vasti therapy, ajwan is pungent in taste and heating in energy.

Asafoetida (*hingu*)

The resin of the fleshy root of the perennial hingu or as it is commonly called, asafoetida plant, is collected from the mature plant, which is over five years old. Sometimes called "devil's dung," due to its highly pungent and pervasive sulphurous smell, asafoetida is one of the most potent digestive stimulants in Ayurveda and is generally used in very small quantity. It is used for Vata and Kapha disorders such as constipation, indigestion, flatulence, abdominal distension, intestinal pain, arthritis, whooping cough, convulsions, epilepsy, intestinal parasites, hysteria and palpitations.

Contra-indicated for Pitta conditions, asafoetida is also used in vasti therapy. While strengthening the intestinal flora, asafoetida helps to break down constricted fecal matter, accumulated from extensive eating of animal or unwholesome foods, and to destroy worms in the large intestine. Asafoetida is highly heating in energy.

Ashwagandha

Ashwagandha is the Sanskrit word for the smell or vitality of a horse—in short, that which gives the body its "horse power." Known as winter cherry in English, the root of the ashwagandha plant is used to alleviate Vata conditions such as sexual debility, nervous exhaustion, emaciation, problems relating to old age, loss of memory, spermatorrhea, tissue deficiency, insomnia, paralysis and infertility. Kapha disorders such as difficulty in breathing, coughing and anemia also respond to ashwagandha. When Pitta is not high in the body, skin diseases and glandular swellings are also treated with ashwagandha.

Similar to ginseng in nature, ashwagandha is an excellent herb for increasing semen and fertility. Also used in vasti therapy, which is administered through the vagina or penis, ashwagandha serves to alleviate urinary tract or bladder conditions as well as infertility or insufficiency of semen or sperm.

Ashwagandha is an excellent stabilizer for the fetus during pregnancy. It also regenerates the hormonal system, while promoting tissue healing. Although sweet, astringent and bitter in taste, ashwagandha is heating in energy.

Bala

Commonly known as the country mallow, bala, as it is called in Sanskrit, is that which gives strength and vitality. An excellent tonic for all three doshas, bala is sweet and cooling in nature. It works on all the dhatus, especially the marrow and nerves. Three main varieties of the mallow family are used in Ayurveda: bala, atibala and mahabala. Bala is a revitalizing tonic and is especially effective in curing Vata disorders. Healing to the heart, bala feeds the nerves, has a calming influence on the muscular system, and relieves inflammation of the nerve tissue.

Externally, oil made with bala is used to mollify nerve pain, numbness, and muscular cramps. Bala is also used as one of the mild ingredients in vasti therapy to tone the colon, while strengthening intestinal flora and regulating proper peristaltic action.

The Use of Ghee in Abhyanga and Snehana Therapies

Promotive of health, memory, intelligence, vital fire, vital essence and nourishment, ghee is a curative for Vata and Pitta disorders.

— *Charaka*

Ghee, which is clarified butter made from pure cow's milk, increases the bodily essence of rasa and helps to soothe the senses and vital tissues. Ghee cools the mind, memory and digestion, and induces self-cognition, intelligence, and clarity of complexion and voice. A most important substance in Ayurvedic healing, ghee is used as a vehicle to transport herbs and medicinal substances deep into the vital tissues of the body. Ghee is also applied externally, its deeply penetrating action swelling the skin, invigorating internal tissues and promoting the idyllic emotion of calmness.

In snehana therapy, ghee is used alone or in medicated form by blending it with Ayurvedic herbs. Taken internally, ghee facilitates the cleansing of bodily tissues and the elimination of excess doshas. Medicated ghee is used for conditions such as peptic ulcers, blood disorders, skin diseases, insomnia, mental disorders, epilepsy, paraplegia, and tumors.

Renowned Ayurvedic Medicated Ghee Preparations for Snehana Therapy

In Ayurveda pure cow's ghee is called *accha peya*, or *ghrita* and medicated ghee is called vicarana sneha. (See Ghee Making, p. 493.)

For skin and blood disorders	tikta ghrita mahatikta ghrita
For mental disorders	brahmi ghrita mahakalyana ghrita
For muscular disorders	guggulu tikta ghrita

444

AYURVEDIC OILS
Glossary of Snehana and Massage Oils

Sanskrit	Latin	English
abhisuka	pistacia vera	pistachio
akshota	jugullans regia	walnut
arjuna	terminalia arjuna	arjuna
aruka	prunus domestica	bokhara plum
ashoka	saraca indica	ashoka
atsi	linum usitatissimum	linseed
bakuchi	psoralea corylifolia	babchi seeds
bhallataka	semecarpus anacardium	nut tree
bhringaraja	eclipta alba	bhringaraja
bhucanaka	arachis hypogaea	peanut
bibhitaki	terminalia belerica	beleric myrobalam
bilva	aegle marmelos	bael tree
brahmi	hydrocotyle asiatica	Indian pennyworth
char	buchanania lanzan	cuddaph almond
eranda	ricinus communis	castor
graha-druma	terminalia catappa	Indian almond
guduchi	tinospora cordifolia	guduchi
haritaki	terminalia chebula	chebulic myrobalam
kala sarshapa	brassica campestris	black mustard
karanja	pongamia pinnata	Indian beech
khadira	acacia catechu	catechu tree
kharjur	phoenix dactylifera	date palm
kumari	aloe barbadensis	Indian aloe (aloe vera)
kusumbha	carthamum tinctorius	safflower
masha	phaseolus mungo	mung bean
mulaka	raphanus sativus	radish (daikon)
narikela	cocos nucifera	coconut palm
nimba	azadirachta indica	neem
pippali	piper longum	long pepper
shak	tectona grandis	teak nut
sigruka	morniga oleifera	horseradish
supari	areca catechu	betel nut palm
suria-mukhi	helianthus annuus	sunflower
tila	sesamum indicum	sesame (gingelly)
vacha	acorus calamus	sweet flag (calamus)
vatama	prunus amygdalus	almond
yasti madhu (madhuka)	glycyrrhiza glabra	licorice

445

Glossary of Ayurvedic Essential Oils

Sanskrit	Latin	English
ahiphena	papaver somniferum	poppy plant
ajaji	nigella sativa	black cumin
apamarga	achyranthes aspera	prickly chaff flower
ardraka	zinziber officinalis	ginger
bakul	mimusops elengi	Indian medlar
bhustrina	cymbopogan citratus	lemon grass
bramha dandi	argemone mexicana	prickly poppy
champaka	michelia champaca	yellow champa
chandana	santalum album	sandalwood tree
dhanyaka	coriandrum sativum	coriander
ela	amomum subulatum	large cardamom
ela	elettaria cardamomum	cardamom
garjar	daucus carota	carrot
guggulu	commiphora mukul	Indian bedellium
haridra	curcuma longa	turmeric
jati	jasminum officinale	jasmine
jatiphala	myristica fragrans	nutmeg
jiraka	cuminum cyminum	cumin
kali maricha	piper nigrum	black pepper
kamala	nelumbo nucifera	lotus
karpura	cinnamomum camphora	camphor
karpura-haridra	curcuma amada	mango-ginger
katukumbi	lagenaria siceraria	bitter gourd
kesar	crocus sativus	saffron
ketki (keora)	pandanus tectorius	screw pine
krishnatil	guizotia abyssinica	nigeri
kusthapa	gynocardia odorata	chaulmugra
lasuna	allium sativum	garlic
lavanga	syzigium aromaticum	clove tree
madhuca	madhuca indica	mohwa
mahanimba	melia azedarach	lilac
maricha	capsicum annum	red chili-pepper
mathika	jasminum sambac	Arabian jasmine
medica	lawsonia inermis	henna
narangi	citrus reticulata	orange
nila pushpa	viola odorata	violet
nilika (nilini)	indiofera tinctoria	indigo
nilpuspi	ipomoea hederacea	morning glory
nimbuka	citrus aurantifolia	lime/lemon
nirgundi	vitex negundo	Indian privet

Glossary of Ayurvedic Essential Oils (continued)

Sanskrit	Latin	English
parijutika	nyctanthes arbortristis	coral jasmine
pippali	piper longum	long pepper
pudina	mentha longifolia	mint
rakta chandana	pterocarpus santalinus	red sandalwood
rohisa	cymbopogan martini	rusa oil
saptala	acacia concinna	cassia flower
sarpadanshta	peganum harmala	Syrian rue
sevanti	chrysenthemum indicum	chrysanthemum
shali	oryza sativa	rice
shatapushpa	pimpinella anisum	anise
shatpushpa	anethum sova	dill
shatpushpa	foeniculum vulgare	fennel
somalata	ruta graveolens	rue
somaraji	centratherum	wild cumin
sukasa	cucumis sativus	cucumber
surasa	ocimum basilacum	sweet basil
sushavi	carum carvi	caraway
taruni(shatapatri)	rosa damascena	rose
tulsi	ocimum sanctum	holy basil
twacha	cinnamomum zeylanicum	cinnamon
valuka(ushira)	vetiveria zizanioides	khus-khus grass (vetiver)
vanharidra	curcuma aromatica	wild turmeric
zupha	hyssopus officinalis	hyssop

AYURVEDIC WOODS, HERBS AND SUBSTANCES
Description of a Few Woods Used in Svedana Therapy

Sandalwood, champa, ashoka and bael wood are considered sacred and irreplaceable in this ancient art of health and are well worth importing to use in these therapies. A few varieties of the flame tree, found in the Western hemisphere, may be used instead of the widely used palasha tree.

The woods used in the sveda therapies are mostly native to India, although some comparable Western hemisphere woods may be substituted. These include the kindling from a variety of small pepper tree; the wood from fruit trees such as the fig, apple, pear, peach, plum and mango; and the wood from flowering trees such as the lilac and jasmine. White pine kindling may be used in the construction of snehana and svedana treatment tables, benches, and so on. You may find it worthwhile to visit the botanical gardens in your area and familiarize yourself with the comparable trees and bushes available in your natural terrain. The Latin and, when available, English names will prove helpful to you in your inquiry.

Glossary of Woods Used to Construct Treatment Tables

Several woods are used in Ayurveda for the construction of sweat lodges, benches, and treatment tables. These woods may also be used for kindling on the stone and earth surfaces and in the sveda furnaces to produce heat for the sauna-type therapies, namely: jentaka, kuti, karshu, ashmaghna and bhu svedas.

Sanskrit	Latin	English
agnimantha	clerodenronphlomidis	the arni tree
amra	mangifera indica	mango tree
asana	terminalia tomentosa	sain tree
ashoka	saraca indica	ashoka tree
bakula	mimusops elengi	Indian medlar tree
bilva	aegle marmelos	bael tree
champaka	michelia champaca	yellow champa tree
chandana	santalum album	sandalwood tree
devadaru	cedrus deodara	deodar tree
khadira	acacia catechu	catechu tree
mahanimba	melia azedarach	Persian lilac tree
palasha	butea monosperma	flame tree
pippali	piper longum	long pepper tree
purnarnava	boerhaavia diffusa	spreading hog weed
udumbara	ficus racemosa	country fig tree
varuna	crateva nurvala	garlic pear tree

Common Sweat-Producing Herbs

Sweat-producing herbs and substances used in svedana therapies are called svedapagana. Certain common herbs available in the Western hemisphere may also be used in the sveda therapies, i.e., mistletoe, rue, sage, rosemary, sassafras, savory, skunk cabbage, spikenard, stillingia, valerian, mugworth, oregano, basil, bayberry, burdock, camphor, catnip, eucalyptus, galangal, grindelia, ground ivy, sesame seeds, chia seeds, juniper berries, pennyroyal, wild ginger, angelica and ephedra.

The following herbs are most suitable for the mild svedana treatments used for Pitta disorders: lemon balm, motherworth, birch, borage, chamomile, coriander, echinacea, elderflowers, horsetail, kudzu, lemon grass, peppermint, spearmint, stoneroot, yarrow and chrysanthemum.

Glossary of Ayurvedic Herbs Used with Kindling

The following herbs are generally burned with the kindling in preparation for the ashmaghna, bhu, karshu, kupa and holaka svedas.

Sanskrit	Latin	English
arka	calatropis procera	arka plant
eranda	ricinus communis	castor oil plant
japa	hibiscus rosasinensis	hibiscus or shoe flower plant
purnarnava	boerhaavia diffusa	spreading hog weed (white variety)
shobhanjana (shigru)	morninga oleifera	horseradish or drumstick tree
utkataka	echinops echinatus	camel's thistle plant

Oils used to burn kindling

ashvakarna
khadira

Glossary of Herbs and Substances for Svedana Poultices

Sanskrit	Latin	English
atasi	linum usitatissimum	linseed seed
badri	zizyphus jujuba	jujube leaves, root & fruit
chanaka	cicer arietinum	chick pea
eranda	ricinus communis	fruit of the castor plant
kala sarshapa	brassica campestris	black mustard seed
karanja	pongamia pinnata	Indian beech
kulitha	dolichos biflorus	the horse gram
maricha	piper nigrum	black pepper corns
masha	phaseolus radiatus	urad or black gram
methica	trigonella foenumgraecum	fenugreek seed
mugda	phaseolus mungo	mung or green gram
pippali	piper longum	long pepper
rasna	vanda roxburghii	rasna root
suradaru	cedrus deodara	deodara leaves (turpentine tree)
tila	sesamum indicum	sesame seed
yava	hordeum vulgare	barley grain

Note: For Vata disorders, these herbs may be used with molasses, ghee and vinegar or tamarind paste added to the legumes.

449

AYURVEDIC HERBS AND SUBSTANCES FOR THE HEALING DIET
Glossary of Herbs and Substances Used in The Healing Diet

Sanskrit	Latin	English
adhaki (turvi)	cajanus cajan	pigeon pea
ajaji	nigella sativa	black cumin seeds
ajwan	apium graveolens	celery seeds
amra	mangifera indica	mango fruit
anjira	ficus carica	figs
ardraka	zinziber officinalis	ginger root
atibala	abutilon indicum	country mallow root
bala	sida cordifolia	country mallow root
barahikand	dioscorea bulbifera	yam
bhinditaka	hibiscus esculentus	okra
bhringaraja	eclipta alba	bhringaraja (leaves, root, seeds)
chincha (imli)	tamarindus indica	tamarind fruit
chitraka	plumbago zeylanica	chitraka root
dadima	punica granatum	pomegranate fruit
dhanyaka	coriandrum sativum	coriander (leaves, seeds, cilantro)
draksha	vitis vinifera	grapevine (fruit, juice, raisin)
ela	elettaria cardamomum	cardamom (seeds, pods)
gargar	daucus carota	carrot
gaurani	cyamopsis/tetragonoloba	cluster bean (string bean)
goghuma	triticum aestivum	wheat
gotu kola (brahmi)	hydrocotyle asiatica	gotu kola root
gur	saccharum officinarum	brown palm sugar
haridra	curcuma longa	turmeric root
hinguka	ferula narthex	asafoetida (resin)
ikshu (jaggery)	saccharum officinarum	brown cane sugar
jatiphala	myristica fragrans	nutmeg
jiraka	cuminum cyminum	cumin seeds
kaladi	musa paradisiaca	plantain
kamala	nelumbo nucifera	lotus (root, seeds)
kapitha	feronia limonia	wood apple tree (fruit)

Glossary of Herbs and Substances Used in The Healing Diet
(continued)

Sanskrit	Latin	English
katukumbi	lagenaria siceraria	bitter gourd
kesar	crocus sativus	saffron
kharjur	phoenix dactylifera	dates, date sugar
kulitha	dolichos biflorus	horse gram
lashuna	allium sativum	garlic root
lavanga	syzigium	cloves bud
mahayavanala	zea mays	corn
maricha	piper nigrum	black pepper
masha	phaseolus radiatus	urad (black gram)
mudga	phaseolus mungo	mung (green gram)
narangi	citrus reticulata	orange
narikela	cocos nucifera	coconut, oil
nimba	azadirachta indica	neem leaves
nimbuka	citrus aurantifolia	lime, lemon
parusha	grewia asiatica	parusha fruit
pippali	piper longum	long pepper
pudina	mentha longifolia	mint
rajika	eleusine corocana	millet grain
raktapurka	garcinia indica	kokum butter tree (kokum fruit)
shali	oryza sativa	rice (red & brown variety)
shatavari	asparagus racemosa	asparagus (leaves, root)
sukasa	cucumis sativus	cucumber
sushavi	carum carvi	caraway seeds
tila	sesamum indicum	sesame (seeds, oil)
Triphala:		
amalaki	emblica officinalis	emblic myrobalam (dried fruit)
bibhitaki	terminalia belerica	beleric myrobalam (dried fruit)
haritaki	terminalia chebula	chebulic myrobalam (dried fruit)
tulsi	ocimum sanctum	sweet basil
twacha	cinnamomum zeylanicum	cinnamon bark
yava	hordeum vulgare	barley grain

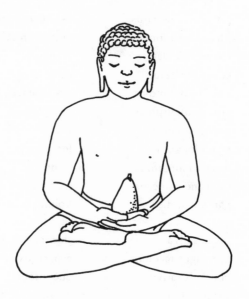

The Buddha Holding a Heritaki Fruit

APPENDIX B

GLOSSARY OF INGREDIENTS

UNCOMMON INGREDIENTS

Aduki- Also known as adzuki or feijao, this small dark red bean is native to Japan and China. Rich in nutrients, it is considered, like mung, to be a tridoshic bean.

Agar agar- A buff-colored, translucent seaweed available in 12-inch bars or in flakes. Indigenous to India, agar-agar has been used since Vedic times as a food thickener and to make gels. Use warm water or other liquid to dissolve. Available in most health food stores and in Indian and Oriental grocery stores. May be used by all types.

Ajwan (ajwain)- Also known as bishopweed, this tiny spice seed is related to caraway and cumin. Its delicate flavor resembles the combined tastes of lemon, pepper and thyme. Available in Indian and Oriental grocery stores and occasionally in health food stores. Good for Kapha and Vata types.

Aloe vera- Called kumari in Sanskrit, aloe vera is bitter, astringent, sweet and cooling in nature. It is used in pancha karma therapy as a tonic, blood cleanser, mild laxative, and for douching. Excellent for Pitta, it may be used by all types.

Aragvadha (purging cassia)- A family of the senna plant, the fruit, bark and pods are used in Ayurvedic purgative therapy. Pungent and bitter in taste and cooling in energy, the fruits, bark and pods are used primarily by Pitta and Kapha types.

Arka (sadapushpi)- The root, leaves and flowers are known for their extensive use in Ayurvedic purgative and emesis therapy. The "milk" of the plant is known for its sharp potency, and a few drops of it is used to alkalize purgative decoctions. Arka is bitter and pungent in nature and is heating in energy. Good for Kapha, Pitta and Vata disorders.

Ashwagandha- Bitter, astringent and heating in nature, this herb may be used primarily by Vata and Kapha types as a tonic, nervine, aphrodisiac and a rejuvenative.

453

Atibala- This herb, like bala, is sweet and cooling and may be used by all three doshas, although it is most suitable for Pitta and Kapha types. Atibala is used as a mild laxative as well as a tonic and calming agent.

Ayurvedic formulated oils- Amavathahara, anu taila, bilva, brahmi, chakra, dashamula, dhanvantari, kaseesadi, ksheerabala, masha, Narayana, nirgundi, pinda, padmaka, shatavari, sidda, yasti madhu. (See Appendix G for Ayurvedic Resources and Suppliers. If oils are not available, follow instructions in Chapter Four to make oils by using the appropriate herbal powders, more easily available.)

Ayurvedic formulated pills- Avipattkar, icchabhedhi, drakshadi, jalodharari, kutajaghana. (See Appendix G for Ayurvedic Resources and Suppliers.)

Ayurvedic medicated ghee- Tikta ghrita, maha tikta ghrita, brahmi ghrita, matikalyana ghrita, guggulu tikta ghrita. (See Appendix G for Ayurvedic Resources and Suppliers.)

Bala- Sweet and cooling in nature, this herb may be used for all three doshas as a rejuvenative tonic and nervine.

Besan- Chickpea flour. Good for Pitta and Kapha types and maybe used occasionally by Vata types.

Bhringaraja- Bitter, sweet and cooling in nature, this herb may be used for all three doshas as a nervine, blood cleanser and tonic.

Black cumin- Called kala jeera in Sanskrit, the black cumin is a relative of both the cumin and caraway plants. Used extensively in Vedic cooking, black cumin, like cumin, is considered good for all three doshas. It is pungent and bitter in taste and is used as a stimulant, blood cleanser and carminative. Available at Indian grocery stores.

Brahma dandi (Mexican poppy)- Pungent, astringent and sweet in taste with heating energy, the root, seeds and flowers are used in pancha karma to soothe Vata disorders, and sometimes Pitta disorders.

Brahmi (Indian pennyworth or thyme-leaved gratiola)- Also called gotu kola, the whole plant is used Ayurvedically. Bitter, pungent, sweet and cooling in nature, brahmi is used to promote memory, sleep, and longevity. It is used as a blood cleanser, to reduce internal bleeding and to alleviate heart disease and diabetes. Good for all doshas but excellent for Pitta disorders.

Burdock root- This dark brown root of the burdock plant is long, thin and wiry and has medicinal properties. Bitter, pungent, sweet and astringent in taste with heating energy, this root is good for Pitta and Kapha types. Available in health food stores.

Cardamom- Known as ela or elachi in Sanskrit, the cardamom pods and seeds are used extensively in both Vedic cooking and Ayurvedic medicine. Cardamom is sweet, pungent and heating in nature and may be used primarily by Vata and Kapha types as a carminative and stimulant, as well as to relieve mucus. It may also be used occasionally by Pitta types.

Chana dhal- A variety of small chick pea, which is husked and split, this buff-yellow dhal is very popular in Indian cuisine. Best for Pitta and Kapha types.

Chitraka- Pungent and hot in nature, this herb is used by Vata and Kapha types to promote digestion, regulate menstrual flow, and as a tonic for liver, spleen and intestine.

Coconut- The whole coconut fruit is used extensively in India to make many wholesome products. Sweet in taste, the fresh and dried coconut as well as the coconut oil are used in Ayurveda as a neutralizing tonic and diuretic by Pitta and Vata types. Available at Indian and Oriental grocery stores.

Dadima (pomegranate fruit)- Sweet, bitter and astringent in nature, the pomegranate fruit is used extensively in pancha karma therapy as a tonic and blood cleanser. It is also used to destroy bacteria, parasites, fungus and yeast in the body. Good for Pitta and Kapha types.

Dashamula- A combination of ten Ayurvedic herbs, namely: ashwagandha, shatavari, yasti- madhu, punarnava, arjuna, bala, bilva, gokshura, vidari and kumari, generally used in pancha karma therapy for Vata disorders.

Dhanyaka (coriander leaves and seeds)- Used extensively in Vedic cooking as well as in Ayurveda, coriander is bitter, pungent and cooling in nature. It is good for all three doshas.

Draksha- Sweet and cooling in nature, the grape powder, juice or medicinal wine is generally used in pancha karma therapies. Good for Vata and Pitta types, although Kapha types may use occasionally.

Echinacea- A relative of the camel's thistle (utkataka), this herb is bitter, pungent and cooling in nature. Used for its antibiotic quality, echinacea also helps to induce sweating. Good for Pitta and Kapha types.

Eranda (castor root and oil)- Pungent, sweet and heating in nature, castor root and oil are used in purgation therapy as a strong laxative causing rapid evacuation. Castor root and oil also calm the tissues and relieve pain. Good for Vata types.

Fruits used in pancha karma (fresh fruit, fruit juice and dried fruit powder)- pilu, draksha, palasha, bilva, badri kanchanara (red and white variety), dadima, amalaki, bibhitaki, and haritaki. (See Appendix A for English names).

Ghee- Best made fresh (see recipe, pg. 493), this clarified butter is also available in health food stores and Indian grocery stores. Ghee is excellent for Vata and Pitta uses.

Gokshura- Sweet, bitter and cooling in nature, this herb may be used mostly by Pitta and Kapha types as a diuretic, tonic and aphrodisiac.

Gotu kola- See Brahmi.

Gourds used in pancha karma- Dokshi, koshataki (torai), koshaphala (bidali), katukumbi (bottle gourd), mahajali (kadwi torai). Generally the seeds, which are pungent and bitter, and fruits, which are cooling, are used in emesis therapy to relieve excess Kapha. Fresh gourds are available at Indian grocery stores.

Gum arabic- Sweet and cooling in nature, gum Arabic is used as an emollient to the tissues as well as a tonic to calm the internal membranes. Good for Pitta and Vata types.

Japa (shoe flower, or hibiscus)- The leaves, roots, flowers and buds are used in pancha karma therapy. Sweet, astringent and heating in nature, hibiscus is used as a blood cleanser, to relieve thirst and stop internal bleeding. Good for Pitta and Kapha types.

Honey (madhu)- In Ayurveda, honey is known as yogavaha, since it enhances the therapeutic effects of the medicines which are added to it. Its unique qualities of sweet and astringent tastes, yet heating energy, make honey an excellent vehicle for carrying medicines deeply into bodily tissues, allowing penetration through the subtle tissues and pores. Adding to its uniqueness is the effectiveness of naturally aged honey in reducing obesity and diabetes. For obesity, honey is mixed in hot water. This is the only circumstance in which honey is combined with heat, since when heated or used in hot substances, honey becomes highly toxic in the body.

Honey is excellent for Vata and Kapha disorders. Even though sweet, it reduces Kapha due to its dry, rough and heavy attributes. Although heating in nature, it may be used discriminately by Pitta types, especially as a medicinal carrier. Honey is used to alleviate conditions such as ulcers, bronchitis, asthma, hiccoughs, nausea, excessive thirst, bleeding, diabetes, eye diseases (when applied topically) and sore throat. Honey also promotes intelligence, strength and determination.

Hot chili pepper- Native to tropical and semi-tropical climates, chili peppers come in an infinite variety of hotness. Those recommended in this book are the medium-hot variety, such as the one-inch long red or green chilies found in Indian, Oriental, and Latin American grocery stores. You can reduce the heat of a pepper by deseeding it. Cut off the stem and slice the pepper in two lengthwise. Use a dinner knife to scrape the seeds off. Alternatively, remove the stem by cutting around it and twisting or pulling it out of the pepper; most of the seeds should come out with the stem intact. Good for Kapha types although it may be used occasionally by Vata types.

Unrefined brown sugar (jaggery and gur)- For millennia, jaggery and gur, both unrefined sugars, have been culled and preserved in India's villages. Jaggery is made from the juice crushed from the sugar cane, while gur is made from the sap drained from the coconut, date and palmyra palm trees. Much in demand in India, gur is made into several types of confections and offered at religious ceremonies. The season's first batch of gur is a sought-after delicacy.

Jaggery and gur, available through Indian grocers, may be used interchangeably in the formulas and recipes in this book, along with unrefined brown sugar and Sucanat, available through health food stores.

When used in milk preparations, unrefined sugars should be added towards the end of the cooking process. Jaggery, gur and Sucanat share smooth, heavy, oily, sweet and cooling qualities and are used primarily to reduce excess Vata and Pitta conditions. Kapha types should use these sugars sparingly since all sugars increase body fat.

Jatamansi (Indian spikenard)- The root of this plant is used to relieve Pitta and sometimes Kapha conditions. Sweet, bitter and astringent in taste, jatamansi is cooling in nature.

Karanja (Indian beech)- The leaves, seeds, bark and root are used extensively in pancha karma as an emetic, to relieve nervous tension, skin diseases and ulcers, and remove parasites from the body. Karanja is pungent and bitter with a heating energy, and is good for Kapha, Pitta and Vata disorders.

Katuki (gentian plant and root)- Bitter, pungent and cooling in nature, gentian is used as a bitter tonic, blood cleanser, and to reduce bodily heat. Good for Pitta and Kapha disorders.

Kudzu- The root of the kudzu plant is best known for its medicinal starch, which may also be used as a food thickener. Kudzu starch is similar to guduchi starch used in Ayurveda. Good for Pitta and Vata types, although it may be used occasionally by Kapha types.

Lemon grass- Pungent, bitter and cooling in nature, lemon grass is good for all three doshas. Generally used to cool the system, or as a diuretic and sweat inducer.

Lotus root- Known as kamala in Sanskrit, the lotus plant is native to ponds and lakes of Kashmir, China and Japan. Every part of the lotus plant is used medicinally in Ayurveda. The roots may be used fresh or dried for cooking, whereas the root powder may be used medicinally as a nutritive tonic and nervine for Pitta and Vata conditions.

Madana (emetic nut)- Known for its extensive use in Ayurvedic emesis therapy, both the kidney-shaped fruit and seeds are used. Madana fruits and seeds are sweet, bitter and astringent in taste and cooling in energy, and may be used by both Pitta and Kapha types.

Masoor dhal- Commonly called French lentil, this small bean when split resembles the red lentil. Traditional to North Indian cooking, this legume is best for Pitta and Kapha types, although seasoned appropriately, Vata types may use occasionally.

Matar dhal- Common split peas, yellow and green. Best for Pitta and Kapha types.

Mung dhal- Also known as mudga or green gram, this legume used since Vedic times is considered queen of the legumes because of its alkalizing and healing properties. May be used by all types, although Vata types need to spice appropriately.

Musta- Bitter, astringent, pungent and cooling in nature, this herb is used to alleviate fever, thirst, diarrhea, as well as disorders and burning sensation of the skin. A natural blood cleanser, musta is good for Pitta and Kapha disorder uses, and may be used occasionally by Vata types.

Neem- Also called nimba in Sanskrit, the neem tree grows predominantly in arid regions of Punjab and Rajasthan. The entire tree is used medicinally in Ayurveda. Neem leaves are also used in Vedic cooking. Bitter in taste, neem is used primarily by Pitta and Kapha types to reduce conditions such as fevers and blood disorders, and as a bitter tonic. Fresh neem leaves, commonly called curry leaves, are available at Indian grocery stores.

Nilini (indigo plant, root or dye)- Bitter, pungent and cooling, indigo is used in pancha karma therapy as an antibiotic and mild laxative. Good for Pitta and Kapha disorders.

Padmaka (wild cherry bark)- this bark is used extensively in Ayurveda to relieve cough, bronchial spasm, palpitations, and skin and eye problems. Bitter, astringent and sweet in taste with cooling energy, padmaka is good for all types, but in particular for Pitta and Kapha.

Pippali- A hot and pungent red pepper, two to three inches long, and one of the three ingredients in the Ayurvedic formula known as trikatu. It is excellent for Kapha types, and occasionally for Vata types, to provide heat to the body and to stimulate digestion.

Plantain- Known as green banana in the United States and kacha kela in India, plantain is actually considered a vegetable. Used in the cuisines of South India and South and Central America, it is available in most Indian and Latin American grocery stores. Astringent, pungent and bitter in taste, plantain is a natural diuretic and may be used by Pitta and Kapha types.

Pudina- The Sanskrit term for mint, pudina is mentioned as a vital tridoshic herb in ancient Ayurvedic texts. Especially pleasing to Pitta types, it is available fresh or dried in health food stores and farmers' markets.

Punarnava- Bitter and cooling in nature, this herb may be used mostly by Pitta and Kapha as a diuretic, laxative and a rejuvenative.

Rock Salt- Primarily mined in crystalline form from the seabeds of the Sindh mountain region in Pakistan, where it is known as senda namak; this salt has been used since ancient times in Ayurvedic foods and medicines. It may be used by all the types and substituted for sea salt in any of the recipes in this book. Its sister salt, known as kala namak, is a deep purple, highly pungent rock crystal that has a volatile taste and a smell resembling hard boiled eggs. It may be used occasionally (in small quantity) by Vata and Kapha types. Rock salt may be ordered through Ayurvedic Resources and Suppliers (see Appendix G).

Saffron- Known as kesar in Sanskrit, saffron threads are handpicked from the saffron crocus cultivated in India, China, the Mediterranean and Asia Minor.

459

Carmine red in color with an exquisitely delicate taste, saffron is used in Ayurvedic medicine to tone the colon, cleanse the blood, regulate menstrual flow and as a rejuvenative. Saffron is also used extensively in India for making sweet drinks and desserts. It may be used by all three doshas. Available at Indian and Middle Eastern grocery stores, as well as through health food stores.

Shatavari- Sweet, bitter and cooling in nature, this herb is used as a nutritive and calming agent, to regulate menstrual flow and to boost the hormonal system. Good for Pitta and Vata disorders.

Soybean- Native to India, China and Japan, the soybean is a medium-sized bean, either black or white in color. This bean is highly nutritive, as well as cooling, making it an excellent choice for Pitta types. Seasoned appropriately, both Kapha and Vata types may use occasionally. The derivatives of the soybean, tofu and soy milk, may also be used accordingly.

Sucanat- Trademark for a natural sugar made from sugar cane juice. Excellent for Vata and Pitta use. Kapha types may use sparingly.

Tamal patra (Indian cassia)- A family of the cinnamon plant, the dried leaves and bark are used extensively in Ayurveda as a stimulant, blood cleanser and to promote perspiration through the skin. Pungent, astringent and sweet in taste with heating energy, the tamal patra is good for Vata and Kapha types, although Pitta types may also use occasionally.

Tamarind- The pulp of the tamarind pod, used since ancient times in India. The tamarind tree is considered auspicious in Indian mythology, and its fruit is known as imli. Fresh tamarind is available in the tropics. Dried tamarind is packed in the shape of small bricks or slabs that can be prepared as a pulp. Dried tamarind, tamarind pulp (or paste), and a gel-like tamarind concentrate are all available in Indian grocery stores. Sour and sweet in taste, Tamarind is a natural stimulant and may be used by Vata and Kapha types, although Pitta types may also use occasionally.

Trikatu- A combination of the three pungent herbs, ginger, pippali and black pepper, trikatu may be used primarily by Vata and Pitta types to boost digestion and to stimulate the system.

Triphala- A combination of three ancient Ayurvedic fruits, amalaki, haritaki and bibhitaki, triphala is an excellent tonic for all three doshas. It is used to detoxify the system, as well as a mild laxative and sleeping aid.

460

Turmeric- Also known as haridra in Sanskrit, turmeric comes from the underground rhizome of a perennial plant native to the humid regions of South India and Southeast Asia. Used extensively in both Vedic cooking and Ayurvedic medicine, turmeric is bitter, pungent and heating, but may be used for all three doshas as a blood cleanser, stimulant, and antibacterial agent. Available at Indian grocery stores and health food stores.

Urad dhal- Also known as masha, or black gram, this small, black legume has been used since ancient times. When husked and split, the bean is white. Traditionally used in many South Indian vegetable dishes, urad is considered a tridoshic bean.

Uva ursi- Astringent, bitter, pungent, and cooling in nature, this herb may be used by Pitta and Kapha types for its antiseptic and diuretic properties.

Vacha (calamus, or sweet flag root)- Pungent, bitter and heating in nature, vacha may be used mainly by Vata and Kapha types as a stimulant, rejuvenative and decongestant.

Valerian- Pungent and heating in nature, the herb valerian is used primarily as a sedative, nervine, and to tone the colon. Good for Vata and Kapha disorders.

Vamsha rochana (bamboo)- Sweet, astringent and cooling in nature, this herb is excellent for Pitta and Vata disorders. It relieves mucus and acts as a tonic and calming agent to the tissues.

Vidanga (embelia)- Pungent, astringent and heating in nature, the berries are used in Ayurveda to reduce appetite and fat and to destroy parasites, bacteria and fungus. Good for Kapha disorders.

Wood powders used in pancha karma- Sandalwood, agaru and khadira.

Yastimadhu (madhuka)- Sweet, bitter, and cooling in nature, licorice root and root extract are generally used in both emesis and purgation therapies. Good for Pitta and Vata disorders.

Glossary of Oils for the Healing Diet

True to the Sanskrit term sneha, which means "fat" as well as "lavish love," oil provides essential lubricating love to the dhatus. Some people, such as Kapha types, are born with plentiful love in terms of natural bodily oils; and they need less lubrication from foods. Others, such as the Vata types, have the least amount of bodily love/fat and need a profusion of warmth and lubrication from nature as well as from foods. Pitta types are endowed with intense, hot bodily oils from birth and need less lubrication and more coolant to balance their nature.

All foods contain natural oils to varying degrees. In addition to their warming and lubricating attributes, oils fortify and build tissues, soothe bodily membranes, and to some extent activate the digestive fire.

Oils should never be used excessively by any of the body types, although Vata types are allowed ample amounts for their cooking, bathing, and massaging needs. According to the density, taste, and energy of the different kinds of oil, each body type is allowed a good and variable selection from which to choose. Primarily for simplicity's sake, and because these are the most nourishing of oils, sesame, sunflower and ghee are used in the healing diet recipes. To provide variety in your daily diet, choose oils most harmonious to your body type from the list of oils below.

Do not use oils that have been commercially processed, hydrogenated, refined, treated with coloring agents, or mixed with other types of oil. Quality oils can be purchased at health food and gourmet food stores.
Store your oils in a cool, dark place. After opening, do not use for more than one month as oils easily turn rancid.

Almond oil: A delicate, sweet oil pressed from almond nuts. Rich and warming in character, it is used in many Ayurvedic health formulas and massage therapies for Vata types. It should be used as an accent rather than a daily cooking oil. Best for Vata types; Kapha types may use sparingly.

Avocado oil: A thick, rich oil pressed from the pulp of the avocado fruit. It is warming in character and, like olive oil, lends itself as a base to salad dressings and herbal pasta sauces. Best for Vata types; Pitta types may use sparingly.

Canola oil: A recently popular oil pressed from rape seeds. It is light and soothing in character, closely resembling sunflower oil. Recommended for occasional use by all body types.

Coconut oil: An oil extracted from the coconut flesh and used extensively in South Indian cuisine. While it is the most cooling of all oils, it is also very high in fat. Pitta and Vata types may use occasionally.

462

Corn oil: A golden-colored oil pressed from the germ of the maize grain, corn oil has the longest history of use, next to sesame oil. It is light and drying in nature and has a high smoking point. Best for Kapha types as a routine oil; Vata and Pitta types may use sparingly.

Mustard oil: An oil pressed from either the amber-colored or the purplish-brown variety of mustard seeds. It is used extensively in East and North Indian cuisines and has been valued since ancient times in Ayurvedic oil massage therapies. Highly pungent in taste and heating in nature, it is a traditional ingredient in chutneys and pickles. Best for Kapha types, as an accent rather than a daily cooking oil; Vata types may also use as an occasional cooking oil by first heating to near-smoking point to decrease pungency.

Olive oil: A rich, thick, and mildly pungent oil pressed from ripe olives. Introduced by Mediterranean, Spanish, and Italian cuisines, it has gained tremendous popularity throughout the world. Olive oil is available in a wide range of colors, densities, and qualities. The greenish "virgin" or "extra-virgin" varieties may be used, unheated, by Vata and sparingly by Kapha types in salad dressings, herbal pasta sauces, and chutneys. The blond-colored varieties may be used occasionally for cooking by Vata types and sparingly (because of its richness) by Kapha types.

Safflower oil: A light and mild flavored oil pressed from the seeds of the safflower plant, or the flowering saffron thistle. Because of its high smoking point, it is good for deep-frying. May be used occasionally by all body types.

Sesame oil: A rich, thick, and warm oil pressed from sesame seeds. It has been used since ancient times in both China and India, where it is known as tila oil, or gingelly oil. It is available in a light amber color, pressed from the buff-colored seeds, or a deep brown when pressed from the black seeds. When pressed from roasted seeds, it is a deep tan color. Sesame oil is used extensively in Ayurvedic medicine and is considered the main cooking oil for Vata types. May also be used sparingly by Kapha and Pitta types.

Sunflower oil: A golden oil pressed from the seeds of the sunflower plant. It is hailed as the best all-round oil for all body types, and especially for the Pitta types because of its gentle, cooling nature and mildly sweet taste.

Walnut oil: A deep amber-colored oil pressed from walnuts. It is delicate, nutty, and aromatic and may be used sparingly by all types to accent salads, dressings, greens, and desserts. Like almond oil, it is best for Vata types.

463

Glossary of the Holy Grains for the Healing Diet

It is said in the Vedas that the entire universe is held within each grain. The components of a grain—the husk, bran/germ, and endosperm—symbolize the cosmic gunas of sattva, rajas, and tamas, reflecting the harmony or protection, dynamism, and inertia of the living universe, respectively. The grain endures the seven stages of life, from seed to sprout, to seedling, to young plant, to mature plant, to flowering plant, to fruitful plant.

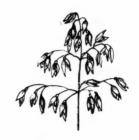

Amaranth: Amaranth was discovered in the crevices of fallen caves of Mexico; it is believed that this grain was harvested by the indigenous people of Mexico more than six thousand years ago. A natural herbicide and insecticide, the Amaranth plant fares well in arid soil and in India is grown around other plants to protect them. A relative of the tumbleweed, it has similar properties to quinoa but is smaller in size. Sweet and astringent with a heating energy, amaranth is excellent for Vata and Kapha types and may be used occasionally by Pitta types.

Barley: Known as jawar, barley has been cultivated in India since the Vedic period. Once the husk is removed, the remaining grain—referred to as hulled barley, or "pot" or "scotch barley" in the West—is nutritionally intact. It consists of a layer of germ and protein known as aleurone. When the aleurone layer is stripped, the ivory colored pearl barley remains. In India, the silken, freshly ground barley flour, which has a low-gluten content, is often mixed with whole wheat flour to make chapati. Barley flour performs like white flour, except it is much more nutritious and wholesome.

Barley is best for Pitta types and also supports Kapha types. Although cooling in energy, Kapha does well with this grain due to its dryness.

Buckwheat: This edible fruit seed has been used as a cereal grain for centuries in Asia and Europe. Related to rhubarb, garden sorrel, and the dock family, buckwheat is known as kutu or phaphra in India. Much like a wheat berry, buckwheat has a hard outer shell which when removed yields a seed called a groat. In India this is traditionally ground fine and used in pakora or tempura style batter, used as a dough for poori (a thin fried chapati), and for making sweets, such as halva.

Buckwheat groats are best suited to Kapha types, due to their somewhat pungent nature. However, mixed with wheat and a natural sweetener, both Pitta and Vata types may indulge occasionally.

Corn: Native to India and the American continents, corn is a special grain. In India the freshly ground flour is known as makkai atta. Low in gluten, it is mixed with whole wheat flour to lend a different texture to flatbreads. Like millet and barley, corn is used mainly by the peasants in rural India.

Corn is excellent for Kapha types, and if cooked porridge style or fresh as corn-on-the-cob, slathered with organic butter or ghee, an occasional repast of this food will also be good for Vata types.

Millet: Known as bajra in North India and raji in South India, this delicious buff-colored grain is widely harvested from several cereal grasses. The two most popular kinds are finger millet and pearl millet, the kind found most often in natural food stores. Millet is the third most used grain in India, after rice and wheat. It grows well in sandy and poor soil, and in hot, harsh climates, thriving where wheat may be too frail. Freshly ground millet flour is often mixed with other flours into flat breads or mixed with vegetables.

Millet is best for Kapha types. If it is cooked softly, it may be used occasionally by Vata types. This grain is heating in energy.

Oats: Of the common grains, oats are among the highest in nutritive value and creates happiness in the tissues. This wonderfully sustaining food is available in many forms today. The whole grain is threshed to remove the inedible husks. The remaining grain, with the bran and germ left intact, is referred to as groats. These groats, or whole kernels, may be further reduced by being split with a sharp steel blade to make steel-cut oats, also called Scottish or Irish oatmeal.

To make old fashioned rolled oats, the groats are slightly softened by steaming and then flattening with steel rollers; this makes for a faster cooking cereal. As a result of intensive processing, dehydrated instant oats have little nutritive value.

Although heating in energy, best for Vata types, the rich, sweet taste of oats supports Pitta as well as Vata.

Quinoa: Called the Mother Grain by the Incas, quinoa was first harvested more than 3,000 years ago in South America but little used by the Incas for more than four centuries after the Spanish conquest. Quinoa is a distant relative to the beet, spinach, and Swiss chard family. In fact, the leaves of the quinoa plant are cooked and used like spinach.

Quinoa is sweet, astringent, and pungent, with a heating energy. An excellent grain for Vata and Kapha types, it may also be used occasionally in the fall and winter by Pitta types.

Rice: Rice is the primary food for most ancient cultures; it is the most widely consumed grain in the world, with more than thirty thousand varieties of rice currently being cultivated. Eighty percent of the rice in the world is grown in India, China, and Japan.

Basmati Rice: An aromatic, nutty flavored rice, basmati has been cultivated for centuries in North India and Pakistan. Some villages in northern India conduct a harvest ritual of hulling and winnowing the grain by hand, with all the villagers sharing in this sadhana. Basmati is renowned for its long, slender shape, which lengthens instead of swelling when cooked. The word basmati translates literally as the "queen of fragrance." This sattvic grain remains unrivaled among the aromatic rices, due to its exquisite scent, which has been likened to the jasmine flower and the exotic walnut.

Basmati is available in both white and brown. White basmati is easy to digest, cooling the digestive fires, and is held in high regard Ayurvedically as a cleansing and healing food for all body types, although Kapha types may use only occasionally. Brown basmati is also considered nutritive and healing, especially for Vata types.

Black Japonica Rice: This medium-grain rice, which has a black bran, is grown in small quantities on the Lundberg farms in California. It is used in many gourmet rice blends because of its flavor. Black Japonica is sweet and slightly pungent in taste. Good for Vata types, it may be used occasionally by Pitta and Kapha types.

Brown Rice: Brown rice comes in long, medium, and short grains. This rice has only the hull removed; both the bran layer and germ layer are left intact, clinging to the kernels. Brown rice has a cream color and a chewy texture, due to its high gluten content. It is superbly rich in minerals and vitamins and has three times the fiber of white rice. Generally, the medium and short grains have more amylopectin, a waxy starch, which gives them a chewier and stickier character than long-grain rice; they also take longer to cook. The long-grain brown rice is fluffier and lighter when cooked. All types of brown rice must be well-cooked and chewed properly to facilitate proper digestion. Brown rice is best for Vata types. On rare occasions, Pitta and Kapha types may indulge.

Calmati Rice: Basmati has recently been cross-seeded with an American long-grain variety in northern California to produce this popular brown basmati. This rice should not be used interchangeably with the Indian Basmati rice for the cleansing diet. Good for Vata types, it may be used occasionally by Pitta and Kapha types.

Italian Rices: Arborio, vialone nano, carnaroli, and padano, the most popular rices in Italy, are grown in the regions of Piedmont and Lombardy. Most Italian and Spanish rice is medium-grain and high in starch, which makes the grains stick together. When cooked, these varieties become soft, translucent, and yet retain a firm central core; they also yield a top layer of rice cream. Arborio is often used to prepare the well known Italian rice dish called "risotti." Italian rice may be substituted occasionally in any recipe calling for short- or medium-grain rice. These are good for Vata types, may be used occasionally by Pitta types, and seldom by Kapha types.

Jasmine Rice: Native to Thailand, this rice resembles the basmati grain. It has a rich fragrance and is silken to the touch. Unlike basmati, this rice is not aged and usually expands into a moist and medium-grain shape when cooked. Jasmine rice is now grown successfully in the United States. Due to its cooling energy during digestion, it may also be used for cleansing by those of all types on a healing diet. As part of a regular diet, like most rice, Jasmine is suited to the Vata types.

Sushi Rice: This short-grain white rice, used in Japan for making sushi, can be found in most Oriental food stores and some natural food stores. When cooked, it is softer and stickier than most other types of rice due to its high starch content. Best for Vata types, sushi rice may be used occasionally by Pitta and Kapha types.

Sweet Brown Rice: This sticky cream colored short-grain rice is used in East Asian cuisines for making desserts. Its taste is naturally sweeter than short-grain brown rice. Native to both India and Japan, it can be found in some Oriental or natural food stores. Best for Vata types, sweet brown rice may be used occasionally by Pitta and Kapha types.

Texmati Rice: A hybrid of Indian basmati rice and American long-grain white rice, it is also called American basmati. Its aroma and popcorn flavor favor the basmati, but its cooking texture is softer and stickier. The rice is named after the state in which it grows, Texas, and its resemblance to the basmati rice. Available in both white and brown, Texmati may sometimes be substituted for basmati rice, except in the cleansing diet. As a regular diet, Texmati is best for Vata types and may be used occasionally by Pitta and Kapha types.

Valencia Rice: A medium-grain rice native to Spain, this rice is soft and flavorful. It is similar to the Italian rices in that it retains a firm central core after being cooked. Valencia is used in the traditional Spanish rice dish known as paella. This rice is good for Vata types and may be used occasionally by Pitta and Kapha types.

Rye: Among the grains produced by grasses or cereal grains, rye, along with millet and barley, is sorely underestimated. Rye grows better in cold, wet climates where wheat fares badly. Rye is also available in its cracked form, which is similar to cracked wheat and steel cut oats. Through a drying, steaming, and flattening process the rye berries are made into rye flakes, which make a gentle and nutritive breakfast dish. Rye is a deliciously pungent food suited to Kapha types.

Wheat Berries and Processed Wheat: Like rice, wheat is an ancient grain which has been a staple of Indian cuisine for over 5000 years. In India, wheat is used in as many ways as there are dialects. The ancient flatbread, known as chapati, is still the primary grain served with meals in North India. Chapati is made from a low gluten, soft-textured, cream-colored wheat flour, known as atta. In this flour the whole kernel—bran, germ, and endosperm—is milled to a fine powder, which offers no resistance to being rolled into a dough. An even finer strain of flour, known as pisi lahore, is sometimes used to yield a soft, silken chapati. Semolina, known as sooji in India, is a granular meal made from the endosperm of the durum wheat. Its glutinous character makes it a perfect ingredient for a South Indian dish, called uppama. Sooji is available in three textures—fine, medium, and coarse; it is used in sweets, such as halva, and in breakfast porridge.

Although it is cooling in energy (best for Pitta types), wheat is a rich, vital, and sweet grain which supports Vata as well as Pitta.

Cracked Wheat: This split whole kernel of wheat is slightly different from bulgur. The cracked wheat is not pre-cooked or parched in the sun before it is broken. However, both bulgur and cracked wheat may be used interchangeably. Farina is a finely ground wheat kernel that generally is used for breakfast porridge.

Couscous: This grain is made from semolina, the endosperm of durum wheat. To make couscous, semolina flour is mixed with salted water, then tossed and rubbed into tiny pellets. The pellets are then steamed on a cotton sheet over simmering water until they swell. This step can also be accomplished by steaming pellets twice over a hot, bubbling pot of stew.

Couscous is native to the diets of Moroccans, Algerians, Tunisians, and Egyptians. In North Africa, the term couscous describes a variety of dishes.

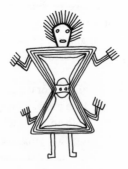

Corn Goddess

KITCHEN EQUIPMENT

Ideally, a few stainless steel pots and pans, as well as accessories such as spoons, spatulas, ladles, colanders or sieves, and a tea strainer are kept exclusively for preparing your formulas and recipes for the various treatments. Always dip your treatment utensils in boiling water before using. Earthenware and ceramic pots and bowls, also recommended for treatment preparations, help provide the formulas with the earth's warming energy.

For wholesome cooking, it is wise to vary your cooking utensils. Use enamel, copper, glass, cast iron, earthenware and stainless steel to enjoy a variety of benefits.

COOKWARE AND ACCESSORIES:

Pressure Cooker: A large, stainless steel pressure cooker is invaluable for cooking the grains and legumes called for in the poultices and healing diet recipes. Pressure cooking produces a much more nutritious meal or effective poultice. If you do not have a pressure cooker, grains and legumes may be cooked in a clay pot, an enamel coated cast-iron pot, or a heavy stainless steel pot.

Ceramic Bowls: Available through most natural food stores, Japanese groceries, and pottery stores, ceramic bowls are highly recommended for storing your massaging and aromatic oils just prior to use. Ceramic maintains the oils' natural energies as well as the desired temperature.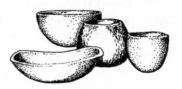

Ceramic Hand Grater: This ideal tool for grating ginger, garlic or nutmeg can be found in natural food stores or Japanese groceries. See Appendix G for Ayurvedic Resources and Suppliers.

Cheese Cloth: To promote harmony and the development of your natural sadhana instincts, cheese cloth and cotton towels are suggested in this book as an alternative to paper towels.

Hand Grinders: These old fashioned hand food grinders, available in varying sizes, are recommended for grinding wet legumes (dhals), grains, nuts, and seeds, as well as for pureeing vegetable soups and for pulping fruits. The larger sizes (six inches and eight inches in diameter) are best suited to grinding legumes and grains, for pureeing vegetables, and so on. The smaller size (four inches in diameter) is recommended for grinding nuts and seeds. See Appendix G for Ayurvedic Resources and Suppliers.

Hand Stone, Stone Mortar and Pestle: Originating in the ancient cultures, the grinding of grains, legumes, spice seeds, and nuts, with a hand stone and a stone mortar and pestle, is an indispensable sadhana to awaken and sustain cognition of and harmony with nature. This stone equipment is still used profusely in India and Mexico and in many South American countries. In India the hand stone is called batta and the stone bed sil. The large bowl-shaped stone mortar and pestle is called himan dasta. See Appendix G for Ayurvedic Resources and Suppliers.

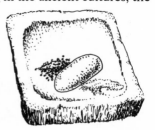

Figure 1C: Hand Stone

Indian Sieves: This eight-inch round, drum-shaped sieve, called chalni, is excellent for a number of sifting and straining tasks. Made with either a stainless steel or tin rim, the chalni is sold with five interchangeable mesh sieves of varying gauges, from very fine to very coarse, excellent for straining herbal powders, as well as roots and so on. See Appendix G for Ayurvedic Resources and Suppliers.

Suribachi: Japanese bowl-shaped earthenware mortar and wooden pestle. These bowls are wide and grooved inside, naturally conducive to a meditative clockwise or counter-clockwise grinding motion. They are available in three or four sizes. See Appendix G for Ayurvedic Resources and Suppliers.

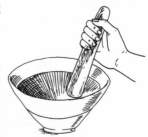

Figure 2C: Suribachi

Cautionary Note: Modern Utensils and Cooking Appliances

We have come a long way from the original cookware, an animal's stomach lining. Pressure cookers and enamelware pots are definite improvements; however, our modern stand-up work tables and stoves have deprived us of working in various crouching positions, an essential sadhana so beneficial to our overall health and sense of wellbeing. Crouching provides excellent stimulation to the vital organs and tissues and is a means of receiving the earth's energies through the womb and solar plexus.

Gas and electric stoves deprive us of the direct exchange between our food and the fire of transformation that occurs when we cook on a wood burning stove.

However, of the two, a gas burning stove is far better than electric because there is direct flame involved. Electrical appliances are drying to the internal and external organism and generate noise pollution. Also, electricity passing through food damages the tanmatra or energy quanta of the food, which aggravates all three doshas, Vata in particular.

Microwave cooking is hazardous to one's health, as it transmutes and distorts the energy structure of a food. It depletes food of its ojas-producing potential, its energy and its memory.

Food processors, electric blenders, dough-kneading machines and so on have removed the most important aspect of food sadhanas from our lives: the transformation of fresh grains, beans, vegetables and spices which occurs when we process them with our own hands and feet. Dissonant machinery cannot refuel and refine the exchange of energy between the human body and nature.

Because our hands are still engaged to a certain degree, hand grinders are valid kitchen tools. They certainly generate results more quickly than the hard-to-find giant mortar and pestle. Of course, the occasional use of a blender or an electric coffee mill is acceptable. The point here is not that we revert back to 500 B.C., but that we make conscious choices which allow for the maximum amount of human exchange with nature. The sadhanas reaped from preparing foods with hand tools are irreplaceable. These are the peaceful weapons that were given to humans so that we could live in harmonic vigor with nature. Therefore, please walk gingerly through the maze of cooking inventions. Consider what portion of your vital and cognitive memory (topics discussed in Chapters One and Two) you are willing to sacrifice to the so called conveniences of modern life.

The principle of sadhana is so simple, so subtle, that we need to deliberately, consciously set about retrieving our innocence. We need to learn through remembering—to embrace our ineffable nature. We need to find our stillness amid the clatter and clamor of daily life. And most importantly, perhaps, we need to ponder on all of these things.

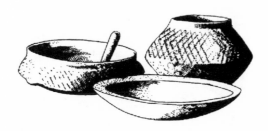

471

PANCHA KARMA ACCESSORIES, EQUIPMENT AND UTENSILS

ACCESSORIES

Emesis Bib

Fold a piece of cotton muslin cloth, 15 inches wide and 36 inches long, width-wise, leaving a 24-inch length on the bottom side and a 12-inch length on the top side of the fold.

Cut a semi-circle, 8 inches in diameter, in the center of the folded side. Turn under 1/2 inch around the outside edge of the bib and stitch. Do the same around the cut-out neck or use a 1/2 inch bias piping. When wearing the bib, the neck opening is placed over the head so that the long side is in front.

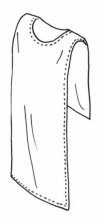

Figure 1D: Emesis Bib

Treatment Gown

Using a light cotton cloth, approximately 4 feet long by three feet wide (depending on the size of the person), make a loosely fitting gown that ends below the knees and has elbow length sleeves (see sketch at right). The gown should open in the back and have two sets of ties to secure it.

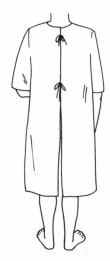

Figure 2D: Treatment Gown

Practitioner's Clothing

Select moderate weight cotton clothing in white or pale, pleasing colors. The pants, shirt, and top should be loose, comfortable and easy to pull on or off. The top should have a pocket in the front, as well as sleeves which extend just below the elbows.

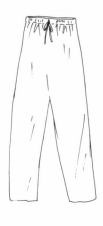

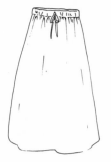
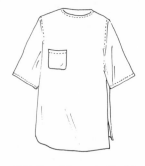

Figure 3D: Practitioner's Clothing

ACCESSORIES FOR SVEDANA

Heart Protection

Pearls

- Put an authentic pearl necklace in a soft, thin, wet cotton pouch.
- Place the pouch directly over the area of the heart, on the chest slightly to the left.
- Leave the pouch in place throughout the therapy.

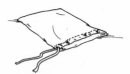
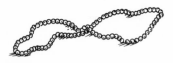

Figure 4D: Heart Protection

Fresh Lotus Flower

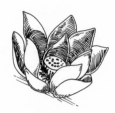

- As an alternative to the pouch-encased pearl necklace, a fresh, stemless lotus flower may be placed on the chest directly over the heart.
- Leave the lotus in place throughout the therapy.
- To maintain freshness before use, keep the lotus in a bowl of water. Each flower is to be used only once.

Figure 5D: Lotus

Sandalwood Paste
- As an alternative to the pearls or lotus flower, mix 5 tablespoons of sandalwood paste and 3 tablespoons of cold water into a soft paste.
- Put the paste into a thin, wet cotton pouch, approximately 4 inches square.
- Place the pouch directly over the heart and leave in place during treatment.

String Bandage for the Heart Pad
- Use a thin strip of cotton, 2 inches wide and 4 feet long, to secure the heart pad, if necessary. Place the string bandage over the pad and secure it around the chest in a knot.

Eye Protection
Soft Whole Wheat Dough
- Mix 5 tablespoons of freshly ground whole wheat flour and 3 tablespoons of cold water into a soft dough. The same amount of sandalwood powder may be substituted for the whole wheat flour.
- Divide the dough into two equal pieces. Roll each piece into a ball in the palms of the hands.
- Place each ball of dough into a thin, wet cotton pouch 2 inches square.
- Plop the wet pouches gently over the closed eyes.
- Leave these pouches on the patient's eyes for the duration of the therapy.

String Bandage for the Eye Pads
Use a thin strip of cotton, approximately 2 inches wide and 3 feet long, to secure the eye pads, if necessary. Place the string bandage over the eye pads and secure it around the head in a knot.

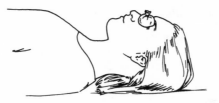

Figure 6D: Eye Protection

Groin and Vaginal Protection
Loin Cloth
- Cut light cotton cloth into two pieces, 8 inches wide and 12 inches long. Stitch the two long edges and one short edge of each piece, leaving the remaining short edge unstitched.

- Fold the unstitched edge of each piece of cloth over 1-1/2 inches, then stitch the edge so that there is a one inch seam to draw a string through.

- Run a flat cotton strip (1/2 inch wide by 48 inches long) through this casing.

- Before using, soak the loin cloth in cold water for 10 minutes. Squeeze to semi-dry and sprinkle approximately 2 tablespoons of sandalwood powder on each flap.

- Have the patient tie the loin cloth around the waist, tucking the front flap under to cover the groin or vaginal area.

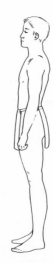

Figure 7D: Loin Cloth

Bolus Wrapping
- Lay out four 18-inch-square cotton napkins and place a ladle of porridge in the center of each.

- Take two opposite ends of each napkin and tie into a single knot. Be careful not to burn your hands on the hot porridge.

- Take the remaining two ends of each napkin and tie into another single knot on top of the other knot.

- Take the bottom knot ties and re-knot over the top knot ties.

- Then take the top ties and create a double knot.

The double knot is to allow a secure grip of the bolus, without burning the hands on its hot contents while applying the bolus.

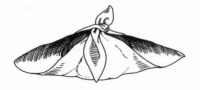 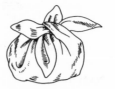

Figure 8D: Bolus Wrap

476

ACCESSORIES FOR SNEHANA

The Head Wrap

A head wrap of unbleached cotton cloth is recommended for wear following the head treatment procedures in order to protect the shaved head from cold, wind and excess heat.

Assembling the Head Wrap

- Take a piece of unbleached, medium-weight cotton fabric, 24 inches square, and sew the edges, if you wish. Fold into a triangle.
- Take the folded side of the triangle and fold it over to form a 2-inch band.
- Cover the head with the triangular cloth by placing the center of the 2-inch band low on the forehead, allowing the pointed end of the cloth, which is at right angles to the band, to fall back along the head.
- Cover the ears with the other two ends of the triangular wrap and tie them behind the head in a double knot, ensuring that the center back end is secured beneath the knotted ends.

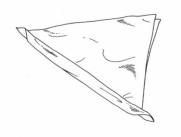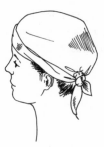

Figure 9D: Head Wrap

Pichu Cloth: Folding and Dipping Techniques

- Fold a 12-inch-square piece of cotton cloth into three even layers.

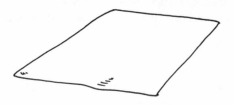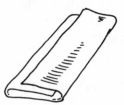

Figure 10D: Pichu Cloth

- Hold both ends of the folded cloth and dip the "belly" of the cloth into the bowl of oil.

- Let go of the cloth, leaving the ends hanging over the rim of the bowl.

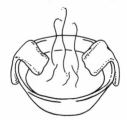

Figure 11D: Pichu Cloth

Shirovasti: The Leather Treatment Cap

Leather is used for the shirovasti cap because it is oil proof, fairly pliable, and can be stretched to fit most head sizes.

- Cut a piece of leather as follows: top edge, 11 inches; bottom edge, 9-1/2 inches; side edges, 8 inches.

- Take the cut leather to a tailor and have the two 8-inch sides sewn together with a 1/4 inch merrow (overlock) stitch. The result is a tall cap with two open ends.

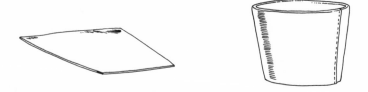

Figure 12D: Shirovasti Cap

Cleaning directions: After the cap has been used, turn it inside-out and use a clean rag to thoroughly remove the oil and plaster. If plaster stains remain, use a wet rag and rub the stains until they are gone. Dry the cap by placing it in direct sunlight for an hour. Finally, to maintain suppleness, rub a small amount of sunflower oil into the cap after it dries, and store it in a dry place until you are ready to use it again.

EQUIPMENT AND UTENSILS

Traditional pancha karma apparatus is still not readily available in the United States. Therefore simple equipment designs and assembly instructions are given

478

below, along with information about alternative pancha karma equipment, which may be purchased domestically. Seek the help of a local carpenter, blacksmith, tailor, craftsperson and so on, to assist you in assembling these extraordinary pieces of equipment. Bear in mind that these measures will also help you reclaim these wholesome activities, sadhanas, which braid you with nature's ways.

Creating your own Dhara Patra for Shirodhara Treatment

To assemble your dhara patra, the following items are necessary: a long piece of rope, a metal urn, a small metal bowl, a small piece of wooden dowel, and a piece of fine cotton string.

Hanging rope

Enough rope is needed to suspend the metal urn from the ceiling to approximately 3 inches from the reclining patient's forehead, i.e., approximately 12 inches from the surface of the treatment table. You will also need enough rope to encircle the pot securely.

Metal urn: the main vessel

- The urn should be made of brass for Kapha and Vata disorders, and silver for Pitta disorders. Its dimensions should be 8 inches in diameter across the bottom, 6 inches in diameter across the top, and 6 inches tall. The rim of the urn should be approximately one inch high, so that the rope can be fastened around it to enable the pot to hang, like a potted plant, from the ceiling.

- Take the pot to a welder or blacksmith, and have a 3/4-inch round hole drilled in the center of its base.

The small metal bowl (to be placed upside-down inside the main vessel)

- The bowl should be brass for Kapha and Vata disorders, silver for Pitta disorders, and 3 inches high with a diameter of 4 inches.

- Take the bowl to a welder or blacksmith, and have a 3/4-inch round hole drilled in the center of its base.

The cotton string and the wooden dowel

- Purchase a ball of cotton string, 1/8 inch thick, and cut a 9-inch piece from it.

- Secure a 2-inch piece of wooden dowel, 1/4 inch in diameter, from your local hardware store. You may have to ask the proprietor to cut the dowel for you.

Assembly

- Tie the 9-inch piece of string to the 2-inch piece of wooden dowel, using approximately 2 inches of string to tie around the dowel.

- Turn the small metal bowl upside down and, placing the dowel in the center of the upturned bowl, pull the string to the inside of the bowl through the hole in its base.

- Holding the bowl, along with the dowel and the string, in the inverted position, place it in the main vessel, the metal urn; pull the string in the small bowl through the hole of the main vessel. If you have difficulty getting the string through the hole, a small piece of wire tied to the loose end of the string will make it easier to direct the string through the hole.

Securing the hanging rope to the dhara patra

- Cut one 10-inch piece and three 24-inch pieces of rope.

- Tie the 10-inch piece firmly around the neck of the main vessel, securing it firmly with a double knot.

- Tie the three 24-inch pieces to the rope around the neck of the main vessel, allowing an equal distance between each of the three pieces of rope (i.e., if the circumference of the neck is 12 inches, the ropes should be tied 4 inches apart from each other).

- Tie the three loose ends of rope into one big knot.

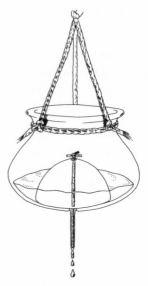

Figure 13D: Dhara Patra

Note: Broken lines show the upside-down bowl with its dowel and string coming through the bottom of main vessel.

Hanging the dhara patra

- After assembling the dhara patra, hang it from a hook secured in the ceiling so that the dhara patra is suspended over the head end of the treatment table, either 12 inches from the surface of the treatment table, or 3 inches from the center of the patient's forehead. This is done by fastening a bolted hook into the ceiling where the dhara patra is to be hung. Use the same type of hook as for a heavy hanging plant. Then take a long piece of rope (the length depends on the height of your ceiling) and pull one end underneath the big center knot of the dhara patra, tying the two ends together to form a loop.

- Hang the looped rope onto the ceiling hook, pulling on it to make sure that it is secure.

480

Using the dhara patra

- After assembling and hanging the dhara patra, move the small wooden dowel to rest slightly off the center of the hole in the small bowl inside the dhara patra. Uncover the bucket of oil and have your assistant remove the oil from the bucket with a small cup and pour it into the dhara patra. Leave the bucket uncovered during treatment.

- Be sure that both you and your assistant assume a comfortable sitting position throughout the treatment.

- After assuming this position, take hold of the dhara patra firmly, holding the rim with one hand. Keep it still until the oil is poured, then gently rock the vessel back and forth, but no more than 2 inches in either direction. Set up a "tick-tock" rhythm in your mind and move the vessel forward on the "tick" and backwards on the "tock."

- Maintain this momentum for the entire duration of the treatment.

- The oil will funnel through the hole in the small bowl on to the string and seep down, dropping methodically as directed on to the center of the patient's forehead.

- The assistant must maintain an even flow while pouring the oil directly over the hole in the small bowl. Try not to interrupt the flow while refilling the cup. There is approximately ten seconds of oil flow remaining on the string after the previous cup has been emptied, which means the assistant has ten seconds to refill the cup.

- After the prescribed time of treatment has elapsed, use both hands to still the dhara patra, while your assistant simultaneously stops pouring the oil and removes the rope loop from the hook in the ceiling.

- As soon as the flow of oil retained by the string begins to slow down, the dhara patra is quickly removed. Cover the bottom of the urn with your hands to prevent leakage, and hand it to your assistant as soon as he/she has removed the hanging loop from its hook.

- The assistant takes the dhara patra to the sink and cleans it while you continue with the post-shirodhara procedure.

Note 1. You may perform this treatment without an assistant by filling the suspended dhara patra with oil immediately before treatment.

Note 2. A separatory funnel with a ring and stand may be used instead of the dhara patra for shirodhara treatment. This equipment, requiring only one attendant, is available through chemistry equipment suppliers.

Cleaning the dhara patra

- Keep one hand under the dhara patra to cover the hole while taking it to the sink.
- Gently dismantle the dhara patra, removing the small bowl inside, along with the string and the dowel.
- Use a clean rag to wipe the oil from each piece. If medicated buttermilk or cream is used, wash the pieces with warm water.
- Use another dry, clean rag to re-wipe the pieces and squeeze the string tightly with the rag to remove any excess oil.
- After drying all the pieces, place the bowl, string, and dowel inside the main vessel. Cover with a clean cotton rag and store until needed again.

Note: Pour the unused portion of oil from the bucket into a clean glass container. This oil may be used once more on the next day. Thereafter, fresh oil needs to be prepared. If the treatment substance is medicated buttermilk or cream, do not re-use leftovers. It is best to freshly prepare the precise quantity of oils, buttermilk or cream needed for each treatment.

ASSEMBLING A NADI SVEDA VESSEL

Items required:

- A stainless steel or enamel kettle, approximately 12 inches in diameter and 18 inches in height, with a 2-gallon capacity.
- A rubber hose, 1 - 1 1/2 inches in diameter and 40 inches long.
- A rubber band, one inch in diameter and 1/2 inch wide.

Assembly:

- Stretch the opening of one end of the rubber hose so that it can be slipped over the spout of the kettle.
- Draw the rubber hose over the spout until at least 2 inches of the spout is covered.
- If necessary, use the rubber band to secure the hose to the spout. This is done by slipping the rubber band over the unattached end of the hose and moving it up and over the attached end. Make sure the hose is securely fastened to the spout before pouring the hot decoction into the nadi vessel.
- Close the open end of the hose with a 3-inch-long cork. Leave at least 2 inches of the cork exposed, so that you may unplug the hose without burning your hand.

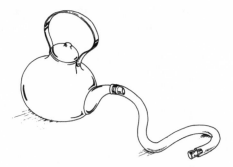

Figure 14D: Nadi Sveda Vessel

Note: A distillery apparatus, available through chemistry equipment suppliers, may also be used for nadi sveda instead of a kettle.

Assembling a Parisheka Pitcher

1. Secure two stainless steel pitchers, one 10 inches tall and 6 inches in diameter, and the other 6 inches tall and 4 inches in diameter. The large pitcher is used to pour decoction on the body, and the small pitcher is used when treating the head.

    Traditionally, gold, bronze or brass pitchers were used for Vata types; silver or pewter for Pitta types; and copper, bronze, or gold for Kapha types.

    Take the pitchers to a blacksmith or a fine woodwork carpenter and have 25 holes drilled in the bottom of the large pitcher and 16 holes in the small pitcher, the holes to be drilled at equal distances apart. The size of each hole made in both containers should be 5/8 inch in diameter.

2. Secure a 7-foot tall piece of bamboo, approximately 3/4 inch in diameter, or two shorter pieces equivalent to 7 feet.

    Take the bamboo to a fine woodwork carpenter and have it cut into 41 pieces, each 2 inches long. Advise the carpenter to cut the bamboo pieces close to but not on the joints, using a small carving knife to remove the membrane surrounding the inside of the bamboo joints. Twenty-five pieces are to be inserted in the holes in the large pitcher and 16 pieces in the small pitcher, the smaller ends inserted into the holes so that the bamboo pieces can act as spouts. The bamboo pieces must be securely fastened, so that almost half of the length of each piece is inside the container and the rest is evenly extending outside of it. Test their evenness by standing the pitcher on the surface of a table. If the pitcher is wobbly, adjust the length of the pieces until they are even.

483

If bamboo cannot be found, metal piping of the same metal as your pitcher may be used instead. Follow the same procedures as above.

Note: Alternatively, you may use appropriately-sized stainless steel watering cans as your parisheka pitchers. The decoction will then be poured from the watering can's showering spouts.

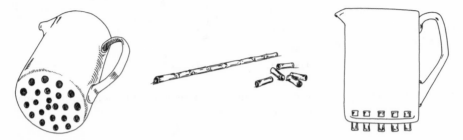

Figure 15D: Parisheka Pitcher

The Rope Cot

Traditionally, a rope cot 6 feet long, 4 feet wide, and 3 feet high is used for svedana treatment when heat or steam is to be generated from below the patient. Rope cots are easily assembled by tying pieces of rope over a sturdy wooden frame. (See sketch below.)

Alternately, you may use a cot with a canvas cover.

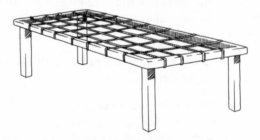

Figure 16D: Rope Cot

Droni: Grooved, Wooden Massage Table

Traditionally, the massage table or droni used in pancha karma treatment is carved from wood such as khadira or sandalwood. A 1-inch deep and 2-inch wide gutter is carved out in the rim of the outer edge of the table's surface, with a 3-inch opening at the center of the foot end of the table. This allows the oils which are poured on the subject in therapies such as shirodhara and parisheka to flow off and

484

away from the table. A container is placed under the opening at the foot of the table to receive the used oil or decoction.

Generally, the droni is approximately 6 feet thick, with a gradual slope, the head of the droni being one inch higher than the foot end, allowing the fluids to flow down and away. Without the support of legs, the droni is usually placed directly on the floor, and the attendants perform the oil therapies in a squatting or kneeling position. A modern droni may be constructed with 3 1/2 foot legs.

A wooden dowel, approximately 4 inches in diameter, is generally placed as a head rest for the patient to prevent the face from being immersed in oil while lying on the stomach.

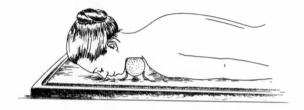

Figure 17D: Droni Table and Neck Rest

APPENDIX E

TECHNIQUES AND PROCEDURES FOR PREPARING FORMULAS AND RECIPES

Cleaning and Washing Grains and Legumes

Cleaning:

1. Spread a clean piece of cloth or natural burlap on a clean kitchen or dining room floor. If these cloths are not available, you may use a shallow, flat basket.

2. Place no more than a fortnight's worth of unwashed grain or legumes in the center of the cloth, and squat or sit in a comfortable position.

3. Spread out a few handfuls of grain or legumes and sift to find debris such as stones, husks, and stems. Place the debris in a container until you can return it back to the earth. While you may invite your family or friends to join you in this activity, be alert and maintain quiet. Do not allow children to play with the grain or legumes, or fight and become excited. You may also choose this as your still time and perform this sadhana alone.

4. When finished, brush and fold the cleaning cloth and store in a clean place until your next use. Place the sorted grain or legumes in a glass jar with a tight-fitting lid and store in a cool, moisture-free location.

Washing:

1. Grains and legumes should not be washed before meal preparation time. Fill a large bowl with cold water and the amount of grain or legumes you need. Wash the grains or legumes with your hands, and remove any remaining bran or husks that float to the surface.

2. Drain and rinse several times until the water runs clear.

Grinding Grains and Legumes

Use a large hand grinder that clamps on to the kitchen counter or table. Place approximately one cup of grain or legumes at a time into the mouth of grinder. Position a bowl under the large open-spouted end and begin grinding by turning the handle. If a fine, smooth consistency is needed, grind once more.

Legumes and grains may also be ground in a very large mortar with a pestle. This method takes about thirty minutes to grind two to three pounds of legume or grain. Grains and legumes may be ground dry or wet to prepare your ubtans.

Juicing Fresh Ginger

To do this by hand, all you need is a ceramic hand grater and a piece of plump, fresh ginger. Peel half a finger-length of fresh ginger and grate to a fine pulp. Wash your hands and, placing the grated ginger in your stronger hand, squeeze the pulp firmly over a small bowl. Retain the pulp, using it for cooking or to make fresh ginger tea. Half a finger-length of ginger makes approximately two tablespoons of juice.

Making Fresh Coconut Milk

To select a fresh coconut, shake it to be sure there is water inside; fresh coconut is also usually heavier than it looks. Preheat oven to 400 degrees F. Using a sharp knife or ice pick, pierce the two "eyes" and let the water drain out of the coconut. Place the coconut in the pre-heated oven for ten minutes, or until the shell begins to crack. Break open the coconut with a hammer and let cool for ten minutes. Pry nut pieces away from the shell with a small knife, and scrape off the thin brown film. Using a hand grinder, grate the coconut pieces; then place one cup of the grated coconut in a stainless steel bowl with two cups of warm water and let sit for thirty minutes. With clean hands, gather the grated coconut and place in the center of a clean cloth over the same bowl. Wrapping the cloth tightly around the coconut, twist both ends in opposite directions; continue to squeeze until all of the milk is released into soaking water.

Pour coconut milk into a jar and use fresh. For a thicker milk, use less water. The grated coconut may be used in a salad or for soups.

Making Fresh Almond Milk

In a large bowl, combine four cups of hot water and one cup whole almonds and let sit for thirty minutes, until skins loosen. Slip skins off with your fingers and discard, along with the soaking water. Place skinned almonds and two cups of cold water in a hand grater and puree for three to five minutes, until the nuts are completely dissolved and the milky liquid is smooth. Pour into a jar and use right away. For a thicker milk, use less water.

Making Tamarind Paste from Dried Tamarind

Cut a two-inch piece from a slab of dried tamarind and place it in two cups of boiling water. Remove from heat and let soak for four hours. Remove the softened tamarind from the water and squeeze it with clean hands into a bowl, releasing the pulp from the roughage. Rub the roughage inside a fine sieve and scrape whatever pulp comes through the sieve into the bowl. It is best to prepare tamarind just before using, allowing for sufficient preparation time. The roughage is a good addition to dhals and soups, but should be removed and discarded before serving.

Preparing Vegetables for the Healing Diet

The ancient Vedic cultures approached food and the preparation of food with great reverence. For any food to retain its vital power and taste depends completely upon how we handle it. Unruly scrambling, tossing, chopping or throwing does not lend itself to a splendid meal. Each vegetable is to be approached with utmost respect for its universal nature.

The natural grain of each and every vegetable will tell you how it is to be cleaned and cut. Vegetables that grow on a stalk, such as broccoli and celery, are first to be cut lengthwise and then, if smaller pieces are needed, horizontally. Leafy greens are to be cut along the grain of their leaves; their stems may be diced horizontally. Avoid using the coarse or purplish parts of the stems. Elongated root vegetables, such as carrots, daikon, and parsnips, may be cut in many ways. The initial cut needs to be a horizontal one, on a slant. Each cut of the root vegetable should incorporate the air/space (top) energy, the earth/water (bottom) energy, and the fire (middle) energy. Round root vegetables, such as rutabagas, potatoes, and onions, have a grain that runs along their center length. Onions and potatoes in particular endure the most unjust handling—they are generally cut opposite their grain. Cut in lengthy slices, these vegetables taste better.

Cutting Techniques

Cabbage:

Shredding: Cut cabbage in half, lengthwise, along center grain, and then again in quarters. Remove core from all four quarters. Place each quarter lengthwise on cutting board and slice thinly along the grain.

Matchsticks: To produce matchsticks, cut cabbage cores in pieces 1/4 inch thick. Place pieces in stacks one inch high and cross-cut at a thickness of 1/16 inch.

Large leafy greens:

Diagonal slice: Fold each leaf lengthwise along its spine and cut off the stem. Open the leaves and stack them ten to twelve pieces high. Fold the stack over along the spine and slice thinly on the diagonal, along leaf grain. Gather the stems and cut finely on the diagonal as well.

Half-moon stem: Whenever possible use your stems. Cut lengthwise down the center of stems. Place center face down on cutting board. Cut on the diagonal, or straight across for a half-moon effect, 1/4 inch thick.

Broccoli/Cauliflower:

Flowerettes: Cut below the flower and hold flower face down on cutting board. Cut into the stem toward the flower. Do not cut through flower. Gently pull flowers apart with your hands.

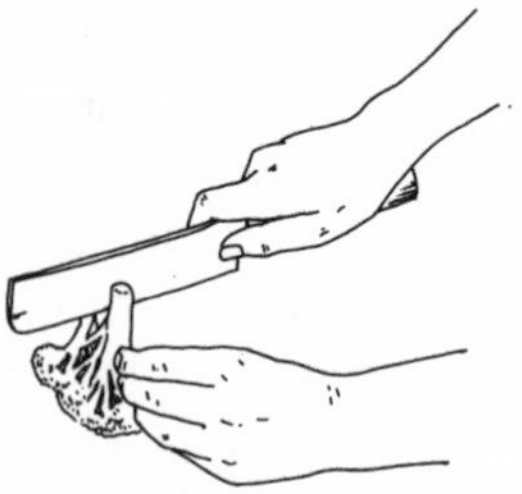

Long root vegetables:

Shavings: Hold root vegetable in your hand, away from your body. Shave the vegetable by chipping away in thin or thick shavings.

Figure 1E: Broccoli Cutting

Matchsticks: Slice root vegetable on the diagonal, 1/8 inch thick. Place the slices in stacks one inch high and cross-cut 1/16 inch thick to produce a matchstick effect.

Half-rounds: Slice root vegetable in half lengthwise. Place center down on cutting board. Cross-cut in half-rounds to desired thickness.

Quarter-rounds: Slice root vegetable in half, then again in quarters, lengthwise. Place center down on cutting board. Cross-cut in quarter-rounds to desired thickness.

Log-cut: Cut root vegetable in pieces two inches long. Cut each piece into vertical slabs. Slice each slab lengthwise at a thickness of 1/4 to 1/2 inch.

Roll-cut: Cut root vegetable once on the diagonal at the one inch point. Roll the vegetable 90 degrees away from you and cut again in the same way. Continue rolling vegetable back and forth, repeating the process until the whole vegetable is cut.

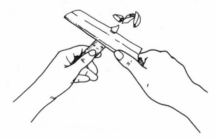

Figure 2E: Shavings

Small round vegetables:

Cubes: Slice vegetable into three vertical slabs. Slice each slab into vertical logs. Cross-cut in cubes of desired size.

490

Onions:

Crescents: Cut onion in half, lengthwise, along center grain. Place each half face down on cutting board. Slice lengthwise along the grain in crescents of desired thickness.

Minced: Cut onion in half, lengthwise, along center grain. Place each half face down on cutting board. Turn the cutting board and cross-cut against the grain to desired size.

Squash:

Halves: Remove stem with a paring knife and cut squash in half, lengthwise, along center grain. Remove fibrous innards and seeds with a spoon.

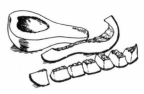

Chunks: Prepare as for halves, then place halves face down on cutting board. Cut each half lengthwise down the center. Turn cutting board and cross-cut against the grain to desired size.

Figure 3E: Squash Cut

STERILIZING PROCEDURES FOR TREATMENT UTENSILS

These measures are to be used in all snehana and svedana therapies involving the application of pastes, poultices, or plasters directly to inflamed, ulcerated, open sores and for other physical conditions which could easily become contaminated.

Before making the paste or poultice, sterilize all utensils used in its preparation and application, as well as all containers that will hold the ingredients.

To sterilize, place containers and accessories—including scissors, spoons, and so on—in a large pot of boiling water. Cover and boil over medium heat for two hours. Remove from heat and let cool. Remove equipment with stainless steel tongs and place in large zip-lock plastic bags until they are to be used.

If bandages and towels are to be used, these materials must be soaked in hot water for two hours and dried in a dust-free area under direct sunlight before using. Immediately after drying, they must be placed in a zip-lock plastic bag until used. Alternatively, sterilized bandages available in medical supply stores may be used.

Use only sterilized gauze, available in medical supply stores, for cleaning areas to be treated.

Before beginning treatment, wash your hands in the warm witch hazel solution and dry with a clean cotton hand towel.

Sterilize surgical rubber gloves so that your hands are not in contact with the affected area nor with the herbal paste and other formulas.

Use only stainless steel containers and accessories, e.g., spatulas, that are new or have been used specifically for making formulas under sterilized conditions.

If a suribachi and pestle, food grinder, or mortar and pestle and rubber spatula are used, sterilize them in the same way as the stainless steel containers.

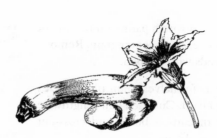

APPENDIX F

MILK PRODUCTS RECIPES

Ghee (ghrita or sarpi)

Ghee is one of the most ancient and sattvic foods known. Good for all doshas, it is a specific for Vata and Pitta, with minimal use recommended for Kapha types.

Ghee keeps indefinitely without refrigeration, the elements that cause butter to spoil having been removed. It simply needs to be kept covered and free from water or contaminants. Always dip into your ghee jar with a clean spoon.

Maintain a calm mind and clean appearance while preparing your ghee. Making ghee is one of the most healing food sadhanas, giving grace to our lives when done regularly.

Ghee Making

1 lb unsalted organic butter

1 heavy stainless steel saucepan

1 stainless steel spoon

Sterilize the storage jar, saucepan, and spoon in advance by filling with or immersing in boiling water. Cook the butter gently over moderate heat for approximately fifteen minutes. The foam that surfaces during the heating process will settle on the bottom of the pan as sediment. Watch carefully to avoid burning and stir occasionally. When the ghee begins to boil silently, with only a trace of air bubbles on the surface, it is done. Let cool and then pour into the clean container, making sure that the sediment remains on the bottom of the saucepan.

Note: The sediment may be taken as a snack. Vata and Pitta types may take it mixed with one-half teaspoon of brown sugar; Kapha types may also use it occasionally but without the sugar.

Fresh Butter *(makhan)*

    2 qt organic milk
    1 heavy stainless steel pot
    1 stainless steel spoon
    1 cool clay or enamel coated cast-iron pot

Sterilize your butter-making utensils by filling with or immersing in boiling water. Bring milk to a boil and let cool; bring it to a boil twice more. Skim cream off the top and store in a covered pot at 60° F for one week. (In India it is kept in an earthen pot known as a ghara.) Store the remaining milk in a cool place.

Place the cream in a large wooden or stainless steel bowl and whip briskly with a whisk until it thickens. (In India, butter is whipped with several chopsticks tied together with strings.) When the butter begins to emerge and separate into flakes, add two handfuls of crushed ice, which will make it lumpy. Mold the butter firmly with your hands, allowing the buttermilk to separate. When no more buttermilk remains, rinse the butter with ice cold water. If you are not going to go on to make ghee, add a few pinches of fine rock salt, if desired. Garnish butter with fresh herbs, according to type, just before serving. Make fresh butter as needed for a fortnight's use.

Yoghurt *(dadhi)*

    2 qt organic milk
    6 tbs plain organic yoghurt (as starter)
    2 heavy stainless steel saucepans
    1 long stainless steel spoon
    1 cooking thermometer

Sterilize one of the heavy saucepans by filling it with boiling water. In it, heat the milk over medium-low heat until it comes to a boil. Stir constantly to avoid sticking or burning. Let the milk boil for fifteen minutes, until it has reduced by one-eighth and is fairly thick. Set aside until the temperature reaches about 118° F.

Sterilize the second saucepan and spoon. When the milk has cooled to 115° F, pour one cup into the newly sterilized pan. Add starter (be sure it contains acidophilus culture from organic brand of yoghurt) and whip until smooth. When remaining milk has reached 112° F., add it to the starter mixture and blend well with the long spoon.

Cover pan with a clean heavy cotton cloth and quickly move yoghurt to a warm place, 90 - 100° F. If the temperature is too warm or too cool, yoghurt will not form. An oven with a gas pilot light is an ideal place; the best temperature is 100° F.

Let the yoghurt sit for six to seven hours. If it is not firm enough, let it sit for a few hours more. Remove and keep in a cool place. Use yoghurt within three days.

Vata types: serve with warming spices, such as cardamom, cinnamon, and black pepper, and dilute with water, if desired.

Pitta types: serve with turmeric or neem leaves, or sweeten with dried fruits, jams, jaggery, maple syrup, or Sucanat; dilute with water, if desired.

Kapha types: use only occasionally and add pinches of turmeric, black pepper, cardamom and other Kapha-reducing spices.

Fresh Buttermilk *(chaach)*

When cream is churned into butter, the milky whey left in the container is buttermilk (see above). After you mold the butter, gather the buttermilk into an earthenware, stainless steel, or glass jug. Store in a cool place and use within forty-eight hours.

This natural buttermilk can be used as a starter to make curd cheese. Pure buttermilk is most beneficial for Vata types.

Milk Dough *(khoa)*

When milk is boiled until most of its water has evaporated, the soft mass of dough that remains is called khoa. It is usually sweet due to the natural sugars in lactose. Often, jaggery is added to the milk when the dough is to be used to make sweets.

AYURVEDIC RESOURCES AND SUPPLIERS

The resources and suppliers herein listed are not necessarily endorsed by the author. Use the guidelines set out in Chapter Nine, Part One to screen any Ayurvedic resources, and in particular the treatment centers, to your personal satisfaction.

AYURVEDIC STUDIES

Nutrition and Sadhanas
Teachers trained by Bri. Maya Tiwari

Wise Earth Foundation
Bri. Maya Tiwari
25 Howland Road, #R8
Asheville, North Carolina 28804
(704) 258-9999
(Re-opens Spring 1996, for Teachers and Practitioners Training Programs only.)

Ayurvedic Center of New Jersey
Gandharva Sauls
263 Teaneck Road
Ridgefield Park, NJ 07660
(201) 440-3106

Omaha Yoga Center
Aparna Susan Gillespie
6105 Maple Street, Suite A
Omaha, NE 68104
(402) 553-8250

Prem Leena Dillingham
1705 14th Street
Boulder, CO 80302
(303) 449-0295

Rasa Yoga Studio
Ketul
246 West 80th Street
New York, New York 10024
(212) 875-0475

Rasmali Rosemary Jordan
166 2nd Avenue, #3D
New York, New York 10003
(212) 228-7926

Vandita Teresa Bradford
4150 Darley Street, Suite 6
Boulder, CO 80303
(303) 499-9374

General Ayurvedic Studies

American Institute of Vedic Studies
P.O. Box 8357
Santa Fe, NM 87501
(505) 983-9385
Correspondence Course in Ayurveda by Dr. David Frawley

Ayurvedic Healing Arts Center
16508 Pine Knoll Rd.
Grass Valley, CA 95945
(916) 274-9000

Ayurvedic Institute & Wellness Center
P.O. Box 23445
Albuquerque, NM 87192-1445
(505) 291-9698
Correspondence Course "Lessons and Lectures in Ayurveda" by Dr. Robert E.
Svoboda

Himalayan Institute
RR1, Box 400
Honesdale, PA 18431
(800) 822-4547

Institute for Wholistic Education
33719 116th St., Box SH
Twin Lakes, WI 53181
(414) 889-8501
Correspondence Course in Ayurveda

Lotus Ayurvedic Center
4145 Clares Street, Suite D
Capitola, CA 95010
(408) 479-1667

Ayurvedic Treatment Centers

Ayurveda at Spirit Rest
P.O. Box 3537
Pagosa Springs, CO 81147-3537
(970) 264-2573

Ayurvedic Institute & Wellness Center
P.O. Box 23445
Albuquerque, NM 87192-1445
(505) 291-9698

Center for Mind, Body Medicine
P.O. Box 1048
La Jolla, CA 92038
(619) 794-2425

Diamond Way Health Associates
214 Girard Boulevard, N.E.
Albuquerque, NM 87106
(505) 265-4826

Integrated Health Systems
3855 Via Nova Marie, #302D
Carmel, CA 93923
(408) 476-5130

Dr. Lobsang Rapgay
2206 Benecia Avenue
West Los Angeles, CA 90064
(310) 282-9918

Lotus Ayurvedic Center
4145 Clares Street, Suite D
Capitola, CA 95010
(408) 479-1667

Ayurvedic Herbal Suppliers

Auroma International
P.O. Box 1008-SH
Silver Lake, WI 53170
(414) 889-8569

Ayur Herbal Corporation
P.O. Box 6390 SH
Santa Fe, NM 87502
(414) 889-8569

Ayurveda Center of Santa Fe
1807 Second St., Suite 20
Santa Fe, NM 87505
(505) 983-8898

Ayurvedic Institute & Wellness Center
11311 Menaul N.E., Suite A
Albuquerque, NM 87112
(505) 291-9698

Ayush Herbs Inc.
10025 N.E. 4th Street
Bellevue, WA 98004
(800) 925-1371

Bazaar of India Imports, Inc.
1810 University Avenue
Berkley, CA 94703
(800) 261-7662

Devi Inc.
Shivani Ayurvedic Beauty Products
P.O. Box 377
Lancaster, MA 01523
(508) 368-0066

Frontier Herbs
P.O. Box 229
Norway, Iowa 52318
(800) 669-3275

Kanak
P.O. Box 13653
Albuquerque, NM 87192-3653
(505) 275-2469

Khenpa Co.
Ayurvedic Beauty Products
17595 Harvard, Suite C-531
Irvine, CA 92714
(714) 778-0222

Lotus Brands, Inc.
P.O. Box 325-SH
Twin Lakes, WI 53181
(414) 889-8561

Lotus Ayurvedic Center
4145 Clares Street, Suite D
Capitola, CA 95010
(408) 479-1667

Lotus Fulfillment Service
33719 116th Street-SH
Twin Lakes, WI 53181
(414) 889-8501
Retail mail order supplier of Ayurvedic books and herbal products.

Lotus Light
P.O. Box 1008-SH
Silver Lake, WI 53170
(414) 889-8501

Tej Beauty Enterprises, Inc.
162 West 56th Street, Room 201
New York, NY 10019
(212) 581-8136

For hard to find herbs, oils or substances contact the Ayurvedic Institute of New Jersey at (201) 440-3106 (open: Spring 1996).

Pancha Karma Kitchen Equipment

Bazaar of India Imports, Inc.
1810 University Avenue
Berkley, CA 94703
(800) 261-7662
Carries a full line of Indian kitchen equipment, including the interchangeable stainless steel sieve (chalni), stone mortars and pestles (sil batta), and the hand stone with stone bed (himan dasta); cast-iron frying pans (tava) for chapati making; tapered rolling pins in many sizes. Will ship throughout the U.S.

Earth Fare
Attn: Roger Derrough
66 Westgate Parkway
Asheville, NC 28806
(704) 253-7656
Carries hand grinders and suribachi clay pots and bowls.
(Also check Japanese food stores for these items.)

Garber Hardware
49 Eighth Avenue
NY, NY 10014
Carries hand grinders, but no mail order.
(Also check old-fashioned hardware stores.)

Sesam Muhle Natural Products
R.R. #1
Durham, Ontario
Canada, NOGIRO
(519) 369-6326
Carries a line of hand grinders and flakers for grains and legumes, made in Germany.

Taj Mahal Imports
1594 Woodcliff Drive, N.E.
Atlanta, GA 30329
(404) 321-5940
Carries a full line of Indian kitchen equipment, including the interchangeable stainless steel sieve (chalni), stone mortars and pestles (sil batta), and the hand stone with stone bed (himan dasta); cast-iron frying pans (tava) for chapati making; tapered rolling pins in many sizes. Will ship throughout the U.S.
(Also check traditional Mexican stores for large grain-grinding stone mortar and pestle.)

Organic Milk/Certified Raw Milk Suppliers

Organic milk comes from cows that are given grain feed free of antibiotics, pesticides, and growth hormones. It is pasteurized at the minimum allowable temperature but is not homogenized. Certified raw milk is equally healthful. It is neither pasteurized nor homogenized. Most health food stores will order these products for you if they don't already carry them. The following suppliers can be contacted by your local health food store. In some cases, they can deliver to you directly.

Alta Dena Certified Raw Milk
P.O. Box 388
City of Industry, CA 91747
(818) 964-6401
(non-pasteurized, non-homogenized milk)

Natural Horizons, Inc.
7490 Clubhouse Road
Boulder, CO 80301
(303) 530-2711
(organic /pasteurized, non-homogenized milk; whole, low-fat, skim buttermilk and cream)

Organic Valley Family of Farms
c/o Cropp Cooperative
La Farge, WI
(608) 625-2602
(organic butter, non-homogenized low-fat milk)

GLOSSARY OF SANSKRIT TERMS

Although all Sanskrit terms have been explained when first introduced within the text, the following extensive glossary is provided to facilitate learning of the many important Sanskrit terms used in Ayurveda.

abhyanga - anointing body with oil or ghee

accha peya - pure cow's ghee

agni - bodily fire, particularly digestive fire

ahamkara - ego; the "I" notion; cosmic memory recorder of all lives

ahara rasa - ingested nutrients, before they are digested

aja - goat; one who transcends the cycle of births

ajna - limitless power; name of sixth chakra

akasha - space; principle of vacuity

akshitarpana - herbal decoction used to revive eyes

alambusha - one of fourteen nadis; starts at anus and ends in mouth

alepanam - application of astringent plaster

alochaka - fire of eyes; one of five fires of Pitta

ama - undigested, foul-odored remnants of food in bodily channels

anahata- fearless, unafflicted; nature of the black antelope, symbol and name of fourth chakra

anna lepa sveda - fomentation therapy where poultice is applied to whole body

annam - literally, "that which grows on the earth"; food

annavaha srotas - digestive system or channels

antahkarana - inner or psychic instrument, referring to the mind (manas), intellect (buddhi) and ego memory (ahamkara)

anuvasana - decoction generally used in enema therapy

apana - one of five bodily airs; air controlling ejection of bodily wastes

artava - menstrual fluid

artava dhatu - ovum

artavavaha srotas - menstrual system or female reproductive channels

ashmaghna sveda - sudation on a hot stone slab

ashtapana - another term used for decoction enema therapy

Astanga Hridaya - Ayurvedic text written by Vagbhatta

asthi dhatu - bone and cartilage tissue

Atharva Veda - one of four principle Vedas

Atman - indwelling spirit; soul within body; Conscious Self

avagahana sveda - sudation in a hot tub

avalambaka - water dosha of heart; one of the five waters of Kapha

avapeda nasya - introduction of soft paste into the nasal passages

Ayurveda - knowledge of life; Vedic science of health

bala - strength

bandhana sveda - fomentation therapy where poultice is applied to a localized area of the body

baspa sveda - fomentation occurring in a traditionally designed wooden box, whereby the head of the person remains outside of the box

Bharata Bhumi - ancient name of India, land of Bharata; land of dharma

bhasma - literally, "ash"; incinerated metal or mineral used as potent, powdered remedy

bhrajaka - heat of the skin; one of the five fires of Pitta

bhu sveda - sudation on heated surface of the earth

bija - seed mantra

bodhaka - water of the tongue; one of the five waters of Kapha

brahmacarini - student of the Vedas; observing a monastic life

Brahma Randhra - most sacred aperture of the body, situated at the center of the cranium

brahmin - spiritual caste; one of the four castes delineated in the Hindu scriptures

brhmana - tonification or strengthening therapy

buddhi - faculty of personal wisdom; resolve of the mind; the intellect; Buddhi - Mercury, son of Shiva; deity who rules Wednesday

chai - Indian tea mixed with milk

chakra - wheel; seven energy centers of consciousness in the body

Charaka - ancient Ayurvedic scholar

Charaka Samhita - Charaka's treatise on Ayurveda

churna - powder

collyrium - Ayurvedic salves for eyes

darbha - type of grass used in Ayurvedic medicine

deva (devata) - generic name for the gods in the Hindu scriptures

devadatta - one of the five subsidiary airs

Devanagari - means of communication between the gods; later, translated as Samskritam (Sanskrit); one of several scripts in which Sanskrit may be written

dhanamjaya - one of five subsidiary airs

dhani - audible or imperfect sound

dhara chatti - see dhara patra

dhara patra - treatment pot made from metal or clay used to drop oil on head

dharane - to sustain

dharma - right action according to the laws of nature

dhatu - tissue element of the body

dhmapana - introduction of medicated powders into the nasal passages via a straw or tube

dhoma nasya - inhalation of medicated vapors

dhoti - cloth to wrap the lower body

dosha - literally, "that which can go out of balance"; bodily humor

droni - traditional massage table made from woods such as sandalwood, bilva, khadira, and arjuna

Gaja - Lord of herbivorous animals and keeper of earth's memory of plants and herbs; the elephant that represents the fifth chakra

gandhari - one of fourteen nadis; begins below the left eye and ends at the big toe of the left foot

gandusa - retention of fluid in the mouth

Ganesha - Ganapati; elephant-headed Lord, son of Shiva; one who blesses all beginnings and renders them auspicious; remover of obstacles

garbha-pinda - fluid state of embryo; cosmic womb

ghara - earthen pot

go - cow; sacred scripture

Gopala - protector of the scriptures and of cows; another name for Lord Krishna

grisma - Sanskrit term for summer, one of the six seasons in Ayurveda

guna - attribute or respect, as in the three gunas of Maya

guru - quality of heaviness; spiritual teacher; Guru - Jupiter; deity who rules Thursday

gurukula - traditional school for disseminating knowledge of Vedas

hastajihva - one of fourteen nadis; begins below the right eye and ends at the big toe of the left foot

hemanta - Sanskrit term for early winter, one of the six seasons in Ayurveda

holaka sveda - sudation on a daubed surface of the earth

ida - one of two main nadis; begins in the left genital and ends at the left nostril; breath which flows through the left nostril; lunar nadi

indriyas - five senses

Isvara - Vedic name for the omniscient Lord, when used in association with creation

japa - repetition of mantras

jentaka sveda - sudation in a specially designed sweat lodge

jiva - individual soul

jivana - invigoration; life

kala- nutritional membrane for tissues; "body crystal"

kalari- ancient form of martial arts originating in south India

kala vasti - series of sixteen enemas

kambalika - soup made with yoghurt, urad bean and sesame oil

kapha - biological water humor

karma - bondage to action; cause of rebirth

karma vasti - series of thirty enemas

karna purana - dripping fluids into the ears

karshu sveda - sudation in an earth pit

kavalagraha - holding liquid in the mouth for a comfortable period of time

khada - spicy vegetable or herbal soup generally made with buttermilk

kichadi - mixture of rice and mung bean

kitta - waste

kledaka - water of digestion; one of the five waters of Kapha

krekara - one of the five subsidiary airs

Krishna - Gopala, protector of the scriptures and teacher of self-knowledge in the Bhagavad Gita

krushara- thick grain gruel

kuhu - one of fourteen nadis; begins in the throat and ends in the genitals

kumbhika sveda - sudation from a pitcher of warm decoction

kundalini - primal energy of manifestation symbolized by a coiled serpent at the coccyx of the spine

kupa sveda - sudation on a daubed surface of the earth

kurma - one of the five subsidiary airs

kuti sveda - sudation in a specially designed sweat lodge

langhana - depletion or reducing therapy

lassi - traditional Indian beverage made from yoghurt, milk, and fragrant herbs, generally taken after meals to aid digestion

lepa - plastering body with medicated substances

majja dhatu - bone marrow and nerve tissue

makara - crocodile; symbol of sensual movement and trickery

mala - garland; rosary of beads

malas - bodily wastes

mamsa dhatu - muscle tissue

manas - mind

manda - cooked rice at the bottom of the pot

Mangala - Mars; deity who rules Tuesday

manovaha - channels that carry mental energy

mantha - thin gruel made from rice and ghee

mantra - sacred sounds; group of sounds cosmically designed to stimulate certain physical and physic centers of body

mardana - mild pressure massage

marma - anatomical reflex points of the body; vital seats of pranic energy

marsha nasya - introduction of medicated oils into the nasal passages

masala - combination of spices ground together; spicy mixture

masthiskya - medicinal paste applied to the head

maya - cosmic, creative power; manifestation; relative reality

medas - fat

medas dhatu - fat tissue

moksha - a "state" in which the potential material and vibrations for future rebirths on all planes of existence are completely resolved; liberation from the cycle of birth and death

mutravaha srotas - urinary system

nadi - subtle channel within the nervous system made of fine threads of fluid; refers to the gross form in terms of nerves, veins, and so on; pathways of breath; Ayurvedic name for pulse

nadi sveda - steam application through a hose

naga - one of the five subsidiary airs

nasya - nasal insufflation

navana nasya - insufflation of unctuous substances or powders to clear nasal passages

niruha - oils generally used in Ayurvedic enema therapy

odana- thick porridge

ojas - perfected essence of dhatus when bodily system is in excellent order; glow of health

paca kizhi sveda - sudation with green leaf poultice

pachaka - one of the five fires of Pitta; fire of digestion in the stomach

padabhyanga - Ayurvedic foot massage

padaghata - anointing feet with oil

pancha karma - five cleansing therapies of Ayurveda: emesis, enema (two forms), purgation, and nasal medications

parisheka - fomentation with an affusion of Ayurvedic herbs

Patanjali - founder-renovator of the classical Yoga system

payasam - sweet fluid porridge

payasvini - one of fourteen nadis; located in the right ear lobe and connecting with the cranial nerves

peya - decoction made from rice and ghee

phala - fruit

phanita - sticky candy made from sugar cane juice

pichu - process of placing an oil soaked cloth on the forehead

pinda sveda - fomentation therapy with use of a poultice wrapped in a bolus

pingala - one of two main nadis; begins in the right eye and ends in the right genital; solar power; breath of right nostril

pitta - biological fire humor

prabhava - specific action without regard to the general rule of the three stages of taste; exception to the rule; special action of herbs

pradeha - non-absorbent plaster

prakriti - first creation; individual constitution

pralepa - thin, cold layer of plaster

prana - life breath; first of the five airs of the body; vital force; air of the heart

pranavaha - channels that carry prana; force of prana, or breath

pranayama - yogic breathing exercises

prasthara - fomentation on a bed of poultice

prinana - joy infused from nature

puja - religious ceremony

purana - fullness

510

purishavaha srotas - excretory system

pusha - one of fourteen nadis; begins at the right ear and ends at the big toe of the left foot

rajas (rajasic) - activity or aggressive force of creation; one of the three gunas

rakta dhatu - blood tissue

rakta moksha (mokshana) - therapeutic blood letting

raktavaha srotas - circulatory system (hemoglobin portion)

ranjaka - heat of the blood, operating in liver; one of the five fires of Pitta

rasa - initial taste in the three stages of taste; literally, "external beauty," or "maturity"

rasa dhatu - plasma tissue

rasayana - rejuvenation therapy

Rawal - religious head of the Hindus

rtusandhi - junction between two seasons or two phases within a season

rukshana - dehydration therapy

rupa - form

sadhaka - the third fire found in the heart, central to the activity of Pitta; also the one who performs sadhana (the wholesome activities which bring us into harmony with nature)

sadhana - wholesome activity practiced with presence of mind in harmony with nature; helps to revive and awaken cognitive memory

sadhu - simple person

sahasrara - literally, "a thousand petals"; seventh chakra; spatially boundless dwelling

saindhava (sendha namak) - Ayurvedic rock salt

sama - three doshas in a state of sameness

samadhi - silent breath

samana - air of the stomach; one of the five airs of Vata

samhita - text

samskaras - karmic impressions from past lives carried in the subtle body

samvahana - shampooing the body with a warm decoction

sankara sveda - generic name for fomentation therapy where poultice is used

sarada - Sanskrit term for autumn, one of the six seasons in Ayurveda

Saraswati - goddess of knowledge; one of fourteen nadis; begins at the base of the tongue and ends in the vocal chords; sonority of vocal prowess

sattva (sattvic) - central aspect of the three gunas; cosmic force of balance and contentment

shakti - cosmic feminine force; power, energy, power of consciousness

shamana - therapy which nurtures and adds strength to the body; palliative measure

Shani - Saturn; deity who rules Saturday

shankhini - one of fourteen nadis, begins in the throat and ends on the left side of the anus

shikha - crest of the head

shiro abhyanga (shirobhyanga) - anointing the head with oil; head massage

shirodhara - dripping medicated decoction on the forehead

shiro tarpana - application of oil to the head

shirovasti - applying oil to the shaven head

Shiva - pure being or pure consciousness

shodhana - therapy which consists of elimination procedures; purification measure

shukra - collective refined essence belonging to shukra dhatu; refined emotion of love; semen, reproductive fluid; the ovum of the female; Shukra - Sanskrit name for Venus; deity who rules Friday; giver of happiness or fame

shukra dhatu - sperm

shukravaha srotas - male reproductive system or channels

sisira - Sanskrit term for late winter, one of the six seasons in Ayurveda

sirovirechana - snuff inhalation therapy

slesaka - water of the joints; one of the five waters of Kapha

sleshma - another name for Kapha or phlegm

sneha - extravagant love; lubrication; name of the enema treatment in which only half cup of oil is used

snehana - external oelation of the body; lubrication therapy

snehapana - internal lubrication of the body

snehika dhoomapana - herbs mixed with oil or fat for therapeutic smoking

soma - potent nectar taken by the devas to give eternal strength; pleasure principle at work behind mind and senses

srotas - channels, as in the thirteen channels of circulation

sthambana - retention therapy

suksma - subtle

Surya - Sun; deity who rules Sunday

Sushruta - ancient Ayurvedic scholar

sushumna - central and main nadi, within spinal column, which accommodates all nadis

svedana - sudation or fomentation of body; sweat inducing therapy

swami - renunciate; one who knows Brahman and the Self to be One

taila - oil

Taittiriya - literally, "three birds"; one of the Upanishads which deals with Self-knowledge

takra dhara - medicated buttermilk

tamas (tamasic) - inert aspect of creation; one of the three gunas

tanmatra (tanmatric) - quantum energy aspect of the subtle elements that pervade both subtle and gross bodies

tarpaka - water of the sense organs; one of the five waters of Kapha

tarpana - thick gruel of rice, bean, black pepper and ghee

tejas - cool, refined universal fire; subtle, fire of the mind

tikta ghrita - pure ghee combined with bitter herbs

tridosha - three doshas in a state of balance

ubtan - fresh ground legume or grain flour traditionally used to cleanse the skin

udana - air of the throat; one of the five airs of Vata

udvartana - oil or dry massage for Kapha disorder

upadhatu - secondary tissue of the body

upanaha sveda - generic name for fomentation therapy where poultice is used

Upanishad - ancient Vedantic scripture of India

utkarita - pudding made from milk, yoghurt or cream

uttara vasti - douching enema

Vagbhatta - ancient Ayurvedic scholar

vairechanika dhoomapana - therapeutic smoking of dried herbs

vajikarana - aphrodisiac; virilization therapy

vamana - therapeutic vomiting; emesis therapy

varna - pure vibration; unmanifest sound

varsa - Sanskrit term for rainy season, one of the six seasons in Ayurveda

varuni - one of fourteen nadis, which originates between the throat and left ear and ends at the anus

vasanta - Sanskrit term for spring, one of the six seasons in Ayurveda

vasti - Ayurvedic enema therapy

vasti netra - hose used in enema therapy

vasti putaka - enema bag

vata - biological air humor

vayu - air or wind; another name for Vata

veda - knowledge

Vedanta - culmination of Vedas in the philosophy of knowledge of the Self

Vedas - ancient books of knowledge presenting the spiritual science of awareness; first knowledge on earth

Vedic - belonging to the Vedas

vicarana sneha - medicated ghee

vilepika - mixture of four parts water and one part rice

vipaka - post-digestive effect of herbs

virechana - purgation therapy; one of five cleaning actions used in pancha karma

virya - energetic effect of herbs as heating or cooling

vishvabhesaja - healing secret of the universe; universal medicine

vishvodara - one of fourteen nadis; exists in the umbilicus and energizes bodily prana

vyana - air of circulation; one of the five airs of Vata

vyayama - natural forms of exercise

Yama - Lord of death

Yama damstra - period of time between November 22 and December 9 when the earth begins its northward rotation around the sun

yashasvini - one of fourteen nadis; companion nadi to pingala which runs from the left ear to the big toe of the right foot

yavagu - mixture of six parts water and one part barley

yoga - psycho-physical practices aimed at Self-knowledge

yogavaha - that which enhances the effect of what it enjoins

yoga vasti - series of eight enemas

yogin (yogi) - one whose life is devoted to the practice of sadhanas to attain union with God

yusha - bean soup

Note 1: An English translation for the Sanskrit terms of the forty-three main marma points of the body is given in Chapter Four, where they are first mentioned.

Note 2: The Sanskrit names of the Vedic gods used in the prayers and mantras are explained in Chapter Nine, "The Healing Activities," where they are first introduced.

Note 3: The Sanskrit and English names (when available) of Ayurvedic herbs used in this book are given in Appendix B, the Glossary of Ingredients. In Appendix A, I have also provided some lists of Ayurvedic herbs traditionally used in pancha karma, with their Sanskrit, English and Latin names.

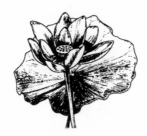

BIBLIOGRAPHY

Berliner, Ann, *Advaita Makaranda (Translation and Commentary)*, New Delhi, Asia Publishing House, 1990.

Bhishagratna, K.L., *Sushruta Samhita*, Varanasi, Chowkhamba, 1968.

Dash, Bhagwan, *Ayurvedic Treatment for Common Diseases*, Delhi Diary, 1974.

Dash, Bhagwan and Junius, Manfred M., *A Handbook of Ayurveda*, Delhi, Concept Publishing Co., 1983.

Devaraj, T.L., *The Panchakarma Treatment of Ayurveda*, Bangalore, Dhanvantari Oriental Publications, 1980.

Feuerstein, Georg, *The Yoga-Sutra of Patanjali (Translation and Commentary)*, Vermont, Inner Traditions International, 1989.

Gandhi, Maneka, *Brahma's Hair*, Delhi, Rupa & Co., 1989.

Govindan, S.W., *Techniques of Massage*, Varanasi, Sarva-Seva-Sangh-Prakashan, 1989.

Lad, Vasant, *Ayurveda: The Science of Self Healing*, Twin Lakes, Wisconsin, Lotus Press, 1984.

Mooss, N.S. (ed. and trans.), *Vagbhata's Astanga Hrdaya Samhita*, Kalpasthana, Kottayam, Kerala, Vaidyasarathy Press, 1984.

Mooss, Vayaskara N.S., *Ayurvedic Flora Medica*, Kottayam, Kerala Vaidyasarathy Press, 1978.

Murthy, Prof. K.R. Srikanta (trans.), *Madhava Nidanam*, Varanasi, Chaukhambha, 1987.

Rajan, Chandra, Kalidasa, *The Loom of Time*, Delhi, Penguin Books, 1990.

Sharma, P.V., *Caraka Samhita, (Sanskrit/English Edition)*, Delhi, Chaukhambha Orientalia, 1981.

Sharma, P.V., *Fruits and Vegetables in Ancient India*, Varanasi, Chaukhambha Orientalia, 1979.

Singh, Prof. R.H., *Pancha Karma Therapy*, Varanasi, Chaukhambha Sanskrit Series, 1992.

Sri Sankaracarya, *Srimad Bhagavad Gita Bhasya, Sanskrit Edition*, Madras Sri Ramakrishna Math, 1983.

Sri Sankaracarya, *Upadesha Sahasri (Sanskrit/English Edition)*, Madras, Sri Ramakrishna Math, 1984.

Svoboda, Robert E., *Ayurveda: Life, Health and Longevity*, Arkana, Penguin Books, 1992.

Svoboda, Robert E., *Prakruti: Your Ayurvedic Constitution*, Albuquerque, Geocom, 1988.

Tiwari, Maya, *Ayurveda, A Life of Balance*, Vermont, Healing Arts Press, 1994.

Tiwari, Maya; Kushi, Aveline and Esko, Wendy, *Diet For Natural Beauty*, New York and Tokyo, Japan Publishing, 1991.

INDEX

air
channels, 24
element, 6, 17, 269
ajwan, 453
in recipes, 354, 358, 360, 366, 378
medicinal uses, 323, 442
akasa, x, 48
akshitarpana, 164-169
alambusha nadi, 29
alcohol, 185
alepanam, 132-134
alertness, 13
allspice oil, 400
almond
essential oil, 209, 372
milk, 351, 369, 372
oil, 117, 462
aloe vera, 116, 179, 337, 340, 375,
442, 453
ama, 14, 17, 19, 22, 70, 181, 182, 397,
439, 440, 441, 442
amalaki, 299, 302, 329, 330, 344, 345,
356, 441
buttermilk, 143, 144
amaranth, 464
amavathahara oil, 198
amethyst, 72, 398, 399
amla, 208, 246, 250
amnesia, 346
anemia, 12, 24, 128, 192, 279, 290,
296, 299, 346, 391, 436, 443
anger, 18, 22, 25, 26, 179, 185, 403
angula, 394
animals, 50-51
anise, 375
anjali, 394
anna lepa sveda, 213-217

anorexia, 14, 24, 141, 146, 151, 155,
159, 160, 192, 205, 221, 236,
238, 245, 249, 252, 256, 259,
279, 290, 296, 440, 442
antahkarana, 37
antimony paste, 392
anu taila oil, 177
anus, 10, 25, 296
anuvasana vasti (see enema therapy)
anxiety, 24, 26, 141, 155, 174, 177,
178, 242
apamarga, 434
apana, 10-11, 30, 73
aphrodisiac, 438
appetite, 34, 42, 43, 142, 192, 221,
318, 441
loss of, 24, 74, 120, 146, 151, 182,
279, 397
apples, 367, 382
apricots, 282
aragvadha (see cassia, purging)
ardraka (see ginger)
arka leaves, 232, 300, 331, 434, 453
arm massage, 106-107
aroma therapy, 71, 72, 74, 76, 398,
399, 400
and massage, 116-118
aromatic mist, 138, 145, 150
artava dhatu, 17, 19
arteries, 7
arthritis, 8, 182, 192, 202, 205, 214,
221, 230, 236, 238, 246, 249,
252, 256, 259, 309, 317, 318,
328, 329, 440, 443
rheumatoid, 126, 182, 192, 202,
205, 214, 217, 235, 238, 245,
249, 256, 259, 309, 318, 441
asafoetida, 116, 365, 442-443

birds, 50
birth, 10, 52
  control, 335, 336, 437
bitter taste, 42, 268
blackberries, 382
blackberry oil, 162
blackouts, 26
bladder, 10, 67, 261, 310, 443
bleeding
  excessive, 25, 132, 146, 151, 229, 279, 397
  from upper pathways, 273, 290, 296
  from lower pathways, 279
  internal, 229, 436
  rectal, 324
blessed thistle, 339
blinking, 11
blood (see also *rakta*), 17
  channels, 25
  disorders, xiv, 74, 132, 139, 141, 146, 151, 192, 279, 346, 435, 436, 444
  fire of, 12
  hemoglobin, 325
  purification, 75, 439, 441, 442
  red corpuscles, 325
  sugar, 279
  to rejuvenate, 126
  tonic, 439
  transfusions, 310
  vessels, 22
blood-letting, 75, 268
blueberries, 382
bodhaka, 14-15, 43
body
  brushing, 74, 392, 398, 399, 400
  cavities, 67
  frame, 34
  temperature, 6, 12
  type (see constitution)

bolus, 195-201
  wrapping, 476
bone
  fractures, 130
  marrow, 17, 25-26, 139
  tissue (see also *asthi*), 17, 25, 309
brahma dandi, 298, 305, 454
Brahma Randhra, 101, 103
brahmi (see gotu kola)
brain, 15, 101, 102, 113, 173, 174, 440
brass, 117
breast
  cysts, 296
  milk, 27, 279, 296, 317
  pain, 318, 328, 329
  tumors, 296
breath, silent, 59
breathing (see also *pranayama*)
  and *nadis*, 29
  and nasal insufflation, 174
  and *prana*, 7, 16
  and *udana*, 8-9
  disorders, 24, 390, 443
brhmana, xiv, xv
broccoli, 371, 381, 490
bronchial disorders, 173, 178, 274
bronchitis, 8, 77, 217, 390, 436, 440, 442
bronze, 117
Brussels sprouts, 371, 382
buckwheat, 344, 378, 464-465
buddhi (wisdom), 8, 37-38, 52
Buddhi (deity), 426
bulgur, 365, 381
bulimia, 14
burdock root, 75, 455
burning sensation, 130, 132, 146, 151, 210, 229, 290, 436

creativity, 12, 29
crouching, 470
cucumber, 325
cumin
 black, 368, 454
 in recipes, 354, 355, 357, 358, 359,
  360, 361, 362, 365, 367, 368,
  370, 376, 377, 379, 380
 medicinal use, 288
cypress oil, 391
cysts, 201, 202, 221

dadima (see pomegranate)
daikon radish, 381
daily
 rituals, 390-400
 transitions, 406
dandelion leaves, 75, 383
dandruff, 139
danti, 268
dashamula, 73, 227, 232, 261, 262, 263,
  301, 455
 oil, 154, 197
dates, 356, 369, 372
 sugar, 365
days of the week, 425
death, 50
 and memory, 53, 55
 fear of, 19
 near-death experience, 41
dehydration, 306
 therapy (see *rukshana*)
deities, 425-427
delusions, 397
depression, 441
devadaru, 73

devadatta, 11
dhanamjaya, 11
dhanvantari oil, 197
dharmas, vii, 420
 sexual, 422-423
dhatus, 5, 16-17
 and tastes, 79-80
 chart, 20
 transformation of, 18-19
dhoomapana (see herbal smoke)
diabetes, 10, 25, 77, 146, 279, 325,
  436, 441
diarrhea, xvi, 10, 11, 26, 279, 324
diet, 343-386, 393
 and memory, 343-45
 energizing, 377-386
 glossary of substances, 450-451
 sattvic, 344, 351, 364-76
digestion (see also *agni*), 6, 10, 12, 13
 disorders of, 10, 12, 24, 146, 151,
  155, 217, 236, 238, 249, 279,
  290, 390, 430
 to improve, 109, 120, 128, 435,
  436, 437, 440, 442
digestive
 fire (see *agni*)
 teas, 289
dill, 218, 379, 382
discernment, 18
disease
 chronic, ii, xv, 23
 process, 68, 69
 stages of, 22-23
diuretic, 436
divination, 49-50
dizziness, 26
dokshi, 282, 285

527

female channels, 27
fennel seed
   in recipes, 362, 363, 366, 373
   medicinal uses, 161, 287, 289,
      320, 323, 325, 328, 340
   oil, 339, 372, 399
fenugreek, 218
fermentation, 352
fertility, 110, 336, 434
fever, 11, 210, 229, 279, 290, 296, 309,
      317, 390, 397, 436, 437, 442
figs, 324, 372
fingernails, 25, 34, 393
fire element (see also *tejas*), 6, 17, 434
flatus, 10, 435, 442, 443
flaxseed, 75
flexibility, 15, 128
flours for *ubtans*, 118-119
flowers, 398
flu, 173, 178, 217, 242, 440, 442
fomentation therapy (see *svedana*)
food
   categories, 344
   channels, 24
   combining, 25, 351
   first, 344
   quantities of, 350
foot massage, 104-105, 112-114, 400
formula preparation, 487-492
Friday, 426-427
fruit
   decoction, 356
   dried, 352
   for *pancha karma*, 456
   gel, 302-303
   shake, 382
   soup, 366-367

fungus, 437
gall bladder, 11, 67, 391
gandhari nadi, 29
gandusa, 159-160
gargling, 128, 159-164, 349, 391
   benefits, 160
   conditions treated, 159
   formulas, 161-164
garlic, 77, 117, 172, 179, 381
garnet, 76, 398, 400
gas (see flatus)
gastro-intestinal disorder, 8, 279, 290,
      296, 300, 317, 318
gems, 71, 72, 74, 76, 117, 398, 399, 400
genital organs, 25, 115
gentian, 298, 299, 306, 458
geranium oil, 209, 398
ghee, xv, 344, 348, 351, 456
   for emesis, 285
   for enemas, 324, 329
   for head treatments, 75, 150, 155
   for massage, 117, 144, 198, 199,
      209, 218, 444
   for nasal insufflation, 77, 179
   for *parisheka*, 226
   for purgation, 303, 307
   in bath, 261
   in herbal smoke, 286
   in plaster, 137
   in recipes, 330, 331, 332, 334
   medicated, 169, 444, 454
   recipe, 493
ginger
   compress, 121-122, 137
   in recipes, 356, 358, 359, 367, 373,
      374, 379, 381
   juice, 116, 383, 488
gynecological disorders, 296, 442

529

judgment, 56-57, 58
jujube (see *badri*)
Jupiter, 426
kala, 18
kalari, xii
kale, 381
kamala (see lotus)
kambalika, 351
Kapha, 3, 139
   cleansing therapies for, 76-77
   colors for, 393, 400
   daily cycles of, 66-68
   domains, 7
   elements of, 6, 32
   essential oils for, 76, 118, 138, 400
   exercise for, 400
   five waters of, 13-15
   functions of, 6
   gems for, 76
   herbs for, 118
   massage for, 93
   massage oils for, 117, 209, 400
   qualities of, 33
   sadhanas for, 400
   seasons and, 69-70, 76-77
   tastes for, 82-83
   ubtans for, 119
karanja leaves, 232, 435
karma, 9, 41, 52
karna purana, 170-172
karshu sveda, 183, 248-251
kaseesadi oil, 156, 157, 262, 263
kashmari, 323
katuki (see gentian)
kavalagraha (see gargling)
kesare oil, 73, 397, 398, 399
khada, 351

khadira
   oil, 235
   wood, 253, 329, 390
kichadi, 351, 360-361, 364, 377
kidneys, 67, 113, 261, 397, 442
   compress for, 121-122
   stones, 309
   to cleanse, 75
kindling, 240, 448-449
kitchen equipment, 469-471
kledaka, 13-14, 182
kottumcukadi oil, 198
krekara, 11
krushara, 351
ksheerabala oil, 198, 228, 262, 263
kudzu, 303, 366, 371, 376, 382, 458
kuhu nadi, 29
kumari (see aloe)
kumbhika sveda, 184, 241-244
kupa sveda, 184, 254-258
kurchi, 298, 304
kurma, 11
kusha grass, 191
kushta root, 251, 323
kuti sveda, 184, 251-254

lachrymal secretion, 164
langhana, xiv
lapis lazuli, 76, 398, 400
large intestine (see colon)
laryngitis, 440, 442
lassi, 351, 372
lavender
   leaves, 373
   oil, 372
laxative (see also purgation), 349, 442
laziness, 14

531

Index of Illustrations

Index of Charts